Treatment of Chronic Pain Conditions

Jason E. Pope • Timothy R. Deer
Editors

Treatment of Chronic Pain Conditions

A Comprehensive Handbook

Springer

Editors
Jason E. Pope, MD
Summit Pain Alliance
Santa Rosa, CA, USA

Timothy R. Deer, MD
The Spine and Nerve Center of The Virginias
Charleston, WV, USA

ISBN 978-1-4939-6974-6 ISBN 978-1-4939-6976-0 (eBook)
DOI 10.1007/978-1-4939-6976-0

Library of Congress Control Number: 2017939135

Printed on acid-free paper

This Springer imprint is published by Springer Nature
The registered company is Springer Science+Business Media LLC
The registered company address is: 233 Spring Street, New York, NY 10013, U.S.A.

To my wife and partner in all things, Emily. Thank you for your steadfast support, grace, generosity, and heart. I am humbled and honored to share this life with you.

To my loving children, Liam, Olivia, and Vivienne. It is a joy to see you experience the world and I am so proud of you.

To my parents, thank you for your sound advice on navigating work–life balance and your unflinching support.

To Dianne and Paul, thank you for your love and support.

To my twin brother, Greg, thank you for your quiet intellect and demeanor.

To brother in practice, Michael Yang, thank you for friendship, trust and support. We will have many more successful and prosperous years to come.

To my practice staff at Summit Pain Alliance, thank you for always exceeding my expectations and always going the extra mile.

To my friends and colleagues in this pain space, Steven Falowksi, David Provenzano, Porter McRoberts, David Kloth, Ash Sharan, Simon Thompson, Leo Kapural, Nagy Mekhail, and so many others. Thank you for your candor, friendship, and support.

To my families at NANS, INS, ASRA, AAPM, and ASIPP. Looking forward to many more years of service.

To Timothy Deer, my mentor and friend, thank you for your support, advice, and partnership. We continue to not be victims of circumstance.

Finally, thank you to God, for making all things possible.

Jason E. Pope, MD

To my patients to whom I have dedicated this book and many hours of work to try to improve the quality of life and suffering of many.

To Missy my wonderful wife and partner in all things. Thank you so much for your support and love. To my children, it has been amazing watching your personal growth and success. Morgan, Taylor, Reed, and Bailie keep up the great work and strive for excellence.

To Jason Pope who has been a brother to me in our goal to improve the global footprint of patient care and excellence in treating the suffering. Brotherly love and friendship is a great thing which I cherish.

To my family in practice in the United States. Chris Kim (my Korean brother); Brian Yee, Warren Grace, Nick Bremmer, Chong Kim, and Doug Stewart; and my incredible clinical team.

To my global partners in research and leadership who have helped me in so many areas: Robert Levy, Simon Thomson, Marc Russo, Fabian Piedimonte, Paul Verrills, Ali Rezia, Konstantin Slavin, Stan Golovac, Lou Raso, Peter Staats, Ramsin Benyamin, David Abejon, Stefan Schu, Jan Vesper, Leo Kapural, David Provenzano, and so many others. Our desire to raise the global standard is so exciting that I am optimistic about the future.

Most importantly my deepest gratitude to God from whom all blessings flow. I am humbled by the ability to continue to work at the wonderful field of medicine.

Timothy R. Deer, MD

Foreword

After over 25 years of working on a daily basis with pain medicine fellows, I came to realize the great privilege I have by working with bright, young doctors who chose the management of acute and chronic pain as their career.

The inquisitive minds of those intelligent and motivated trainees have kept us honest and allowed me personally to enhance my knowledge, as I had to examine the world's literature to be able to answer their intelligent and probing questions and satisfy their eagerness to learn.

To all those fellows in training or going to training as well as all pain management specialists who would like to get comprehensive and practical answers to their burning questions, I am delighted to forward this comprehensive handbook that covers all aspects of the acute and chronic pain management in a complete, easy-to-read manner.

This handbook has 51 chapters that address the basic anatomy and physiology of acute and chronic pain, the fundamentals of clinical examination, and full assessment of radiologic and neurologic studies. This handbook also emphasizes the interdisciplinary aspects of the management of pain from medication to physical restoration and psychological rehabilitation. Finally, there are several chapters that explain the most advanced state-of-the art interventional techniques in a very comprehensive and practical manner.

Congratulations to my friends Timothy Deer and Jason Pope for assembling a great line up of the best pain specialists to contribute to such great book.

Finally, this handbook will be a great asset to those starting their career in pain medicine.

Nagy Mekhail, MD, PhD, FIPP.
Professor of Anesthesiology,
Cleveland Clinic Learner College of Medicine.
Carl Wasmuth professor and Chair.
Director, Evidence Based Pain Management Research.
Cleveland Clinic, Cleveland, Ohio.

Contents

Part XI Advanced Pain Care Therapies: XI. Minimally Spinal Stenosis Treatments

Part XII Selected Chronic Pain Disease XII

Contributors

Syed S. Ali, MD Western Reserve Hospital, Center for Pain Medicine, Cuyahoga Falls, OH, USA

Kasra Amirdelfan, MD IPM Medical Group, Inc, Department of Interventional Pain Management, Walnut Creek, CA, USA

Prin X. Amorapanth, MD, PhD Brain Injury Medicine, Rusk Rehabilitation, NYU Langone Medical Center, Department of Physical Medicine and Rehabilitation, New York, NY, USA

Emil H. Annabi, MD Pima Pain Center, Pain Medicine, Tucson, AZ, USA

Jimmy Arefieg, MD Pima Pain Center, Tucson, AZ, USA

James W. Atchison, DO Rehabilitation Institute of Chicago, Chicago, IL, USA

Justin F. Averna, DO Temple University Hospital, Department of Physical Medicine and Rehabilitation, Philadelphia, PA, USA

Nomen Azeem, MD Sarasota Orthopedic Associates, Sarasota, FL, USA

Alexander Bautista, MD Cleveland Clinic, Anesthesia Institute Pain Management, Cleveland, OH, USA

Brenda Beck, DO Department of Anesthesiology, Division of Pain Management, University Hospitals, Cleveland, OH, USA

Robert Bolash, MD Cleveland Clinic, Anesthesia Institute Pain Management, Cleveland, OH, USA

Randy L. Calisoff, MD Rehabilitation Institute of Chicago, Center for Pain Management, Chicago, IL, USA

Alexios G. Carayannopoulos, DO, MPH Comprehensive Spine Center, Pain and Rehabilitation Medicine, Rhode Island Hospital, Neurosurgery Department, Providence, RI, USA

Jonathan D. Carlson, MD Arizona Pain/Pain Doctor, Glendale, AZ, USA

Gassan Chaiban, MD Interventional Pain Management, Ochsner Medical Center, Department of Anesthesiology, New Orleans, LA, USA

George C. Chang Chien, DO Cleveland Clinic, Anesthesia Institute Pain Management, Cleveland, OH, USA

Jianguo Cheng, MD, PhD Cleveland Clinic, Department of Pain Management, Cleveland, OH, USA

See Loong Chin, MD Cleveland Clinic, Cleveland, OH, USA

Timothy R. Deer, MD The Spine and Nerve Center of The Virginias, Charleston, WV, USA

Armin Deroee, MD Cleveland Clinic, Anesthesiology, Cleveland, OH, USA

Mehul J. Desai, MD MAPS Minnesota Advanced Pain Specialists, Maple Grove, MN, USA

Diedra Dias, MD Ochsner Health System, Department of Anesthesia and Interventional Pain Medicine, Jefferson, LA, USA

Christine El-Yahchouchi, MD University Hospitals Case Medical Center, Department of Anesthesiology, Division of Pain Medicine, Cleveland, OH, USA

Steven M. Falowski, MD St. Luke's University Health Network, Department of Neurosurgery, Bethlehem, PA, USA

Alexander Feoktistov, MD Diamond Headache Clinic, Chicago, IL, USA

Joseph D. Fortin, DO Spine Technology and Rehabilitation, Indiana School of Medicine, Fort Wayne, IN, USA

Enrique Galang, MD Orthopaedic and Rheumatologic Institute, Cleveland Clinic, Cleveland, OH, USA

Ryan Galica, MD Department of Anesthesiology, Pain Medicine, University Hospitals Case Medical Center, Cleveland Heights, OH, USA

Sean K. Graham, MD The Spine Diagnostic and Pain Treatment Center, Department of Pain Medicine, Baton Rouge, LA, USA

Radhika P. Grandhe, MBBS, MD Cleveland Clinic, Department of Pain Management, Cleveland, OH, USA

Michael Grille, MD Cleveland Clinic, Anesthesiology Institute, Cleveland, OH, USA

Maged Guirguis, MD Ochsner Health System, Pain Management, Department of Anesthesiology & Critical Care Medicine, New Orleans, LA, USA

Mayank Gupta, MD American Society of Interventional Pain, University of Kansas Medical Center, Kansas City, KS, USA

Andrew M. Hall, MD Department of Anesthesiology and Perioperative Care, Division of Pain Medicine, University of California, San Francisco, CA, USA

Haroon Hameed, MD KURE Pain Management, Annapolis, MD, USA

John Hau, MD Summit Pain Alliance, Santa Rosa, CA, USA

Salim Hayek, MD Division of Pain Medicine, Department of Anesthesiology, University Hospitals Case Medical Center, Cleveland, OH, USA

Navdeep Singh Jassal, MD University of South Florida, Department of Neurology, James A. Haley VA Medical Center, Tampa, FL, USA

Eduardo Jusino, MD Cleveland Clinic Foundation, Cleveland, OH, USA

Ahdev Kuppusamy, MD LLC, Scottsdale, AZ, USA

Olabisi P. Lane, MD, PharmD University Hospitals/Case Medical Center, Department of Anesthesiology and Perioperative Medicine, Cleveland, OH, USA

Julie Ann Zitterkopf Larson, MD University of Kansas Medical Center, Physical Medicine and Rehabilitation, Kansas City, KS, USA

Imanuel Lerman, MD, MS University of California San Diego, Department of Anesthesiology, Lajolla, CA, USA

Zachary McCormick, MD Northwestern University, The Rehabilitation Institute of Chicago, Chicago, IL, USA

Beth H. Minzter, MD, MS Pain Management, Cleveland Clinic, Cleveland, OH, USA

Hector Miranda-Grajales, MD Medical Injury Rehabilitation Specialists, Gainesville, FL, USA

Ramana K. Naidu, MD Department of Anesthesia and Perioperative Care, Division of Pain Medicine, University of California at San Francisco, San Francisco, CA, USA

Denis G. Patterson, DO Nevada Advanced Pain Specialists, Department of Pain Medicine, Reno, Nv, USA

Joshua Peloquin, DO Midwestern Medica School, Placentia, CA, USA

Jason E. Pope, MD Summit Pain Alliance, Santa Rosa, CA, USA

W. Porter McRoberts, MD Interventional Spine, Pain and Neurosurgery, Holy Cross Hospital, Fort Lauderdale, FL, USA

Rajiv Reddy, MD The Rehabilitation Institute of Chicago, Chicago, IL, USA

Richard M. Rosenthal, MD Regenerative Medicine Applications in Pain, Provo, UT, USA

Stephen Shiller, MD Pima Pain Center, Tucson, AZ, USA

Harpreet Singh, MD Cleveland Clinic Pain Management, Cleveland, OH, USA

Dmitri Souzdalnitski, MD, PhD Western Reserve Hospital, Cuyahoga Falls, OH, USA

Reda Tolba, MD Kenner, LA, USA

Andrea C. Wong, MD, MPH University Hospitals Case Medical Center, Department of Anesthesiology Division of Pain Management, Cleveland, OH, USA

Jiang Wu, MD University of Washington Medical Center, Department of Anesthesiology & Pain Medicine, Seattle, WA, USA

Paul Wu, MD Holy Cross Hospital, Holy Cross Orthopedic/Neuroscience Institutes, Fort Lauderdale, FL, USA

Michael I. Yang, MD Summit Pain Alliance Inc, Interventional Pain Management, Santa Rosa, CA, USA

Sherif Zaky, MD, MSC, PhD Pain Management Service, Firelands Regional Medical Center, Case Western Reserve University, Sandusky, OH, USA

Part I

The Basics: I. Background Focus

Chronic Pain

1

George C. Chang Chien, Eduardo Jusino,
and Armin Deroee

Key Concepts

- Chronic pain is defined as pain that persists beyond the normal tissue healing time and is at least 3–6 months in duration.
- Pain is categorized as being nociceptive or neuropathic. Nociceptive pain is subdivided into somatic and visceral pain. Neuropathic pain is subdivided into peripheral neuropathic pain and central neuropathic pain.
- The sequence of events by which a pain stimulus is perceived involves four processes: transduction, transmission, modulation, and perception.

Definition

The International Association for the Study of Pain defines pain as "an unpleasant sensory and emotional experience associated with actual or potential tissue damage, or described in terms of such damage." Adaptive pain protects the body from injury and promotes healing when injured. Maladaptive or chronic pain represents pathologic operation of the nervous system.

Chronic pain is defined as pain that persists beyond the normal tissue healing time. This time interval is often indicated as 3 months, though some experts have identified the window as 6 months (Table 1.1).

G.C. Chang Chien, DO (✉)
Cleveland Clinic, Anesthesia Institute Pain Management, 9500 Euclid Ave, Dept C-25, Cleveland, OH 44195, USA
e-mail: gchangchien@gmail.com

E. Jusino, MD
Cleveland Clinic Foundation, Cleveland, OH, USA

A. Deroee, MD
Cleveland Clinic, Anesthesiology, Cleveland, OH, USA

Types of pain

Pain is categorized as being nociceptive or neuropathic.

Nociceptive pain arises from a nerve fiber sensitive to a noxious stimulus or to a stimulus that may become noxious. Nociceptive pain is subdivided into somatic (skin, bones, and joints) and visceral (body organs) pain. Somatic pain originates from injury to body tissue and it is well localized, discrete, and intense. Visceral pain results from stimulation of the visceral stretch receptors, and it is diffused and poorly localized.

Neuropathic pain develops from abnormal neural activity due to disease, injury, or dysfunction of the peripheral nervous system (PNS) and/or central nervous system (CNS). It is associated with abnormal sensations (dysesthesia) and pain from normally non-painful stimuli (allodynia). Neuropathic pain may be continuous and/or episodic. The pain is usually described as burning, electric shock, numbness, tingling, and itching.

Neuropathic pain is subdivided into peripheral neuropathic pain and central neuropathic pain. Peripheral neuropathic pain is due to damage to a peripheral nerve with or without autonomic changes (postherpetic neuralgia, diabetic neuropathy, and complex regional pain syndrome). Central neuropathic pain results from abnormal central nervous system activity (thalamic pain syndrome, poststroke pain, and postspinal cord injury pain).

Mechanism

Pain sensation starts in the peripheral nerves through nociceptors. The nociceptor is a receptor of a sensory neuron that responds to potentially damaging stimuli by sending signals to the spinal cord and brain. The pain signal is transmitted from the peripheral nerve to the dorsal horn of the spinal cord and through the CNS where it is processed in the somatosensory cerebral cortex. Nociceptors are categorized as fast conducting myelinated A-delta fibers that signal

J.E. Pope, T.R. Deer (eds.), *Treatment of Chronic Pain Conditions*, DOI 10.1007/978-1-4939-6976-0_1

Table 1.1 Definitions of some of the common terminology in pain medicine

Chronic pain	A pain that persists beyond the normal tissue healing time. This time interval is often indicated as 3 months, though some experts have identified the window as 6 months
Nociceptive pain	A pain that arises from a nerve fiber sensitive to a noxious stimulus or to a stimulus that may become noxious
Neuropathic pain	A pain from abnormal neural activity due to disease, injury, or dysfunction of the peripheral nervous system and/or central nervous system
Neurogenic pain	Pain initiated or caused by a primary lesion or dysfunction or by transitory perturbation in the peripheral or central nervous system
Central pain	Pain initiated or caused by a primary lesion or dysfunction in the central nervous system
Peripheral sensitization	Increased excitability in peripheral nociceptors because of peripheral injury that manifests as primary hyperalgesia
Central sensitization	Increased and prolonged excitability of CNS nociceptors because of peripheral injury that causes promoting increased sensitivity to painful stimuli (secondary hyperalgesia)

immediate, sharp pain and slow conducting unmyelinated C fibers that transmit delayed, longer-lasting dull pain. The five types of nociceptors include the following: thermal, mechanical, chemical, silent, and polymodal.

The sequence of events by which a pain stimulus is perceived involves four processes: transduction, transmission, modulation, and perception. Transduction occurs in the peripheral terminals of nociceptor sensory fibers where different forms of energy (thermal, mechanical, or chemical) are converted into electrical activity. Transmission is the process by which the electrical activity is conducted through the nervous system. This involves three major components: peripheral, synaptic, and central transmission. Nociceptive impulses travel along peripheral nerve fibers through first-order neurons (peripheral transmission) to the dorsal horn of the spinal cord where they synapse with the second-order neurons (synaptic transmission) and further transmit via neurons that cross the spinal cord and ascend to the thalamus and brainstem nuclei where third-order neuron synapsis occurs (central transmission). Modulation is the process where neural activity may be altered along the pain transmission pathway. Perception is the final stage of the pain-signaling process by which neural activity in the transmission pathway results in subjective sensation of pain at the level of the somatosensory cortex.

Chronicity

Many factors may contribute to the development of chronic pain. Peripheral injury leads to increased excitability in peripheral nociceptors (peripheral sensitization) that manifests as primary hyperalgesia. This leads to increased stimuli of the CNS that causes increased and prolonged excitability of CNS nociceptors (central sensitization) promoting increased sensitivity to painful stimuli (secondary hyperalgesia). At least three mechanisms are responsible for central sensitization in the spinal cord: (1) windup and sensitization of second-order wide dynamic range neurons, (2) dorsal horn neuron receptor field expansion, and (3) hyperexcitability of flexion reflexes. Also, peripheral injury is accompanied by many changes including new expression of sodium channels, adrenergic receptors, and cholinergic receptors that contribute to depolarization of injured nociceptors. This depolarization results in sodium and calcium flux that may cause spontaneous action potentials with or without stimulation. Derangements can occur in both the ascending and descending signaling systems at any level. All of these factors may contribute to the development of chronic pain following injury.

Suggested Reading

1. Adler RH. The term 'chronic' with respect to pain should be dropped. Clin J Pain. 2000;16:365.
2. Bennett M. The LANSS Pain Scale: the Leeds assessment of neuropathic symptoms and signs. Pain. 2001;92:147.
3. Chekka K, Benzon HT, Jabri RS. Taxonomy: definition of pain terms and chronic pain syndromes. In: Essentials of pain medicine. 3rd ed. Philadelphia: Saunders; 2011. p. 16–8.
4. Portenoy RK. Mechanisms of clinical pain: observations and speculations. Neurol Clin. 1989;7:205.
5. Raja SN, Dougherty PM. Anatomy and physiology of somatosensory and pain processing. In: Essentials of pain medicine. 3rd ed. Philadelphia: Saunders; 2011. p. 1–7.
6. Wang CK, Myunghae Hah J, Carroll I. Factors contributing to pain chronicity. Curr Pain Headache Rep. 2009;13(1):7–11.

Mechanisms of Chronic Pain

2

Eduardo Jusino, George C. Chang Chien, and Beth H. Minzter

Key Concepts

- Sensitization is a process in which repeated stimulus of a receptor results in the progressive amplification of a response.
- The key excitatory neuromodulators are glutamate, aspartate, and substance P.
- The main inhibitory neuromodulators are GABA, glycine, enkephalins, and somatostatin.
- Mechanisms of persistent pain include the following: peripheral sensitization, central sensitization, ectopic excitability of sensory neurons, physical rearrangement of neurons' circuitry, and disinhibition.
- Research into the mechanisms that generate and maintain chronic pain are necessary to develop new interventions and improved treatment outcomes.

Introduction

After inflammation or tissue injury, pain sensation may continue long after the withdrawal of the noxious stimuli. This transition from acute to chronic pain has been a long-standing medical enigma. Recent advances in the study of pain transmission and processing have begun to unravel the cellular mechanisms that underlie the maintenance of chronic pain. The term sensitization refers to the process in which a repeated stimulus results in the progressive amplification of a response. Sensitization is a key factor in the genesis of chronic pain and a demonstration of plasticity within the nervous system. As an example, repeated stimulation of nociceptive C fibers entering the dorsal root can elicit a progressive increase in the number of action potentials generated. The dorsal root ganglia may become hyperexcitable and display continuous spontaneous electrical activity. This activity results from the expression of many cell-specific molecules in modified cells, which alter the complex neuronal circuits of our nervous system. These neuronal changes are the mainstay of sensitization. Chronic pain sensation can result from such injury. Understanding the changes that follow in neural structures at a molecular level may help lead to new therapeutic interventions.

There are various primary excitatory and inhibitory neurotransmitters implicated in the propagation of chronic pain. The amino acids glutamate and aspartate are the key excitatory neurotransmitters in the somatosensory system. The four types of excitatory amino acid receptors are the N-methyl-D-aspartate (NMDA), alpha-amino-3-hydroxy-5-methyl-4-isoxazolepropionic acid (AMPA), kainite, and metabotropic receptors. Gamma-aminobutyric acid (GABA) and glycine are the key inhibitory neurotransmitters. Substance P is the key excitatory neuropeptide. The enkephalins and somatostatin are the key inhibitory neuropeptides.

Peripheral Sensitization

Nociceptive stimulation of tissue in a neuron's receptive field causes release of inflammatory mediators (prostaglandins, bradykinin, histamine, cytokines, growth factors) that may reduce the threshold for excitation of peripheral receptors. When changes occur in the response characteristics of the primary afferent fibers which transmit pain, the A-delta and C fibers, the peripheral nervous system is said to be sensitized. Peripheral sensitization causes the nerve to be responsive to benign, normally nonpainful stimuli, and this is termed allodynia. This may also provoke an exaggerated response to painful stimuli, known as hyperalgesia. Changes

E. Jusino, MD
Cleveland Clinic Foundation, Cleveland, OH, USA

G.C. Chang Chien, DO (✉)
Cleveland Clinic, Anesthesia Institute Pain Management, 9500 Euclid Ave, Dept C-25, Cleveland, OH 44195, USA
e-mail: gchangchien@gmail.com

B.H. Minzter, MD, MS
Pain Management, Cleveland Clinic, Cleveland, OH, USA

J.E. Pope, T.R. Deer (eds.), *Treatment of Chronic Pain Conditions*, DOI 10.1007/978-1-4939-6976-0_2

in cellular transduction such as increases in the cAMP-PKA mechanism may be involved in further sensitization. Inflammation leads to upregulation of nitric oxide synthase that can cause neuropeptides to be released from nociceptive nerve terminals, and these neuropeptides therein produce inflammatory hyperalgesia. The recruitment of previously silent nerve fibers which become sensitive to stimuli after exposure to inflammatory mediators is another mechanism of peripheral sensitization. The final common pathway for peripheral sensitization appears to involve an increase in intracellular calcium and protein kinase levels.

Central Sensitization

Central sensitization amplifies the synaptic transfer from the nociceptor terminal to the dorsal horn neurons. Initial sensitization is an activity, which is dependent on stimulated nociceptors, but subsequent transcriptional changes at the molecular level sustain the sensitization. Previously subthreshold synaptic input to nociceptive neurons will now generate an augmented action potential output. The NMDA receptor plays an important role as its responsiveness to glutamate is increased, leading to increased excitability of the dorsal horn cell. Inflammation may contribute to both peripheral and central sensitization. Neuroimmune interaction produced by peripheral inflammation causes changes in brain-derived neurotrophic factor, substance P, neurokinin, dynorphin, and cyclooxygenase 2 which may lead to transcription-dependent central sensitization. Also, neuroglial interactions contribute to sensitization by releasing cytokines and chemokines after nerve injury, altering gene transcription. The main causes of central sensitization-maintained pain include neuronal sensitization, reduction in inhibitory interneuron activity, and modulation of descending pathway activity.

Neuronal sensitization is triggered by intense electrical or noxious stimulation of C fibers which promote wide-dynamic-range (WDR) neuron hyperexcitability in the dorsal horn. Repetitive electrical stimulation provokes increased excitability leading to action potential "windup." Windup refers to slow, prolonged depolarization and ultimate burst of action potentials with stimulation. WDR neuron sensitization is associated with excitatory amino acids, tachykinins, and calcitonin gene-related peptide. These neuromodulators affect the dorsal horn neuron by increasing cation fluxes, impinging on intracellular transduction mechanisms, and modulating receptor and transmitter gene transcription. Synaptic transmission augmentation at NMDA receptors is the final common pathway. Adequate depolarization causes an increase in intracellular calcium level leading to protein kinase phosphorylation that antagonizes the magnesium blockade at the NMDA receptor.

Interneurons, as well as descending signals arising from the brain, may be excitatory or inhibitory. Stimulation of some cortical and subcortical areas may cause analgesia. Reduction in inhibitory interneuron activity results in increased WDR neuron excitability consistent with clinical hyperalgesia and allodynia. The loss of GABA and glycerine activity in the dorsal horn produces a state of neuronal hyperexcitability.

Modulation by supraspinal descending pathways is likely due to increases or decreases in several neurotransmitters causing descending facilitation or inhibition. The endogenous opioid, noradrenergic, and serotonergic systems are involved in descending control of nociceptive pain perception. There is evidence that serotonin receptors provoke the release of substance P from the spinal cord. This release of substance P correlates with the receptors' ability to increase nociception at the level of the neurons. Increases in noradrenaline in the dorsal horn may potentiate descending noradrenergic inhibitory circuits, thereby reducing nociceptor stimulation. Diminished cerebral GABA can lead to disinhibition of descending facilitation.

It has been demonstrated that the injured neurons within the DRG are markedly more sensitive to activation, creating the potential for a therapeutic window for treatment of chronic pain with electrical stimulation.

Conclusion

The major causes of hypersensitivity to pain after injury are peripheral and central sensitization. Substances released after tissue injury can be nociceptor sensitizers. NMDA receptor changes can increase dorsal horn excitability. Activated glial cells may produce cytokines that alter gene transcription and contribute to further sensitization. Other mechanisms for persistent pain include but are not limited to the following: ectopic excitability of sensory neurons due to upregulation of voltage-gated sodium channels or downregulation of potassium channels, physical rearrangement of neurons' circuitry in the dorsal horn, and disinhibition due to loss of GABA and glycine-mediated inhibition.

Suggested Reading

1. Cohen SA. Pathophysiology of pain. In: Principles and practice of pain medicine. 2nd ed. Philadelphia: Saunders; 2004.
2. Dougherty PM, Raja SN, Boyette-Davis J. Neurochemistry of somatosensory and pain processing. In: Essentials of pain medicine. 3rd ed. Philadelphia: Saunders; 2011. p. 8–15.
3. Levine JD, Reichling DB. Peripheral mechanisms of inflammatory pain. In: Textbook of pain. Edinburgh: Churchill Livingstone; 1999. p. 59.
4. Woolf CJ, Salter MW. Neuronal plasticity: increasing the gain in pain. Science. 2000;288:1765.
5. Woolf CJ, Thompson SW. The induction and maintenance of central sensitization is dependent on N-methyl-D-aspartic acid receptor activation: implications for the treatment of post-injury pain hypersensitivity states. Pain. 1991;44:293.
6. Woolf CJ; American College of Physicians, American Physiological Society. Pain: moving from symptom control toward mechanism-specific pharmacologic management. Ann Intern Med. 2004;140:441.

Overview of Chronic Pain

3

Denis G. Patterson

Introduction

Chronic pain is a term that defines a set of specific medical conditions in which a patient suffers from pain for extended periods of time. While many interventional treatment options exist depending on the nature of the complaint and the patient's overall well-being, otherwise, many patients are given opioid therapy by primary care and ER physicians. This chapter addresses several key national factors that are currently tied to chronic pain: a growing epidemic of opioid use in the United States which is partially attributable to the lack of physicians who were effectively trained to treat pain, and the result is a significant economic burden on the country.

Opioid Epidemic

The use of using opioids to treat non-cancer pain began in 1986 when Portenoy and Foley published a seminal paper. They treated 38 patients with non-cancer pain for greater than 6 months with a median daily dose of less than 20 morphine milligram equivalents per day. The lack of clinically significant adverse events led them to conclude that physicians could safely and effectively prescribe opioid medications to patients without a history of substance abuse with "relatively little risk of producing maladaptive behaviors which define opioid abuse." The results of this paper began the push for physicians toward a greater acceptance of the use of opioid analgesics to treat non-cancer pain. The movement gained momentum in the 1990s when state medical boards curtailed restrictions on laws governing the prescribing of opioids for the treatment of chronic non-cancer pain. This led to new pain management standards for inpatient and outpatient medical care implemented by the Joint Commission on the Accreditation of Health Care Organizations (JCAHO) in 2000. These new standards lead to an increased awareness of the right to pain relief, which provided further justification for physicians to use opioids to treat non-cancer pain. Other factors that fueled the increase were aggressive marketing by the pharmaceutical industry and the promotion for increased use of opioids in the treatment of non-cancer pain by a myriad of medical organizations.

Unfortunately, the above positions were based on unsound science and blatant misinformation, accompanied by the dangerous assumptions that opioids are highly effective and safe and devoid of adverse events when prescribed by physicians. As a result, opioid use became an epidemic in the United States. The quantity of prescription painkillers (i.e., opioid medications) sold to pharmacies, hospitals, and doctors' offices was four times larger in 2010 than in 1999. Enough prescription painkillers were prescribed in 2010 to medicate every American adult around-the-clock for 5 months. According to the CDC, drug overdose death rates in the United States have more than tripled since 1990. In 2008, more than 36,000 people (approximately 100 people per day) died from drug overdoses, and nearly three-fourths of these deaths were caused by prescription drugs. The misuse and abuse of prescription painkillers was responsible for more than 475,000 emergency department visits in 2009, a number that nearly doubled from the previous 5 years. Almost all prescription drugs involved in overdoses come from prescriptions originally. Most prescription painkillers are prescribed by primary care and internal medicine doctors and dentists, not specialists. The 80/20 rule applies here: 20% of prescribers prescribe 80% of all prescription painkillers.

Lack of Physicians to Treat Pain

Unfortunately, legitimate chronic pain patients who need help have become collateral damage on the recent war on opioid prescribing. Patients who were previously stable on an

D.G. Patterson, DO (✉)
Nevada Advanced Pain Specialists, Department of Pain Medicine, 10715 Double R Blvd, Ste 101, Reno, NV 89521, USA
e-mail: patterson@nvadvancedpain.com

J.E. Pope, T.R. Deer (eds.), *Treatment of Chronic Pain Conditions*, DOI 10.1007/978-1-4939-6976-0_3

effective low dose of painkillers have suddenly been cut off by their physicians for no apparent reason. These chronic pain patients are now paying the price because their physicians fear that law enforcement is "looking over their shoulder."

Meanwhile, public and medical misperceptions are widespread about the nature of pain, its causes, and the way it affects individual patients. Misinformation is fueled by the fact that comprehensive research is lacking, even on basic questions like how many people suffer from disabling chronic pain and how well-existing drugs like opioids treat long-term pain.

The problem is magnified by barriers that exist that allow legitimate chronic pain patients from being able to seek medical care. Traditionally, these patients would seek help from their primary care physicians, but access to primary care physicians in parts of the United States is shrinking due to the dwindling number of primary care physicians. Existing primary care physicians receive little medical education about treating chronic pain and are left to treat most pain with little specific guidance about effective care. In medical school, students receive only a few hours at most of education on pain treatment.

Primary care physicians seeking guidance on treating pain patients might find that they do not have resources to specialists who treat chronic pain. Currently, there are only about 3000–4000 pain specialists in the entire United States. That means that there is only one board-certified pain physician to treat every 25,000–33,000 patients that suffer from chronic pain. Many board- certified pain physicians struggle to keep up with the demand.

Economic Burden

Chronic pain affects 100 million Americans. Pain affects more Americans than diabetes, coronary heart disease, stroke, and cancer combined. The most common chronic pain conditions that patients suffer from are back pain (27%), severe headache or migraine pain (15%), neck pain (15%), and facial ache or pain (4%). Back pain is the leading cause of disability in Americans under 45 years old. More than 26 million Americans between the ages of 20–64 experience frequent back pain.

Chronic pain causes a tremendous cost on our country in health-care costs, rehabilitation, and lost worker productivity. The costs of unrelieved pain can result in longer hospital stays, increased rates of rehospitalization, increase outpatient visits, and decreased ability to function fully leading to lost income and insurance coverage. Chronic pain is a significant public health problem that costs society at least $560–$635 billion annually. This includes the total incremental cost of health care due to pain ranging between $261–$300 billion and $297–$336 billion due to lost productivity (based on days of work missed, hours of work lost, and lower wages).

Suggested Reading

1. Blumenschein K, Fink JL, Freeman PR, Kirsh KL, Steinke DT, Talbert J. Independent evaluation of the impact and effectiveness of the Kentucky All Schedule Prescription Electronic Reporting Program (KASPER). Lexington: Institute for Pharmaceutical Outcomes and Policy; 2010.
2. CDC. Vital signs: overdoses of prescription opioid pain relievers – United States, 1999–2008. MMWR. 2011;60:1–6.
3. Dhalla IA, Mamdani MM, Gomes T, Juurlink DN. Clustering of opioid prescribing and opioid-related mortality among family physicians in Ontario. Canadian Family Med. 2011;57:e92–6.
4. National Centers for Health Statistics. Chartbook on trends in the Health of Americans 2006, Special feature: pain. http://www.cdc.gov/nchs/data/hus/hus06.pdf.
5. Portenoy RK, Foley KM. Chronic use of opioid analgesics in non-malignant pain: report of 38 cases. Pain. 1986;25(2):171–86.
6. Substance Abuse and Mental Health Services Administration. Drug Abuse Warning Network: selected tables of national estimates of drug-related emergency department visits. Rockville: Center for Behavioral Health Statistics and Quality, SAMHSA; 2010.
7. Swedlow A, Ireland J, Johnson G. Prescribing patterns of schedule II opioids in California Workers' Compensation. Cal. Workers' Compensation Update. 1–12 Mar 2011. Available from URL: http://www.cwci.org/research.html (http://www.cwci.org/research.html) (http://www.cdc.gov/Other/disclaimer.html).
8. Volkow ND, McLellan TA, Cotto JH, Karithanom M, Weiss SRB. Characteristics of opioid prescriptions in 2009. JAMA. 2011;305(13):1299–301.

Part II

The Basics: II. Anatomy

Anatomy of the Spine

4

Harpreet Singh, George C. Chang Chien, and Robert Bolash

Key Concepts

- Keen understanding of spinal anatomy is necessary for accurate diagnosis of painful spine conditions and safe undertaking of interventional spine procedures.
- The spinal cord ends at the lower border of the L1 vertebra but may extend as far as the L3 vertebra in select individuals.
- The "safe triangle" approach for transforaminal epidural injections may minimize injury to the nerve root but does not guard against entering the segmental radiculomedullary artery.
- Bony architecture of the spine is best revealed by CT. MRI is the imaging modality of choice for details of bone marrow, ligaments, fascial planes, neural tissues, and soft tissue structures.

Introduction

The vertebral column consists of 33 bony elements joined together by joints and ligaments (Table 4.1). It houses and protects both the spinal cord and proximal portions of the spinal nerves. Detailed understanding of spinal anatomy is essential for accurate diagnosis of painful spine conditions and the safe performance of interventional pain procedures.

H. Singh, MD
Cleveland Clinic Pain Management, Cleveland, OH, USA

G.C. Chang Chien, DO (✉) • R. Bolash, MD
Cleveland Clinic, Anesthesia Institute Pain Management, 9500 Euclid Ave, Dept C-25, Cleveland, OH 44195, USA
e-mail: gchangchien@gmail.com

Osteology

The vertebral column consists of seven cervical, 12 thoracic, and five lumbar vertebrae along with five fused sacral bones that form the sacrum and four fused bones to form the coccyx (Fig. 4.1). Each vertebra consists of a *vertebral body*, a cylindrical ventral mass made of cancellous bone, and a *dorsal vertebral arch* made mostly of cortical bone. The large *intervertebral vertebral foramen*, wherein the spinal cord traverses, is enclosed by the vertebral body and dorsal arch. The body is connected to the dorsal arch by two stout horizontal supports known as *pedicles*. The posterior arch is composed of two flat bones known as *laminae*, which join together in the midline and project posteriorly to form *spinous process*. Near the junction of pedicle and laminae, there are *superior* and i*nferior articular processes* which create a joint with the inferior and superior articular processes of the preceding and succeeding vertebrae, respectively, to form *synovial zygapophyseal joints* (Z-joints, facet joints). At the junction between superior and inferior articular processes, *transverse processes* project laterally on both sides of the vertebra. The junction between the two vertebral bodies consists of cartilaginous end plates of adjacent vertebra, an intervertebral disk, and anterior and posterior longitudinal ligaments.

The size, shape, and sectional contour of the body are variable throughout the spine. However, it is the characteristic elements in the dorsal arch, which gives vertebrae their distinct identity in different areas of the spine (Fig. 4.2).

Cervical Vertebrae

There are seven cervical vertebrae, the first two (*atlas*-C1 and *axis*-C2) and seventh cervical vertebra are unique in morphology. A typical cervical vertebra consists of a bean-shaped body which is relatively small in size. Unique to the cervical spine are the *uncovertebral joints* or the *joints of*

J.E. Pope, T.R. Deer (eds.), *Treatment of Chronic Pain Conditions*, DOI 10.1007/978-1-4939-6976-0_4

Table 4.1 Ligaments supporting the vertebral column

Ligament	Attachment	Function
Anterior longitudinal ligament	Anterior tubercle of C1 to the sacrum, abutting the anterior surface of vertebral bodies	Limits extension
Posterior longitudinal ligament	From C2 to the sacrum, attached to posterior surface of intervertebral disk	Stabilization by limiting spinal flexion. Prevents posterior disk herniation
Supraspinous ligament	Superior to inferior along the tip of the spinous processes	Stabilization by limiting spinal flexion
Interspinous ligament	Connects inferior aspect of the cranial spinous process to the superior surface of the adjacent spinous process	Stabilization by limiting spinal flexion
Ligamentum flavum	Connects the lamina of adjacent vertebra	Stabilization by limiting spinal flexion
Inter-transverse ligament	Connects adjacent transverse processes	Limits lateral flexion

Luschka, formed by the hook-shaped processes of the superior surface of the vertebral bodies of the third to the seventh cervical vertebra and first thoracic vertebra. The transverse process of the cervical vertebra is perforated by the foramen transversarium which protects the vertebral artery. Part of the transverse process dorsal to the foramina creates the posterior tubercle, whereas the ventral end forms the anterior tubercle. The anterior tubercle is most prominent at C6 vertebra where it is also known as *Chassaignac tubercle*. The laminae enclose a relatively large vertebral foramen with a triangular cross section. The superior and inferior articular processes face obliquely superior/posteriorly and inferior/anteriorly, respectively. Notably, the *ligamentum flavum* may not be fused at midline in the cervical spine.

In total, the base of stability in the typical cervical spine vertebra is created by these five points of articulation: the bilateral facets, intervertebral disk, and the uncovertebral joints (above and below).

The atlas, or C1 vertebra Vertebrae, is shaped like a ring and lacks a definite body, consisting only of anterior and posterior arches connected by lateral masses. Lateral masses have superior and inferior articular surfaces. The superior articular surfaces are directed cranially and internally where they articulate with the occipital condyles. The inferior articular surfaces are positioned caudally with a slight medial and posterior tilt. The inferior articular surface of the atlas articulates with the superior articular processes of axis. The axis, or C2 cervical vertebra, is characterized by a prominent anterior odontoid process, which serves as a pivot allowing rotational movement of the atlas and serves to prevent horizontal displacement of the atlas over the axis (Fig. 4.3).

Thoracic Vertebrae

There are 12 thoracic vertebrae, which are characterized by both facet joints and costal articulations. The typical thoracic vertebra (T2–T8) is heart shaped and intermediate in size between the cervical and lumbar vertebra. They have two characteristic demifacets on each side of the body, which articulate with the ribs. The superior demifacet is larger and, in combination with smaller inferior demifacet of the preceding vertebra, articulates with the corresponding rib. Pedicles project from the superior aspect of the body; superior articular processes project from the junction of lamina and pedicle. They are coronal in their plane of articulation, bear an oval articular facet facing backward, and are slightly lateral. The two articular surfaces lie in the arc of a circle permitting limited rotation. Spinous process of thoracic vertebrae angulate downward, gradually increasing in angulation until reaching T7. At T8, their angulation begins to decrease such that the spinous process of T12 is near horizontal. Transverse processes are directed laterally and slight posteriorly. They contain an articular facet on the ventral aspect, which articulates with the tuberculum of the corresponding rib.

Lumbar Vertebrae

The bodies of the lumbar vertebrae become progressively larger to accommodate the increased weight of the trunk and upper body. Transverse processes in the lumbar region vary in length, with the longest at the L4 level and the thickest at the L5 level. True transverse elements are represented by accessory and mammillary processes which are joined by mamillo-accessory ligaments (which may be ossified). Notably, the medial branch of dorsal ramus passes beneath this ligament. The superior lumbar articular processes are widely situated and positioned medially, while the inferior articular processes are reciprocally directed laterally. Laminae in the lumbar region are shorter, and there is less dorsal overlap when compared to the thoracic region. Spinous processes are shorter and nearly horizontally oriented. The vertebral foramen in the lumbar region is triangular in shape and larger compared to thoracic levels but smaller compared to cervical levels (Fig. 4.4).

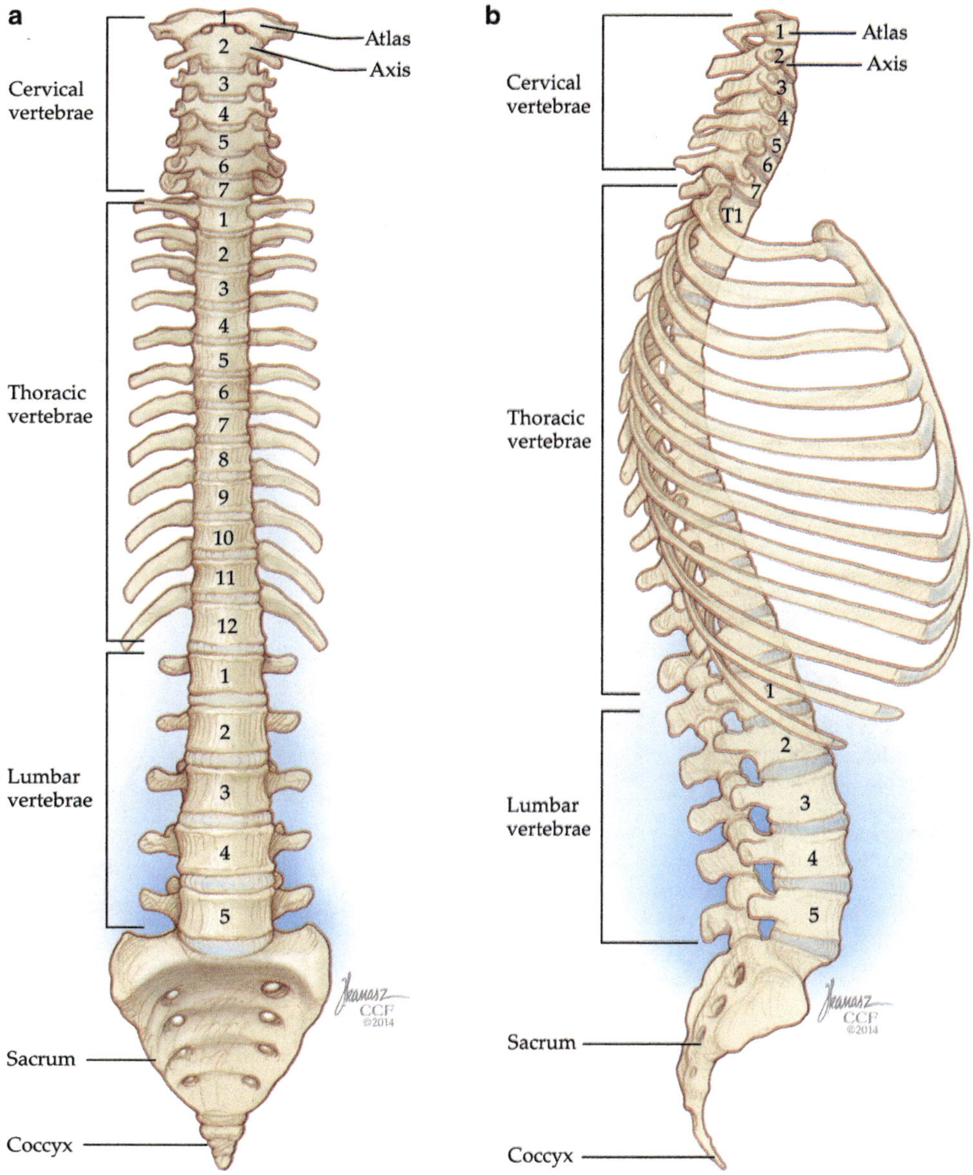

Fig. 4.1 Vertebral column lateral and anterior view (**a**) AP view and (**b**) lateral view (Reprinted with permission, Cleveland Clinic Center for Medical Art & Photography © 2014–2015. All Rights Reserved)

Sacrum and Coccyx

The sacrum is a wedge-shaped bone formed by the fusion of the five sacral vertebrae and their costal elements. The sacrum articulates with two pelvic bones posteriorly forming *sacroiliac joints* on either side.

The sacral canal is the caudal continuation of the vertebral canal. It extends the length of the sacrum and ends at the *sacral hiatus* where the coccyx, a small triangular bone formed by fusion of four coccygeal vertebrae, begins. The anterior and posterior walls of this canal are perforated by sacral foramina, through which the sacral spinal nerves pass. There are four pairs of dorsal and ventral sacral foramina. Sacral spinal nerves divide into dorsal and ventral rami within the sacral canal, and they exit the sacrum via the anterior and posterior sacral foramina, respectively.

Intervertebral Foramen and the Safe Triangle

On the lateral aspect of the posterior elements of the vertebral bodies are foramina created by two adjacent vertebrae. The anterior border of the foramen is formed by the bodies of the vertebrae and the intervertebral disk. The posterior border is marked by the superior and inferior articular processes and facet joints. The superior and inferior borders are formed by the pedicles of the superior and inferior vertebra, respectively. The structures passing through these foramina include the *spinal nerve root*; *dorsal root ganglion*; *segmental spinal artery*; communicating veins between the internal and external plexuses; and *sinu-vertebral nerves*.

The "safe triangle" was initially described by Bogduk and refers to a three-dimensional area lateral to the inferior

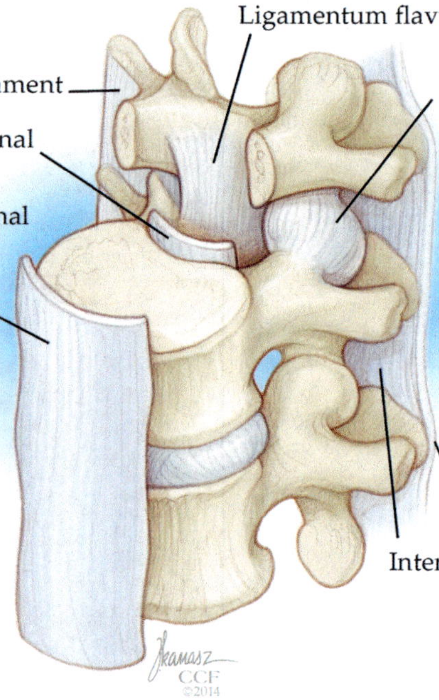

Fig. 4.2 Ligaments of the spine (Reprinted with permission, Cleveland Clinic Center for Medical Art & Photography © 2014–2015. All Rights Reserved)

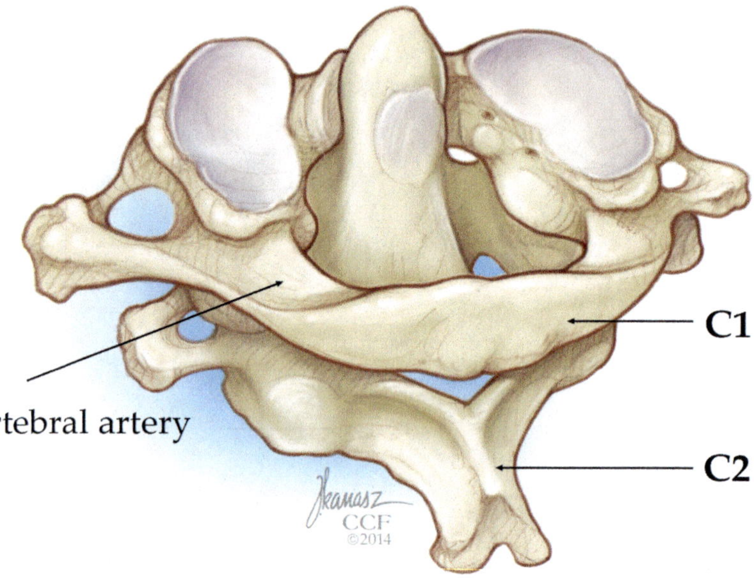

Fig. 4.3 Cervical vertebrae (Atlas and Axis) (Reprinted with permission, Cleveland Clinic Center for Medical Art & Photography © 2014–2015. All Rights Reserved)

margin of pedicle, dorsal to the vertebral body, and cephalad to presumed location of the nerve root (Fig. 4.5). Entering in this area for any interventional procedure (e.g., transforaminal epidural injection) reduces the risk of nerve root injury but does not preclude entering in to the segmental spinal arteries.

Intervertebral Disk

Approximately 80% of the vertebral column's length is due to vertebral bodies, and 20% consists of the intervertebral disk. The intervertebral disk is composed of the cartilaginous end plates, the central *nucleus pulposus*, and the circumferential *annulus fibrosus*. In the adult human, the intervertebral disk is mostly avascular.

Spinal Cord

The central nervous system consists of the brain and spinal cord. The spinal cord extends continuously from the medulla oblongata and terminates at the *conus medullaris*, which is connected by the *filum terminale* to the dorsum of the first coccygeal vertebra. The adult human spinal cord usually ends at the lower border of L1 but may extend as far as L3.

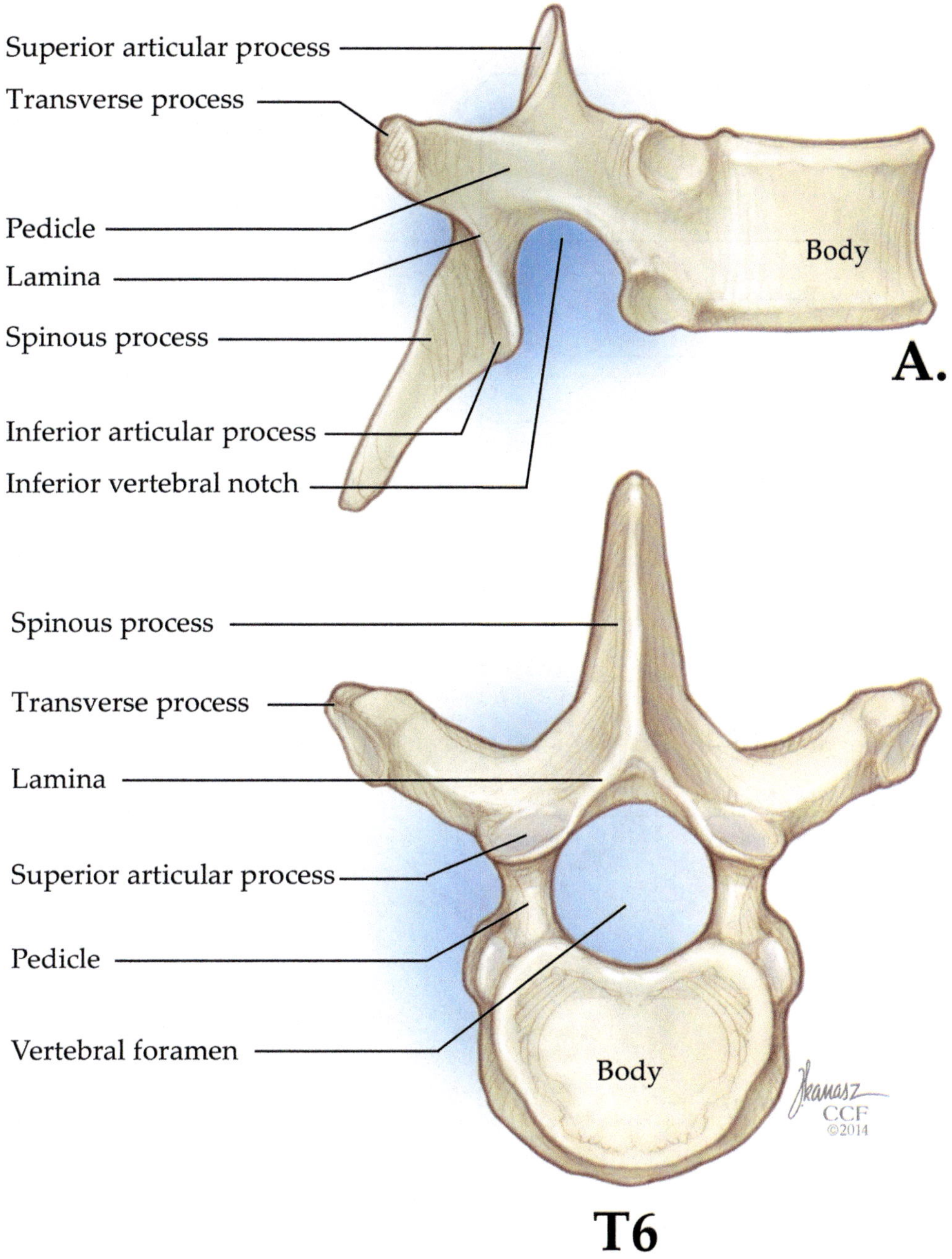

Fig. 4.4 Thoracic and lumbar vertebrae (**a**) AP view and (**b**) lateral view (Reprinted with permission, Cleveland Clinic Center for Medical Art & Photography © 2014–2015. All Rights Reserved)

The spinal cord is divided in half by a dorsal median sulcus and a ventral median fissure. It contains a central canal in the middle and continues cranially with the cerebral ventricular system. As is the case with the rest of the CNS, the spinal cord is composed of white and gray matter. White matter forms the bulk of the deep parts of the brain and the superficial parts of the spinal cord. It is composed of bundles of myelinated nerve cell processes, axons, which carry nerve impulses between the cell bodies of the neurons, which make up the gray matter. Large white matter tracts form descending motor fibers from the brain to the spine, whereas ascending sensory tracts transmit light touch, pressure, temperature, and pain from the spinal cord to the brain (Fig. 4.6).

Gray Matter

The gray matter of the spinal cord surrounding the central canal is "H-shaped," with two dorsal and two ventral horns. The *ventral horn* contains the cell bodies for motor neurons,

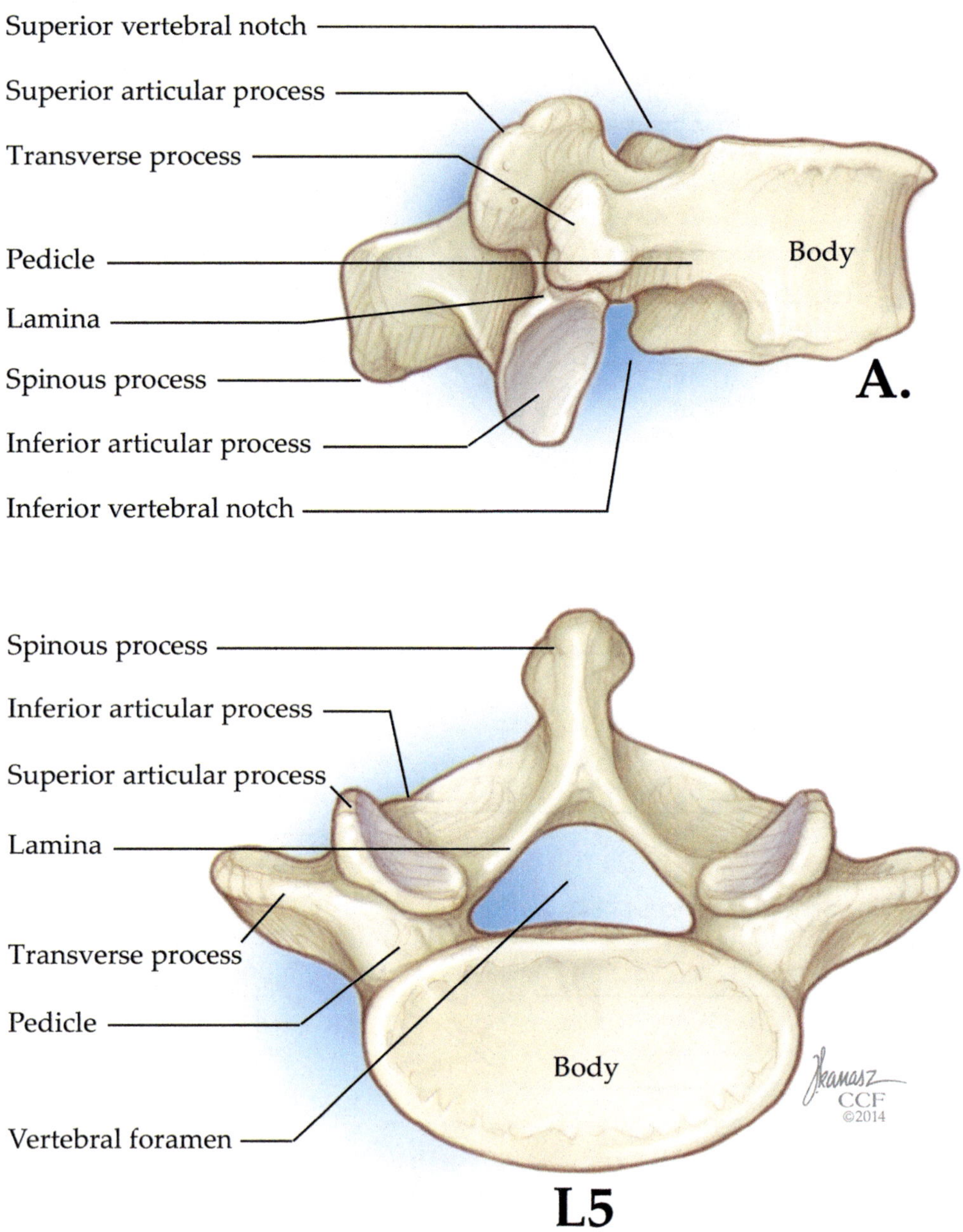

Fig. 4.4 (continued)

and afferent nerves from the dorsal rootlets terminate in the *dorsal horn*. In thoracic and upper lumbar areas, there are small projections in the middle of the dorsal and ventral horn, called *lateral horns*, which contain cell bodies for preganglionic sympathetic fibers. Cytoarchitecturally, the spinal cord gray matter is divided into ten distinct areas known as *Rexed laminae*.

Lamina I to VI is primarily involved with sensory functions and processing. Laminae I and II are the main targets for primary nociceptive afferents. Lamina II, also known as *substantia gelatinosa*, contains mostly interneurons involved with modulation of input from sensory neurons. Aß-fibers, which respond to fine touch, project in laminae III, IV, and V. Aδ nociceptors project to laminae I and V. Lamina V receives both non-noxious (Aß-fibers) and noxious input monosynaptically from Aδ nociceptors and indirectly (polysynaptically) from C fibers. These types of neurons that respond to multiple stimuli are known as WDR (wide dynamic range) neurons and are most abundantly found in lamina V. WDR neurons fire in graded fashion and exhibit phenomenon called windup, wherein repetitive stimulation leads to increased firing and post-discharge.

Rexed lamina VII consists of cell body of preganglionic sympathetic fibers in the lateral horn of the spinal cord. Laminae VIII and IX located in the ventral horn consist of cell bodies of motor fibers to the skeletal muscles.

White Matter

White matter surrounds the gray matter and is divided into ventral, lateral, and dorsal columns by the ventral and dorsal horn. It consists of ascending and descending tracts, consisting of nerve fibers connecting the brain and spinal cord. Their names usually refer to their origin and destination, e.g., corticospinal tract originating from cerebral motor cortex relaying motor signals to the ventral horn of the spinal cord.

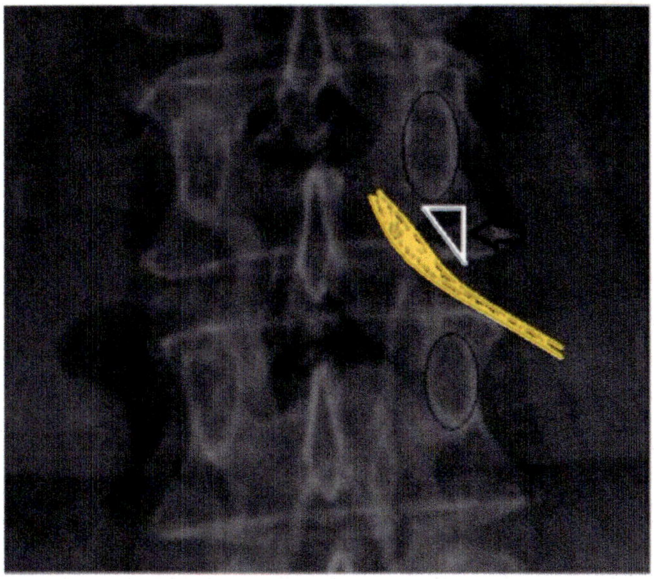

Fig. 4.5 The "safe triangle" – triangular area just superolateral to the nerve root, below the pedicle, and posterior to the vertebral body

Arterial Supply to the Spine

The spinal cord is supplied by three longitudinal arteries, one anterior spinal artery, which forms from the union of the two anterior spinal branches of each vertebral artery at the level of the foramen magnum, and two posterior spinal arteries which may either be direct branches of the vertebral artery or branches from posterior inferior cerebellar arteries (PICA). These longitudinal arteries receive collaterals from segmental arteries which originate from spinal branches of the vertebral, deep cervical, intercostal, and lumbar arteries. They transverse the intervertebral foramina at respective levels and supply anterior and posterior nerve roots, but most not reach the spinal cord. These smaller segmental arteries are called radicular arteries. However, larger segmental arteries primarily situated in the lower cervical, lower thoracic, and upper lumbar regions reach the dura where they divide to form ascending and descending arterioles and anastomose with anterior and posterior spinal arteries. These arteries are also known as *radiculomedullary arteries* to distinguish them from those radicular arteries that supply only the nerve roots. The largest radiculomedullary artery is called the

Fig. 4.6 Cross section of spinal cord demonstrating the Rexed laminae and ascending and descending tracts

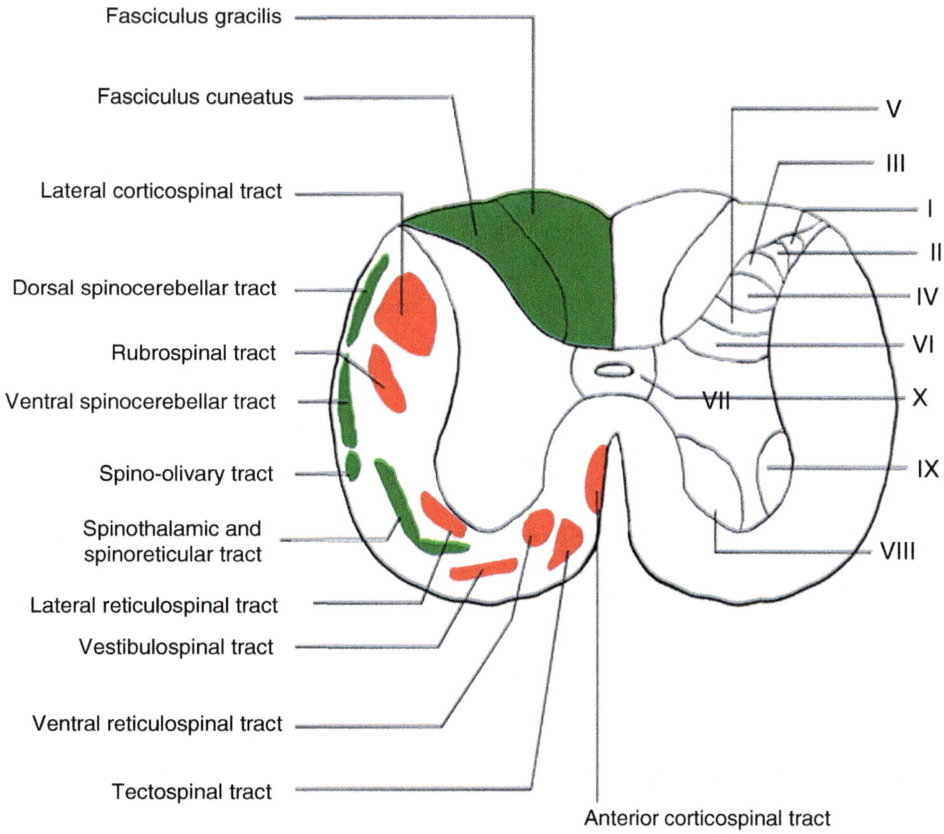

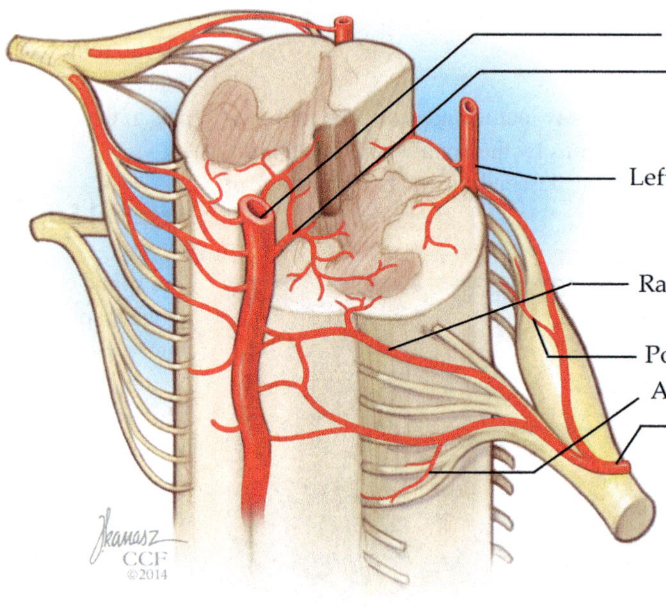

Fig. 4.7 Arterial supply to the spinal cord (Reprinted with permission, Cleveland Clinic Center for Medical Art & Photography © 2014–2015. All Rights Reserved)

artery of Adamkiewicz. It is usually a branch from one of the lower posterior intercostal arteries (T9–11), the subcostal artery (T12), or the upper lumbar arteries (L1 and L2). It most often arises on the left side, above L2 but has been found as low as L5 on the right side. The artery of Adamkiewicz may provide the main blood supply for the thoracolumbosacral part of the spinal cord (T8 to the conus medullaris). The anterior spinal artery supplies the anterior two thirds of the spinal cord, while the posterior one third of the spinal cord is supplied by the posterior spinal arteries (Fig. 4.7).

Venous Drainage of the Spinal Cord

Venous drainage of the spinal cord largely follows the arterial supply. The lower segments of the spinal cord are drained by a venous plexus that continues onward to the anterior and posterior spinal veins and subsequently to the anterior and posterior radicular veins that feed into the internal vertebral plexus of the epidural space, finally emptying into the azygous system.

Ischemia/Infarction of the Spinal Cord

Anterior spinal artery syndrome is caused by occlusion of the anterior spinal artery leading to infarction of anterior two thirds of spinal cord. It may be caused by atherosclerotic/embolic occlusion of the anterior spinal artery and spinal cord hypoperfusion or occurs after major aortic surgeries. Anterior spinal artery syndrome occurs most commonly in the mid-thoracic level because of the paucity of collaterals in this area and is hence termed the watershed area. Clinically the syndrome is characterized by loss of motor function, pain, temperature, and pin-prick sensation below the level of the lesion. Proprioception and fine touch sensation are usually preserved. Cases of spinal cord infraction have been reported with transforaminal epidural steroid injections with particulate steroid injection, even in low lumbar levels, presumably from the occlusion of the anterior spinal artery by the particulate material inadvertently injected into radiculomedullary arteries.

Imaging

Plain radiographs are the most commonly used modality to image the spine. However, information yielded is limited to gross bony abnormalities. Bony architecture of the spine is best revealed by CT. MRI, on the other hand, is less useful for revealing the osseous details; MRI is the imaging modality of choice to reveal details of bone marrow, ligaments, fascial planes, neural tissues, and other soft tissue structures. Common sequences used in spine MRI are T1-weighted and T2-weighted imaging in the axial and sagittal planes. Coronal imaging is useful in diagnosing scoliosis of the spine.

Spinal Pathology

Spondylosis Age-related degenerative changes in the vertebral column are defined as spondylosis. These changes may include loss of intervertebral disk height, uncovertebral

Table 4.2 Grading the level of spondylolisthesis

Grade I – 1–25% slip
Grade II – 26–50% slip
Grade III – 51–75% slip
Grade IV – 76–100% slip
Grade V – complete slip (>100%) also known as spondyloptosis

or facet joint arthrosis, and osteophyte formation. These changes may cause buckling of ligamentum flavum and facet joint hypertrophy resulting in neuroforaminal or spinal canal stenosis.

Spondylolysis Defects in the pars interarticularis are known as spondylolysis. It may lead to axial back pain and instability. In addition, these defects may lead to spondylolisthesis.

Spondylolisthesis Spondylolisthesis is defined as the displacement of one lumbar vertebra over another. Anterolisthesis is a term used to describe anterior displacement of a superior vertebra over an inferior vertebra. Similarly, retrolisthesis is used for posterior displacement of superior vertebra over inferior. The most common etiology in older populations is degenerative change; spondylolisthesis can be traumatic or pathologic in origin as well. The most common location is at the L4-L5 vertebra junction. Spondylolisthesis is graded as a percentage of movement of one superior vertebra over inferior vertebra. Spondylolisthesis can lead to spinal canal or neuroforaminal stenosis. Lateral lumbar radiographs, CT, and MRI can be used to grade the level of spondylolisthesis (Table 4.2). MRI is useful in assessing the canal or neuroforaminal stenosis associated with this condition, though the static image may miss dynamic changes in vertebral body alignment associated with movement (Fig. 4.8).

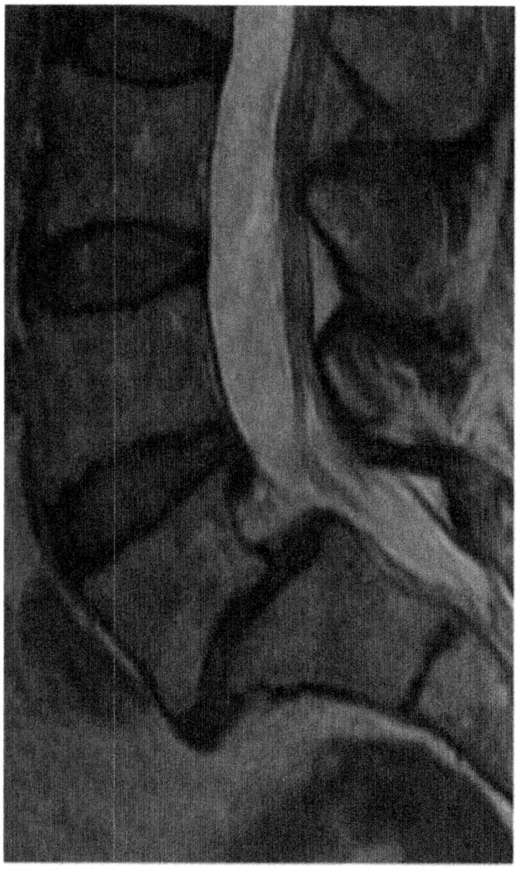

Fig. 4.8 T2-weighted MRI showing grade III anterolisthesis of L5 over S1 vertebra

Spinal Stenosis Spinal stenosis refers to the narrowing of the central vertebral canal resulting in compression of the spinal cord and/or nerve roots. It can be caused by disk degeneration, spondylolisthesis, ligamentum flavum hypertrophy, facet hypertrophy, or mass effect. In the lumbar region, it may manifest as neurogenic claudication. In severe cases it may cause myelopathy.

Myelopathy Myelopathy is referred to as a lesion or dysfunction of the spinal cord. The etiology may be compression caused by spondylosis; infection; neoplastic, vascular, metabolic diseases; etc. Clinical manifestations include gait disturbance, muscle weakness, hyporeflexia at the level of the lesion, spasticity, and hyperreflexia with Babinski sign below the lesion. Severe cases may lead to paresis. MRI is the imaging modality of choice for evaluation of patients with signs of myelopathy. MRI finds include spinal canal stenosis with or without high-intensity cord signals on T2-weighted images. Treatment is usually surgical decompression.

Cauda Equina Syndrome Cauda equina syndrome is caused by compression of the terminal spinal nerve roots. Clinically, the condition is characterized by back pain, saddle anesthesia, bladder or bowel dysfunction, and sexual dysfunction. The most common etiology is compression by a herniated intervertebral disk, but may also be caused by vertebral metastasis, spinal cord tumors, epidural granuloma from intrathecal infusions, traumatic vertebral fracture or dislocation, etc. Cauda equina syndrome is a medical emergency. All suspected cases should be evaluated by lumbar spine MRI, and urgent referral to a spine surgeon should be sought.

Tarlov Cyst Tarlov cyst is a CSF-containing cyst of nerve root most commonly seen in the sacral region. Although these are mostly asymptomatic, larger cysts may cause adjacent bony erosions and nerve root compression, leading to

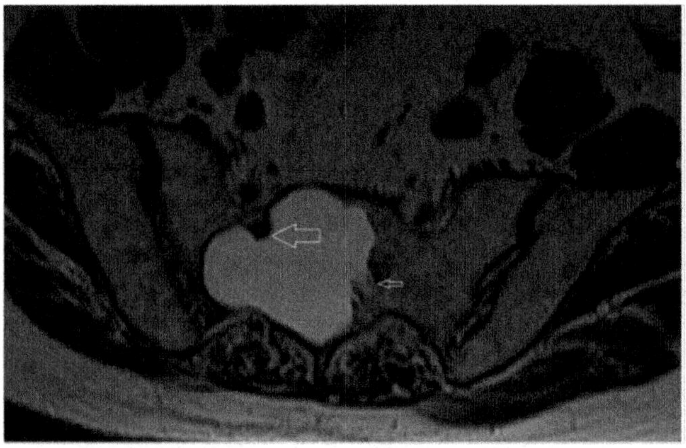

Fig. 4.9 T2-weighted axial section showing Tarlov cyst arising from right S2 nerve root (*large arrow*) causing bony erosion and contralateral nerve root compression (*small arrow*)

pain and radicular symptoms (Fig. 4.9). MRI is the diagnostic modality of choice. Treatment of a symptomatic cyst is drainage.

Suggested Reading

1. Basbaum AI, Bautista DM, Scherrer G, Julius D. Cellular and molecular mechanisms of pain. Cell. 2009;139(2):267–84.
2. Feigenbaum F, Voyadzis JM, Henderson FC. Tarlov cysts. In: Benzel EC, editor. Spine surgery: techniques, complication avoidance, and management, vol. 2. 3rd ed. Philadelphia: Elsevier; 2012. p. 1135–40.
3. D'Mello R, Dickenson AH. Spinal cord mechanisms of pain. Br J Anaesth. 2008;101(1):8–16.
4. Glaser SE, Shah RV. Root cause analysis of paraplegia following transforaminal epidural steroid injections: the "unsafe" triangle. Pain Physician. 2010;13(3):237–44.
5. Hanson JT. Netter's clinical anatomy. 3rd ed. Philadelphia: Saunders/Elsevier; 2014. p. 49–86.
6. Standring S. Gray's anatomy. 40th ed.

Peripheral Pathways and Anatomy of the Peripheral Nerve

5

Michael I. Yang

Key Concepts

- The topography of the sensory and motor bundles is variable related to the surface of the nerve, and therefore cathode stimulation needs to be tested.
- The peripheral nerves have different electrophysiological classifications based on the size and presence of myelin.

Introduction

Ever since Melzack and Wall introduced the gate control theory, the applications for neurostimulation have grown exponentially. First introduced in the intrathecal space, electrical neuromodulation has been advancing into the periphery. Peripheral nerve stimulation (PNS) is the direct electrical stimulation of specific, named nerves outside of the central nervous system, which directly inhibit primary nociceptive afferent fibers.

Background

The peripheral nervous system is composed of the groups of neurons called ganglia and bundles of axons (nerves) that are outside of the brain and spinal cord. The peripheral nervous system has two components, somatic and autonomic. The somatic nervous system consists of the sensory and the motor neurons. Sensory ganglia are unipolar sensory neurons and are in the dorsal root of all spinal nerves as well as many of the cranial nerves. Autonomic ganglia are in the sympathetic chain, or in the associated paravertebral or prevertebral ganglia, or in terminal ganglia within the organs.

The sensory neurons are the peripheral axonal processes of neurons with cell bodies in the dorsal root ganglion. The motor axons are the processes of anterior horn cells of the spinal cord. Peripheral nerves have many layers of connective tissue; axons are encased within the endoneurium and bundled into fascicles and surrounded by the perineurium – the perineurium binding axons into fascicles and the epineurium binding the fascicles into a nerve. The fascicles can divide and fuse to form multiple plexi along the nerve trunk. The nerve axons are then surrounded by Schwann cells, which wrap the axons in myelin. The blood vessels are slightly coiled so as to accommodate for the various movements of the nerves. Smaller capillaries from the epineurial blood vessels course to all inner parts of the nerve, so it is difficult to make any part of a peripheral nerve ischemic. All the above layers of the nerve are innervated and have a complex plexus of nociceptors (Fig. 5.1).

The diameter of the axon and the distance between the nodes of Ranvier determine the speed of conduction of the nerve signal. The function and classification of an axon can be deduced from its diameter and from conduction velocity. Peripheral nerves can be categorized based on their conduction velocity and diameter (Table 5.1).

Nerves are classified as cranial nerves or spinal nerves on the basis of their connection to the brain or spinal cord, respectively. The 12 cranial nerves can be sensory, motor, or a combination of the two. Spinal nerves are all mixed nerves with both sensory and motor fibers. Spinal nerves emerge from the spinal cord and then form plexuses, which give rise to systemic nerves. Thoracic spinal nerves directly become the intercostal nerves.

By better understanding the anatomy of the peripheral nervous system, one can become more comfortable with implantable techniques.

M.I. Yang, MD (✉)
Summit Pain Alliance Inc., Interventional Pain Management,
392 Tesconi Ct, Santa Rosa, CA 95401, USA
e-mail: Michael.i.yang@gmail.com

J.E. Pope, T.R. Deer (eds.), *Treatment of Chronic Pain Conditions*, DOI 10.1007/978-1-4939-6976-0_5

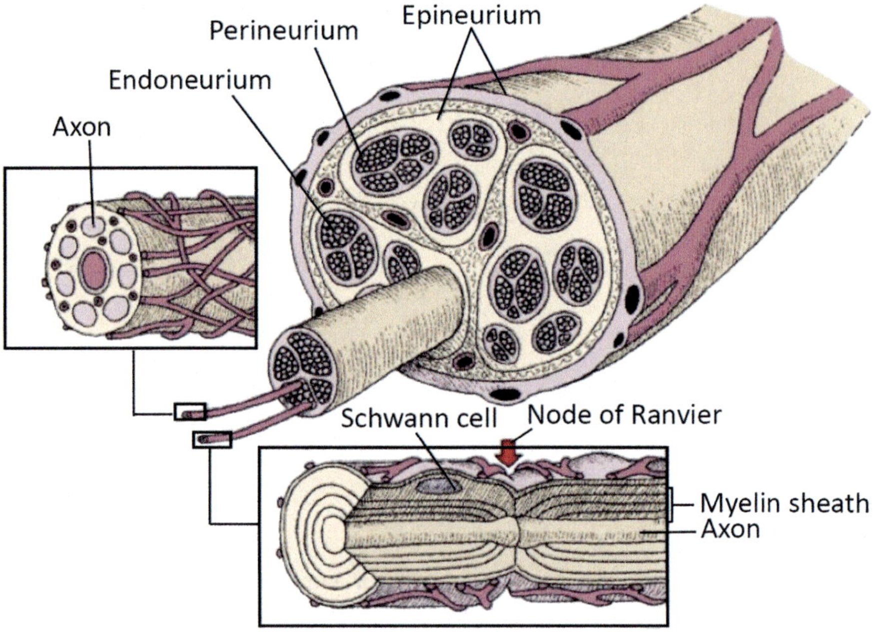

Fig. 5.1 Layers of the nerve

Table 5.1 Nerve fiber classification, diameter and conduction velocity

Electrophysiological classification of peripheral nerves	Classification of afferent fibers only (class/group)	Fiber diameter (μm)	Conduction velocity (m/s)	Receptor supplied
Sensory fiber type				
Aα	Ia and Ib	13–20	80–120	Primary muscle spindles, Golgi tendon organ
Aβ	II	6–12	35–75	Secondary muscle spindles, skin mechanoreceptors
Aδ	III	1–5	5–30	Skin mechanoreceptors, thermal receptors, and nociceptors
C	IV	0.2–1.5	0.5–2	
Motor fiber type				
Aα	N/A	12–20	72–120	Extrafusal skeletal muscle fibers
Aγ	N/A	2–8	12–48	Intrafusal muscle fibers
B	N/A	1–3	6–18	Preganglionic autonomic fibers
C	N/A	0.2–2	0.5–2	Postganglionic autonomic fibers

Adapted from Warren et al. [3]

Suggested Reading

1. Bove G. Epi-perineurial anatomy, innervation, and axonal nociceptive mechanisms. J Bodyw Mov Ther. 2008;12(3):185–90.
2. Esmaeil B, Khorasani MT, Montazeri N, et al. Types of neural guides and using nanotechnology for peripheral nerve reconstruction. Int J Nanomedicine. 2010;5:839–52.
3. Warren S, Capra NF, Yezierski RP. The somatosensory system I: tactile discrimination and position sense. In: Fundamental neuroscience. 4th ed. New York: Churchill Livingstone Inc.; 2012. p. 262–79.

Part III

Evaluation and Assessment: III. History and Physical

6 Evaluation of Headache

Zachary McCormick and Rajiv Reddy

Key Concepts

- A thorough history is the most revealing tool in the evaluation of headaches.
- Screening for health- or life-threatening causes of headache must be performed.
- The most common primary headache disorders include tension-type, migraine, and cluster headache.
- Secondary headaches commonly referred to pain medicine specialists are often related to medication overuse or cervical spine disease/dysfunction.
- Patients often have more than one type of headache. It is helpful to differentiate the most common or primary headache type.
- A headache diary is a useful tool to characterize patterns and triggers.
- The physical examination may provide no positive findings in most patients with primary headaches but can provide vital information in diagnosing health- or life-threatening secondary headaches.
- Imaging is indicated when a health- or life-threatening secondary headache is suspected. The decision to image may be informed by guidelines developed by the American Association of Neurology.

Introduction

According to some sources, headache is the most common complaint that leads people to seek medical care. Thus, the pain medicine specialist must be comfortable with a thorough yet efficient evaluation of headache. The evaluation of headache begins with a targeted history and physical examination. A health- or life-threatening cause of headache must first be ruled out. If the reason for concern is identified, the workup must progress rapidly. If suspicion for a health- or life-threatening headache is alleviated, a reasonable approach involves determining whether symptoms are related to a benign secondary headache disorder versus a primary headache disorder. Headaches may resolve without further need for treatment if a secondary cause of headache can be identified and eliminated. Alternatively, if symptoms appear to be related to a primary headache disorder, establishing a correct diagnosis is vital to subsequently developing a treatment plan.

History

A thorough interview that includes key elements of history (Table 6.1) is necessary to distinguish primary versus secondary causes of headache. Attention to potential "red flags" is important in order to determine the urgency of imaging or other intervention. Elements of history that should provoke concern include a new headache of unusual severity or a sudden change in typical headache patter; a rapid progression to peak symptoms, association with traumatic onset, exertion, or Valsalva maneuver; and nocturnal symptoms, association with recumbent positions, projectile vomiting, neurologic dysfunction, or evidence of other associated systemic illness.

If potential "red flag" symptoms are not present, the focus of interview can shift to distinguishing whether the headache is related to primary or secondary cause. While there are numerous primary causes of headache (Table 6.2), pain medicine specialists tend to encounter tension-type, migraine, and cluster headaches most commonly. Typical features of these headache types are shown in Table 6.3. Likewise, of the numerous types of secondary headaches (Table 6.4), pain specialists are most likely to see patients with cervicogenic

Z. McCormick, MD (✉)
Northwestern University, The Rehabilitation Institute of Chicago, 345 East Superior Street, Chicago, IL 60611, USA
e-mail: zmccormi@gmail.com

R. Reddy, MD
The Rehabilitation Institute of Chicago, Chicago, IL, USA

J.E. Pope, T.R. Deer (eds.), *Treatment of Chronic Pain Conditions*, DOI 10.1007/978-1-4939-6976-0_6

Table 6.1 Key elements of a headache history

Onset
Progression
Temporal pattern (frequency, duration, time of day, menstruation, etc.)
Location
Quality
Severity
Premonitory symptoms
Triggers
Exacerbating and relieving factors
Associated symptoms
Family headache history
Past medical history
Social history – occupation, habits, diet
Medication reconciliation

Table 6.2 Primary headache disorders

Most common	Common
	Paroxysmal hemicrania
Migraine with or without aura	Paroxysmal short-lasting unilateral neuralgiform attacks (SUNCT)
Tension-type headache	Hemicrania continua
Cluster headache	Cold-stimulus headache
	Benign cough headache
	Benign exertional headache

Table 6.3 Typical features of common primary headache

Tension-type headache
Mild/moderate intensity paroxysmal, bilateral "band-like" lasting 30 min to 7 days
Migraine headache
Moderate/severe unilateral paroxysmal "throbbing" headache lasting 4–72 h associated with nausea, vomiting, photo-/phonophobia with or without aura, with predictable environmental or dietary triggers, possible relation to menstrual cycle, aggravated by routine physical activity, improved with sleep, often with a family history of similar headaches
Cluster headache
Severe unilateral orbital/temporal "stabbing/piercing" headache with possible tearing, rhinorrhea, miosis, ptosis, eyelid edema, or facial diaphoresis, lasting 15–180 min occurring more than 5x per day, often a predictable times during the day, in cycles of 2 weeks to 3 months

or medication overuse as the underlying etiology of secondary headache. Typical features of these headache types are shown in Table 6.5.

It is important to recognize that patients may experience more than one type of headache, which may be related. For example, cervicogenic headache may provoke tension-type headache due to reactionary guarding or head, neck, and shoulder girdle postural changes. Any headache type may be associated with independent analgesic rebound headache due to frequent nonsteroidal anti-inflammatory drug (NSAID) use. In cases where headache type is not easily categorize due to symptom overlap or inadequate history, instructing the patient to keep a headache diary may be useful. A sample template for a headache diary useful for clinical practice is shown in Table 6.6.

Table 6.4 Secondary headache disorders

Benign	Health- or life-threatening
Medication-overuse headache	Cerebrovascular dissection, thrombosis, or vasculitis
Cervicogenic headache	Intracranial hemorrhage
Sinusitis	Subdural hemorrhage
Dental	Hydrocephalus
	CSF leak
	Idiopathic intracranial hypertension
	Neoplasm
	Meningitis
	Abscess
	Open-angle glaucoma

Table 6.5 Common, benign secondary headaches most often encountered by pain medicine specialists

Cervicogenic headache
Occipitofrontal unilateral headache with predominant neck pain, worsened by movement of the cervical spine, potentially in the setting of recent trauma/whiplash-type injury or osteoarthritis: cervicogenic headache
Medication-overuse headache
Insidious, progressive onset of frequency and intensity, associated with regular analgesic use, temporally related to the last dose or just prior to the next scheduled dose of an analgesic medication (most often ergotamines, triptans, opioids, or NSAIDs), with possible development of drug-dependence behavior

Table 6.6 Sample headache diary template

Date:
Time started/ended:
Warning signs:
Quality of pain ("stabbing," "throbbing," etc.):
Pain intensity (0–10):
Location:
Other symptoms (nausea, photophobia, etc.):
Treatment or medication tried and effect:
Hours of sleep:
Food eaten today:
Events prior to headache (activity, stress, etc.):
Other comments:

Physical Examination

In general, physical examination in the headache patient will provide less diagnostic information than the history. However, the physical exam can provide vital clues that indicate a health- or life-threatening type of headache. Thus, a thorough but targeted physical exam in the evaluation of headache is necessary and, with repetition, can be performed in approximately 3 min.

A systematic approach to the physical exam will ensure thorough screening and efficiency. Key elements of the targeted headache physical exam are shown in Table 6.7. "Red flag" features on physical exam include Horner's syndrome (arterial dissection, malignancy), oculomotor deficits particularly with pupil asymmetry (aneurysm), combined facial weakness, and numbness (head and neck malignancy). In general, any cranial nerve palsy or neurologic deficit should raise concern for a potentially health- or life-threatening cause of headache.

Aside from screening for potentially sinister causes of headache, a careful examination of the cervical spine and shoulder girdle is often illuminating given that pain medicine specialists often see patients with cervicogenic symptoms. Complete assessment includes postural assessment with attention to cervical spine and scapular position, cervical range of motion in all planes, palpation for tender and trigger points, as well as zygapophysial joint and occipital nerve-regional tenderness.

Table 6.7 Key elements of a targeted headache physical exam

Vital signs
Mental status
Speech
Cranial nerves; particular attention to pupil symmetry, ocular movement, facial symmetry, and strength
Sympathetics; Horner's syndrome (ipsilateral ptosis, miosis, facial anhydrosis)
Fundoscopic exam for papilledema if increased intracranial pressure is suspected
Muscle stretch reflexes, Hoffman's sign, Babinski sign
Motor function
Sensation
Balance
Gait
Musculoskeletal assessment of the cervical spine and shoulder girdle; posture, cervical range of motion, palpation for tender and trigger points
Temporomandibular joint assessment; range of motion, palpation
Palpation of the sinuses and teeth

Imaging

No particular imaging is indicated for a primary headache disorder. However, if there is clinical suspicion for a secondary headache disorder, imaging must be considered. While consensus does not exist, an imaging guideline to inform clinical management of non-acute headache was developed by the American Academy of Neurology (Table 6.8). Imaging may also be considered when cervicogenic headache is suspected, as zygapophysial arthropathy, cervical foraminal stenosis, or other structural findings may provoke such symptoms. Corroborating clinical and imaging findings in such cases may inform the diagnosis as well as identify potential targets for therapeutic intervention.

Conclusion

A thorough, targeted history and physical exam is vital in the evaluation of headache. Pain medicine specialists should be familiar with the commonly encountered types of headache but should also systematically screen for potentially health- or life-threatening causes of headache.

Table 6.8 American Academy of Neurology imaging guideline for non-acute headache

1. Non-contrast-computed tomography
(a) Recommended when urgent neuroimaging is necessary in cases of:
(i) Suspected intracranial hemorrhage
(ii) Suspected elevated intracranial pressure or focal neurologic deficit prior to lumbar puncture
(iii) Headache associated with neurologic changes
(iv) Headache presenting with a substantial change in previously experienced headache characteristics
2. Contrast-enhanced computed tomography
(a) Recommended if abnormality is found on non-contrast CT or a vascular abnormality or tumor is suspected and an urgent evaluation is necessary.
3. Magnetic resonance imaging
(a) Recommended as an initial or urgent diagnostic examination if there is suspicion of venous sinus thrombosis or vasculitis
(b) Recommended when an abnormality is suspected in the posterior cranial fossa or at the craniocervical junction
(c) Recommended when an aneurysm or vascular malformation is suspected and evaluated with magnetic resonance angiography (MRA)
(d) If an abnormality is detected on CT, MRI may further define the abnormality

Suggested Reading

1. Donohoe CD. The role of the physical examination in the evaluation of headache. Med Clin North Am. 2013;97(2):197–216.
2. Frishberg B, Rosenberg JH, Matchar DB, et al. Evidence-based guidelines in the primary care setting: neuroimaging in patients with nonacute headache. www.aan.com/go/practice/guidelines.
3. Waldman SD. Targeted headache history. Med Clin North Am. 2013;97(2):185–95.

Cervical Spine History and Physical

7

Navdeep Singh Jassal

Key Concepts

- The cervical spine history and physical examination of a patient are of utmost importance as diagnostic tools and are the fundamental tools for triage.
- The goal should be to develop your patient's trust, to gain insight of the impact on their level of function, and to identify the likely pain generators.

History

A systematic comprehensive history should follow an inquiry approach into several domains (which can also be relevant to any pain problem), including chief complaint, site, length of illness, intensity, spread/radiation, quality/character, intensity, frequency, duration, time of onset, mode of onset, precipitating factors, aggravating factors, relieving factors, and associated features.

The domain of associated features is the most important, as it may lead the differential toward more serious causes of pain. Refer to "red flags" description and clinical indicators for serious causes of spinal pain in Lumbar Spine H&P chapter, as they also hold true for the cervical spine. After cervical radiculopathy, cervical spondylotic myelopathy is the most common cervical cord lesion after middle age. It typically has an insidious onset; average age set is after 50 years, and it shows signs of bowel/bladder incontinence, weakness/gait instability, and upper motor neuron signs.

Investigating litigation, secondary gain issues, and documenting functional losses should also be included in the history of present illness.

N.S. Jassal, MD (✉)
Florida Pain Medicine, University of South Florida, Department of Neurology, James A. Haley VA Medical Center, Number 127, Tampa, FL 33612, USA
e-mail: navdeepjassal@gmail.com

Physical Exam

The cervical spine traditionally involves inspection, palpation, range of motion, neurologic examination, special tests, and examination of related areas. Emphasis should be placed on the neurologic exam, as cervical spine pathology can be reflected to the upper extremity (weakness, altered reflexes, sensation).

Inspection

This begins as the patient enters the exam room. Check for posture of the head and abnormalities such as blisters, scars (both anterior and posterior), and discoloration.

Palpation

Palpation can be divided into bony and soft tissue palpation.

Bony Palpation

This should be performed as muscles are relaxed in the supine position. Palpate the anterior bony structures of the neck including the hyoid, thyroid cartilage, first cricoid ring, and carotid tubercles. Palpate the posterior aspect including the occiput, the superior nuchal line, the mastoid process, the spinous processes, and the facet joints. The C7 and T1 spinous processes are larger than those above them, and a misalignment can indicate facet dislocation or fracture to the spinous process. The C5 and C6 are the most commonly involved joints in cervical facet arthropathy.

Soft Tissue Palpation

This is divided into two clinical zones including the anterior and the posterior aspect. Palpate the sternocleidomastoid muscle, lymph node chain, thyroid gland, carotid pulse, parotid gland, and supraclavicular fossa in the anterior

J.E. Pope, T.R. Deer (eds.), *Treatment of Chronic Pain Conditions*, DOI 10.1007/978-1-4939-6976-0_7

Table 7.1 Sensory innervation landmarks by dermatome

Dermatome	Landmark
C4	Shoulder
C5	Lateral aspect of the elbow
C6	Thumb
C7	Middle finger
C8	Little finger
T1	Medial aspect of the elbow

Table 7.2 Muscles and action relative to myotomes

Root level	Muscle(s) tested	Action
C4	Levator scapulae	Shoulder shrug
C5	Biceps	Elbow flexion
C6	Extensor carpi radialis L.	Wrist extension
C7	and B.	Forearm extension
C8	Triceps	Middle finger DIP flexion
T1	Flexor digitorum profundus Dorsal interossei	Finger abductors

aspect. Palpate the trapezius muscle, lymph nodes, greater occipital nerves, and superior nuchal ligament in the posterior aspect.

Range of Motion (ROM)

Movements include passive and active flexion, extension, lateral bending, and rotation. Approximately 50% of flexion/extension occurs between the occiput and C1, and 50% of rotation takes place between C1 (atlas) and C2 (axis).

Neurologic Examination

It can be divided into (1) muscle testing of the intrinsic muscles of the neck including flexion, extension, lateral rotation, and bending and (2) neurologic examination of the upper extremity by neurologic levels.

Lesions can be separated into central, spinal nerve root, and peripheral nerve lesions. Comparison of sensory deficits relative to classical dermatome charts (see Tables 7.1 and 7.2) and peripheral cutaneous nerve maps can help localize the lesion.

Table 7.3 Reflexes – cervical spine

Nerve root level	Reflex
C5–C6	Biceps reflex
C7–C8	Brachioradialis reflexTriceps reflex

Muscle strength testing can be used as a tool to grade a specific, symmetric group of muscles (refer to the Table 9.3).

Reflexes

Reflexes are tested by tapping the tendon with a reflex hammer to elicit a muscle contraction. Jendrassik maneuver can be used to optimize the response by distracting the patient by asking him/her to interlock flexed fingers. Hoffman's sign may be indicative of an upper motor neuron disease (Table 7.3).

Gait Testing

Gait testing includes observation of normal ambulation characteristics, heel to toe walk, and tandem gait testing. It is important when considering for cervical myelopathy.

Special Tests

Special tests include the distraction test (effect of neck traction on relieving pain caused by neural foramen narrowing), Spurling's test (radicular pain caused by extending the neck and rotating the chin toward the affected extremity), cervical facet loading (indicative for cervical facet arthropathy), Adson test (determines state of the subclavian artery), and Valsalva test.

Examination of Related Areas

Examination of adjacent, structures including the shoulder and temporomandibular joint, is important, as these areas can all refer pain to the cervical spine.

Suggested Reading

1. Benzon HT, et al. Essentials of pain medicine. Philadelphia: Elsevier/Saunders; 2011.
2. Fishman SM, et al. Bonica's management of pain. Baltimore: Lippincott Williams & Wilkins; 2010.
3. Hoppenfeld S. Physical examination of the spine and the extremities. Norwalk: Appleton & Lange; 1976.

8 Thoracic Spine History and Physical

Reda Tolba

Key Concepts

- Thorough history taking and pain assessment of the thoracic region are essential for proper diagnosis and management of various pain conditions.
- A comprehensive physical exam including inspection and palpation of the thoracic spine including the thorax, abdomen, and back is needed to explore the complaints raised in the history.
- Imaging studies help to correlate findings obtained from the history and physical exam to reach a proper diagnosis.

Introduction

History and physical exam is crucial for diagnosis of chronic pain, specifically for the thoracic spine, as the differential is diverse. We explore the signs and symptoms of common thoracic pain challenges to improve patient outcomes.

History and Pain Assessment

- A detailed history is obtained from the patient with pain in the thoracic region. It includes the onset of pain, duration of the pain, character of the pain, precipitating factors, relieving factors, and intensity of the pain. Asking about the presence of any red flags such as significant motor or sensory deficits, urine or bowel incontinence, fever, and night sweats is essential to rule out any emergent condition that requires immediate attention and intervention.
- The character of the pain can help differentiate between neuropathic pain (burning, shooting) and nociceptive pain (aching).
- The intensity of the pain can be measured by different scales including visual analogue scale (VAS), verbal rating scale (VRS), numerical rating scale (NRS), and others. Other measures can be used to assess the degree of disability caused by the pain such as Pain Disability Index (PDI). Such measures are important to obtain at the initial visit to compare in the future visits the efficacy of the treatment and percentage of improvement the patient is getting.
- It is important to ask about recent history of fall or trauma. Elderly patients with osteoporosis are vulnerable to vertebral compression fractures which can cause severe mid-back pain.
- Previous treatments tried include medications, physical therapy, chiropractor treatment, and interventional pain procedures. Which modality has helped the patient in the past if any.
- Detailed history specific for each common condition that can cause pain in the thoracic region. Thoracic radiculopathy would cause back pain radiating to the chest wall depending on the level involved. Patient with recent history of shingles can develop severe burning pain across the corresponding thoracic dermatome. If the pain lingers more than 3 months, the condition is called post-herpetic neuralgia. Elderly patients with history of falls can develop vertebral compression fracture at the thoracic region causing severe and debilitating thoracic pain. Patients with history of cancer can develop pain in the thoracic spine and ribs due to multiple myeloma or metastatic disease. History of surgery in the thoracic region is important. Patient can develop persistent pain close to the incision, a condition called post-thoracotomy syndrome. History of fever, night sweats, and alarming signs of infection can raise the possibility of more serious conditions like vertebral osteomyelitis. Thorough history is essential to rule out such rare but serious conditions.

R. Tolba, MD (✉)
200 west Esplanade Avenue, Kenner, LA 70005, USA
e-mail: redatolba@hotmail.com

J.E. Pope, T.R. Deer (eds.), *Treatment of Chronic Pain Conditions*, DOI 10.1007/978-1-4939-6976-0_8

Other conditions like osteochondritis can cause pain in the anterior chest wall close to the sternum. Myofascial pain is a common cause of thoracic back pain and is usually confirmed by physical exam.

Physical Examination

- A comprehensive physical examination of the thoracic region including the thoracic spine, ribs, sternum, and chest wall as well as the abdomen is essential to explore the complaints raised in the history.
- Inspection of the thoracic spine for proper alignment and the presence of kyphosis, scoliosis, or angular deformities. Inspection of the chest wall and the thoracic spine for any cutaneous lesions such as herpetic lesions. Inspection of scars of previous surgeries including thoracic spine and thoracotomy scars. Inspection of the thoracic for masses or ecchymosis.
- Palpation of the thoracic spine for spinal tenderness, paraspinal muscle tenderness, and myofascial trigger points as seen in myofascial pain and thoracic facet syndrome. Severe tenderness on range of motion and percussion is noted over the affected vertebral level in patients suffering from vertebral compression fracture. Allodynia and hyperalgesia are sometimes noted over the back and chest wall in patients with herpetic and post-herpetic neuralgia along the affected dermatomes. Tenderness over the costochondral junction is noted for patient with costochondritis. Tenderness over the thoracic spine and over the ribs can be noted in patients with metastatic disease and patients suffering from multiple myeloma. Deep palpation of the abdomen can be performed to rule out any pulsatile masses such as aortic aneurysm which can be presented with thoracic pain. Range of motion of the thoracic spine is usually limited due to its location.
- Imaging studies such as X-rays, CT scans, and MRI should be reviewed. Results interpretation and proper correlation with the history and physical exam are important to adequately diagnose and treat the patients.

Suggested Reading

1. Benzon H, Srinivas NR, Fishman SM, Liu S, Cohen SP, editors. Essentials of pain medicine. 3rd ed. ISBN: 978-1-4377-2242-0. 2011
2. Fishman SM, Ballantyne JC, Pathmell JP, editors. Bonica's management of pain. 4th ed. Philadelphia, Wolters Kluwer/Lippincott, Williams and Wilkins, 2010

Lumbar Spine History and Physical

9

Navdeep Singh Jassal

Key Concepts

- The lumbar spine history and physical examination of a patient are of utmost importance as diagnostic tools and are the fundamental tools for triage.
- The goal should be to develop your patient's trust, to gain insight of the impact on their level of function and to identify the likely pain generators.

History

A systematic comprehensive history should follow an inquiry approach into several domains (which can also be relevant to any pain problem), including chief complaint, site, length of illness, intensity, spread/radiation, quality/character, intensity, frequency, duration, time of onset, mode of onset, precipitating factors, aggravating factors, relieving factors and associated features.

The domain of associated features is the most important, especially with regard to low back pain, as it may lead the differential towards more serious causes of pain. "Red flag" indicators include history of fever/night sweats, trauma, recent surgery, illicit drug use, weight loss, prior history of cancer, occupational exposure, bowel or bladder incontinence and neurological signs/symptoms. This can help to raise suspicion for serious causes for low back pain (see Table 9.1).

Investigating litigation, secondary gain issues and documenting functional losses should be included in the history of present illness. Vocational history including lifting associated with bending or twisting is the most common work activity associated with low back injuries. Nursing, truck driving and machine operations are amongst the occupations with the greatest incidence of back injuries receiving workers compensation.

N.S. Jassal, MD (✉)
Florida Pain Medicine, University of South Florida, Department of Neurology, James A. Haley VA Medical Center, Number 127, Tampa, FL 33612, USA
e-mail: navdeepjassal@gmail.com

Physical Exam

The lumbar spine traditionally involved inspection, palpation, range of motion, neurologic examination, special tests and examination of related areas.

Inspection

Check the back for redness, unusual skin markings, lipoma and birth marks. This may give insight to possible infection, neurologic/bone pathology and spina bifida, respectively. Posture should be checked including assessing for signs of scoliosis, degree of lumbar lordosis curvature or the presence of kyphosis.

Palpation

Palpation can be divided into bony and soft tissue palpation.

Bony Palpation

Locate the L4/L5 interspace by placing your fingers on the iliac crests and your thumbs at the midline of the back. Palpate the spinous processes of other vertebrae superiorly and inferiorly using your L4/L5 reference point. There may indication of spondylolisthesis by a visible or palpable "step off" from one process to the next. Coccydynia can develop after direct trauma and can be assessed via a rectal examination. Examine the posterior superior iliac spines, iliac crests, greater trochanters and ischial tuberosities.

J.E. Pope, T.R. Deer (eds.), *Treatment of Chronic Pain Conditions*, DOI 10.1007/978-1-4939-6976-0_9

Table 9.1 Clinical indicators for serious causes of spinal pain

Pathology	Clinical indicators
Aortic aneurysm	Cardiovascular risk factors, no MSK signs, anticoagulants
Tumour	Prior history of malignancy, age > 50, failure to improve, weight loss, pain not relieved with rest
Infection	Fever, sweating, risk factors including invasive medical procedure/injection, illicit drug use, trauma to skin/mucous membrane, immunosuppression, diabetes, alcoholism
Fracture	Severe trauma
Stress fracture	Sports involving extension and rotation of the spine
Pathologic fracture	Prior history of malignancy, osteoporosis, prolonged uses of corticosteroids

Soft Tissue Palpation

This is divided into five clinical zones including midline raphe (includes superior and interspinous ligaments, paraspinals), iliac crest, posterior superior iliac spine, sciatic area, anterior abdominal wall and inguinal area.

Range of Motion (ROM)

ROM is greatest at L5–S1 and movements include flexion, extension, lateral bending and rotation.

Neurologic Examination

Neurologic examination can be divided into sensation, motor, reflexes and coordination.

Lesions can be separated into central, spinal nerve root and peripheral nerve lesions. Comparison of sensory deficits relative to classical dermatome charts (see Table 9.2) and peripheral cutaneous nerve maps can help localize the lesion.

Muscle strength testing can be used as a tool to grade a specific, symmetric group of muscles (Tables 9.3, 9.4, 9.5, and 9.6).

Coordination and Gait Testing

Coordination and gait testing is a sensitive indicator for cerebellar function (finger to nose, heel to shin) and equilibrium (observation of normal gait, heel to toe walk and tandem gait testing). Gait testing should also include pelvic tilt, motion and drifting.

Special tests include lumbar facet loading (indicative for lumbar facet arthropathy), femoral nerve stretch (indicative for high lumbar radiculopathy), straight leg raise (tests to stretch the spinal cord/sciatic n.), Hoover Test (determine if

Table 9.2 Sensory innervation landmarks by dermatome

Dermatome	Landmark
L1	Halfway between T12 (midline inguinal ligament) and L2
L2	Mid-anterior thigh
L3	Medial femoral condyle
L4	Medial malleolus
L5	Dorsum of foot
S1	Lateral heel
S2	Popliteal fossa at midline
S3	Ischial tuberosity
S4–5	Perianal area

Table 9.3 Lumbar region nerve root testing

Grade	Description
0	No muscle contraction
1	Trace contraction that is visible or palpable
2	Full active ROM with gravity eliminated
3	Full active ROM against gravity
4	Full active ROM against gravity with min-mod resistance
5	Full active ROM against gravity with max resistance

Root level	Muscle(s) tested	Action
L2	Psoas, Iliacus	Hip flexion
L3	Quadriceps femoris	Knee extension
L4	Tibialis	Ankle dorsiflexion
L5	Extensor hallucis longus (EHL)	EHL extension
	Peroneus Longus	Ankle Eversion
S1	Hamstrings	Ankle plantar flexion

Table 9.4 Muscles and action relative to myotomes

Reflexes
Tested by tapping the tendon with a reflex hammer to elicit muscle contraction
Jendrassik manoeuver can be used to optimize the response by distracting the patient by asking him/her to interlock flexed fingers
Clonus and an upgoing great toe (Babinski's sign) may be indicative of an upper motor neuron disease

Table 9.5 Reflexes and grading

Grade	Description
0	No response
1+	Reduced, hypoactive
2+	Normal response
3+	Brisk, hyperactive without clonus
4+	Hyperactive with clonus

Table 9.6 Reflexes – LS spine

Nerve root level	Reflex
L3–4	Patellar reflex
S1–2	Achilles reflex

malingering), Gaenslen's Sign (indicative for SI joint pathology) and Patrick/Faber Test (indicative to detect hip pathology or SI joint pathology).

Examination of Related Areas

Examination of related areas should include the hip, rectum and pelvis, as these areas can all refer pain to the lumbar spine.

Suggested Reading

1. Benzon HT, et al. Essentials of pain medicine. Philadelphia: Elsevier Saunders; 2011.
2. Fishman SM, et al. Bonica's management of pain. Baltimore: Lippincott Williams & Wilkins; 2010.
3. Hoppenfeld S. Physical examination of the spine and the extremities. Norwalk: Appleton & Lange; 1976.

Upper Extremity Physical Examination

10

Enrique Galang and George C. Chang Chien

Key Concepts

- The evaluation of the upper extremity must begin with a detailed history, as this is essential in formulating a differential diagnosis.
- A thorough understanding of the anatomy of the upper extremity is required to effectively perform a physical examination.
- Advanced imaging and electrodiagnostic studies (NCV/EMG) coupled with a thorough history and physical examination can assist the clinician in making a diagnosis.

Introduction

Neck and shoulder pain are common complaints among the general population. They are the second and third most common musculoskeletal complaints after back pain in the primary care setting. Unfortunately, differentiating between neck and shoulder pain can be a challenging task, as both share symptoms. Furthermore, symptoms secondary to upper extremity compressive neuropathies may add to the complexity of achieving a clinical diagnosis. Provocative maneuvers are essential in localizing the site of pathology. During the history and physical examination, the clinician must be cognizant of signs or symptoms that may indicate a more sinister disorder by attending to red flags. The red flags include fever, unexplained weight loss, history of cancer, history of violent trauma, and upper extremity spasticity. A careful history and physical examination are essential in the diagnostic evaluation of the upper extremity (Table 10.1).

E. Galang, MD (✉)
Orthopaedic and Rheumatologic Institute, Cleveland Clinic, 9500 Euclid Ave, Cleveland, OH 44195, USA
e-mail: egalang.md@gmail.com

G.C. Chang Chien, DO
Cleveland Clinic, Anesthesia Institute Pain Management, 9500 Euclid Ave, Dept C-25, Cleveland, OH 44195, USA
e-mail: gchangchien@gmail.com

Anatomy

A thorough understanding of the anatomy of the upper extremity is required to effectively perform a physical examination and is paramount to making the correct clinical diagnosis. The joints of the shoulder include the acromioclavicular joint and glenohumeral joint (GHJ). The glenohumeral joint is a ball and socket type joint. The main components of the GHJ are the glenoid fossa and humerus, labrum, glenohumeral capsule, glenohumeral ligaments, and dynamic shoulder stabilizers (rotator cuff muscles – supraspinatus, infraspinatus, teres minor, and subscapularis muscles). The elbow is a complex hinge joint with three joint articulations: humeroulnar joint, humeroradial joint, and proximal radioulnar joint. The ulnar nerve courses through the cubital tunnel at the elbow and is a common site of pathology for the ulnar nerve. The wrist is a condyloid joint which contains the fibro-osseous tunnel known as the carpal tunnel. Within this tunnel travels the median nerve which is site of the most common entrapment neuropathy.

Innervation

The brachial plexus is comprised of the fifth, sixth, seventh, and eighth cervical and the first thoracic nerve roots. A thorough anatomical understanding of these nerve roots and how they course the upper extremity is of the utmost importance. Specifically, the clinician must familiarize themselves with the anatomical courses of the median, ulnar, and radial nerves as they are at risk for compression at multiple locations of the upper extremity.

J.E. Pope, T.R. Deer (eds.), *Treatment of Chronic Pain Conditions*, DOI 10.1007/978-1-4939-6976-0_10

Table 10.1 Differential diagnosis of upper extremity pathology

Differential diagnosis	
Primary neck pathology	
	Cervical facet arthropathy
	Cervical discogenic pain syndrome
	Cervical sprain/strain
Primary shoulder pathology	
	Rotator cuff tendinopathy/tear
	Acromioclavicular joint arthropathy
Neurologic disorders	
	Cervical myelopathy
	Brachial plexopathy
	Cervical radiculopathy
	Peripheral mononeuropathy
Muscle and connective tissue disorders	
	Myofascial pain syndrome
	Fibromyalgia
Non-neuromusculoskeletal disorders	
	Pancoast tumor
	Ischemic chest pain
	Pneumonia

Table 10.2 Muscle strength grading

Strength grade	Description
0	No movement
1	Trace movement, muscle twitch only
2	Full range of motion with gravity eliminated
3	Full range of motion Against gravity
4	Full range of motion with partial resistance or asymmetric to contralateral side
5	Full strength (appropriate for age/body build)

Note: (+) and (−) may be used in some conventions to denote subtle gradations in strength

Table 10.3 Muscle stretch reflex grading

Reflex grade	Description
0	Absent
1+	Diminished
2+	Normal
3+	Increased
4	Sustained clonus

Physical Examination

The basic elements of the physical examination of the upper extremity include inspection, palpation, range of motion, and a neuromuscular examination. The use of provocative maneuvers targeted at suspected sites of pathology can aid the clinician in determining a diagnosis. With regard to the neuromuscular examination, the clinician should evaluate strength, reflexes, and dermatomal patterns. Muscle strength should be performed in the antigravity position to allow for detection of minimal weakness (Table 10.2).

The symmetry of muscle reflexes implies normalcy. The biceps reflex may be absent or diminished in a C6 (or C5) radiculopathy or a brachial plexopathy. The triceps reflex may be absent or diminished in a C7 radiculopathy, a brachial plexopathy, or a proximal radial neuropathy. The brachioradialis reflex may be absent or diminished in a C5 or C6 radiculopathy, a brachial plexopathy, or a radial neuropathy (Table 10.3).

One should also test for abnormal reflexes such as the Hoffman reflex. A Hoffman reflex is flexion-adduction of the ipsilateral thumb and index finger with passive snapping flexion of the distal phalanx of the middle finger. It is imperative that the clinician understands the motor and sensory points of the upper extremity (Fig. 10.1). In addition to assessing the motor and sensory function of the upper extremity, the clinician can also use provocative maneuvers to further narrow their differential diagnosis (Table 10.4).

Imaging Studies

Imaging studies in combination with the history and physical examination can further help the clinician decipher the diagnosis for the patient. X-ray imaging can assist in the diagnosis of cervical facet arthropathy and shoulder osteoarthritis. Magnetic resonance imaging can help the clinician delineate between a cervical radiculopathy/myelopathy and a cervical muscle strain/sprain. For rotator cuff pathology, magnetic resonance imaging and musculoskeletal ultrasound share comparable sensitivity and specificity.

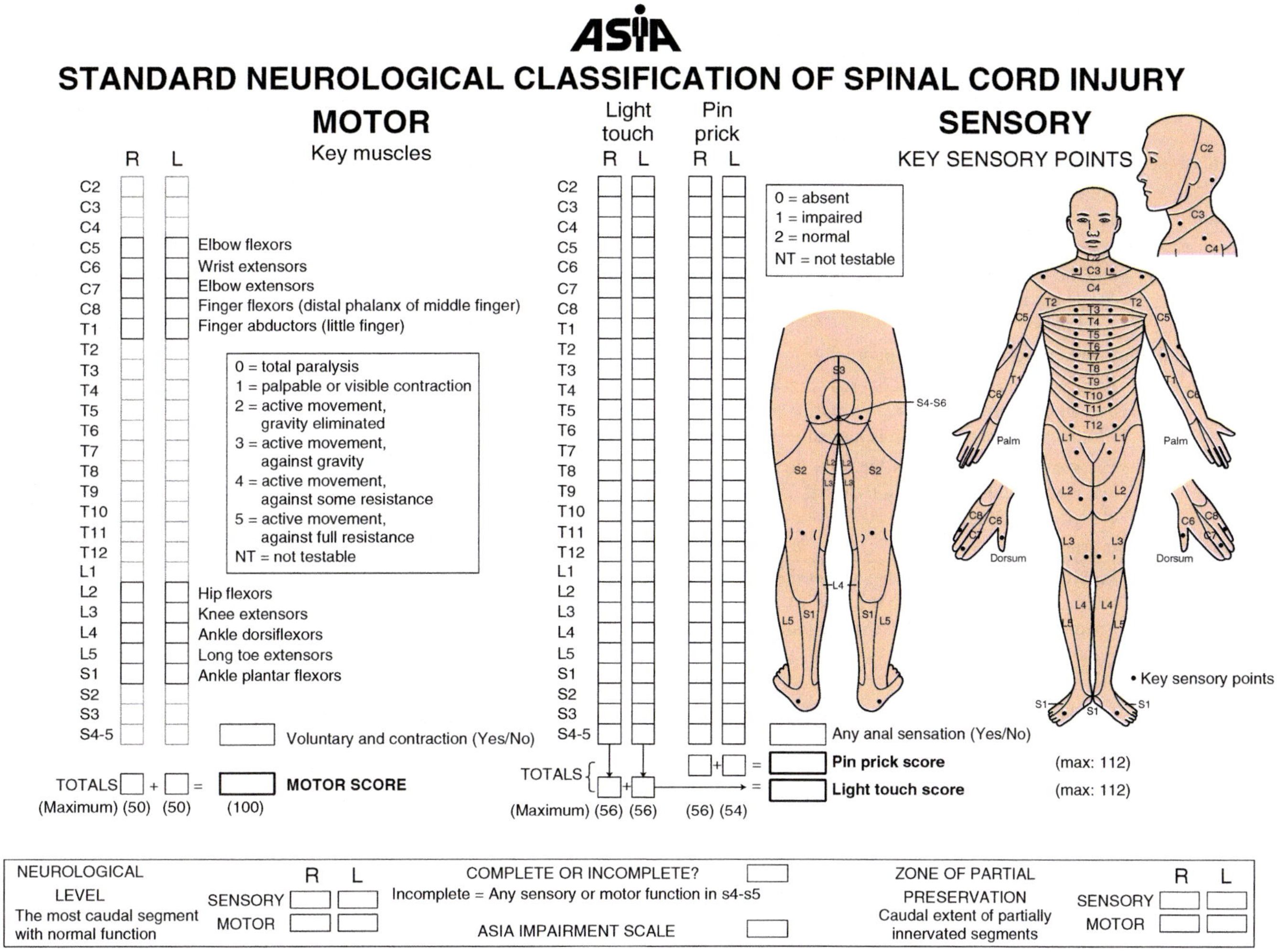

ASIA

STANDARD NEUROLOGICAL CLASSIFICATION OF SPINAL CORD INJURY

MOTOR

Key muscles

	R	L	
C2			
C3			
C4			
C5			Elbow flexors
C6			Wrist extensors
C7			Elbow extensors
C8			Finger flexors (distal phalanx of middle finger)
T1			Finger abductors (little finger)
T2–T12			
L1			
L2			Hip flexors
L3			Knee extensors
L4			Ankle dorsiflexors
L5			Long toe extensors
S1			Ankle plantar flexors
S2			
S3			
S4-5			Voluntary and contraction (Yes/No)

0 = total paralysis
1 = palpable or visible contraction
2 = active movement, gravity eliminated
3 = active movement, against gravity
4 = active movement, against some resistance
5 = active movement, against full resistance
NT = not testable

TOTALS ☐ + ☐ = ☐ **MOTOR SCORE**
(Maximum) (50) (50) (100)

SENSORY

Light touch R L; Pin prick R L (C2, C3, C4, C5, C6, C7, C8, T1, T2, T3, T4, T5, T6, T7, T8, T9, T10, T11, T12, L1, L2, L3, L4, L5, S1, S2, S3, S4-5)

0 = absent
1 = impaired
2 = normal
NT = not testable

Any anal sensation (Yes/No)

TOTALS ☐ + ☐ = **Light touch score** (max: 112)
☐ + ☐ = **Pin prick score** (max: 112)
(Maximum) (56) (56) (56) (54)

KEY SENSORY POINTS

NEUROLOGICAL LEVEL The most caudal segment with normal function		R	L
	SENSORY		
	MOTOR		

COMPLETE OR INCOMPLETE? ☐
Incomplete = Any sensory or motor function in s4-s5
ASIA IMPAIRMENT SCALE ☐

ZONE OF PARTIAL PRESERVATION Caudal extent of partially innervated segments		R	L
	SENSORY		
	MOTOR		

Fig. 10.1 Myotomes and dermatomes of the upper extremity

Table 10.4 Upper extremity physical examination maneuvers

Examination name	Description
Cervical radiculopathy	
Neck compression test	Passive lateral flexion, extension, and compression of the head. A positive test reproduces ipsilateral radicular symptoms distal from the neck
Supraspinatus tear	
Empty can test	With the arm at 90° of abduction, neutral rotation, and 30° of internal rotation; resisted shoulder extension is performed. A positive test is pain and weakness
Subacromial impingement/rotator cuff tendinopathy	
Hawkin's test	Forward elevation of the affected shoulder to 90° and then terminally internally rotating the shoulder. Presence of pain is a positive test
Neer test	Passive forward flexion of the arm. Presence of anterior shoulder pain with terminal forward elevation is a positive test
Acromioclavicular arthropathy	
Apley scarf test	Passive adduction of the arm across the midline attempting to approximate the elbow to the contralateral shoulder. Presence of pain at the AC joint is a positive test
Carpal tunnel syndrome	
Carpal compression test	Gentle but firm, sustained pressure to the median nerve of each hand simultaneously. The reproduction of pain or paresthesias of the symptomatic hand is a positive test

Additional Studies

Electromyography/nerve conduction studies (EMG/NCS): NCS assess the ability of the peripheral nerve to conduct electrical impulses. Needle EMG assesses nerve and muscle function. EMG/NCS may help the clinician elucidate and localize the neurological lesion.

Suggested Reading

1. Alexander E. History and physical examination, and differential diagnosis of neck pain. Phys Med Rehabil Clin N Am. 2011;22:383–93.
2. Fish D, Gerstman B, Lin V. Evaluation of the patient with neck versus shoulder pain. Phys Med Rehabil Clin N Am. 2011;22: 395–410.
3. Hegedus E, Goode A, Cook C, Michener L, Myer C, Myer D, Wright A. Which physical examination test provide clinicians with the most value when examining the shoulder? Update of a systematic review with meta-analysis of individual tests. Br J Sports Med. 2012;46:963–78.
4. King J, Wright T. Physical examination of the shoulder. J Hand Surg [Am]. 2014;39(10):2103–12.
5. Popinchalk S, Schaffer A. Physical examination of upper extremity compressive neuropathies. Orthop Clin N Am. 2012;43: 417–30.
6. Zouzias I, Byram I, Shillingford J, Levine W. A primer for physical examination of the elbow. Phys Sportsmed. 2012;40(1):51–61.

Lower Extremity Physical Examination

11

See Loong Chin, Enrique Galang, and George C. Chang Chien

Key Concepts

- The evaluation of the lower extremity must begin with a detailed history, as this is essential in formulating a differential diagnosis.
- A thorough understanding of the anatomy of the lower extremity is required to effectively perform a physical examination.
- Advanced imaging and electrodiagnostic studies (NCV/EMG) coupled with a thorough history and physical examination can assist the clinician in making a diagnosis.

Introduction

Low back pain is the most common musculoskeletal complaint in the primary care setting. The ability to perform a thorough history and comprehensive physical examination is key to making a diagnosis and initiating a successful treatment plan. Unfortunately, lower extremity pain is often confounded by radiculopathic pain originating from the lumbar spine. Determining the source of the pain can be challenging as multifactorial causes from both the lower extremity and lumbar spine play a role. Furthermore, pathologies of the hip, knee, foot, and ankle add to the complexity of achieving a clinical diagnosis, as these joints are essential in the functional movement and stability of the lower extremity. Provocative maneuvers are useful in localizing painful lesions. During the history and physical examination, the clinician must be cognizant of signs or symptoms that may indicate a more sinister disorder by attending to red flags. The red flags include fever, unexplained weight loss, history of cancer, history of violent trauma, and lower extremity spasticity (Table 11.1).

Anatomy

An intimate understanding of the anatomy is key in performing an efficient and thorough physical examination. This understanding, moreover, allows the clinician to thoughtfully take into account the kinetic movements of the lower extremity as they relate to the patient's chief complaint.

The joints of the pelvis and hip include the bilateral sacroiliac (SI) joints, the pubic symphysis, and the femoroacetabular (hip) joints. The femoroacetabular joint is the most mobile joint in the pelvis. Because of this mobility, hip joint pathology is often manifested during weight bearing and ambulation. There are multiple trochanteric bursas providing cushioning over the greater trochanter. These bursas often become inflamed and are a frequent source of lateral hip pain. The knee joint is a hinge joint, which connects the femur superiorly to the tibia and fibula inferiorly. Because the knee joint is the largest joint in the body, the joint is susceptible to injury. Multiple ligaments of the knee include the anterior cruciate ligament, posterior cruciate ligament, medial collateral ligament, and lateral collateral ligament. These ligaments provide anterior/posterior and valgus/varus stability. The two menisci of the knee are crescent-shaped fibrocartilaginous tissue located medially and laterally. The ankle mortise is compromised of the medial malleolus, the lateral malleolus, and the talus. The lateral malleolus extends more distally then its medial counterpart, therefore making it very important in ankle stabilization. The ankle and foot have multiple joints including talocrural, subtalar, and inferior tibiofibular joints. The main ligaments that provide support are the anterior

S.L. Chin, MD
Cleveland Clinic, Cleveland, OH, USA

E. Galang, MD
Orthopaedic and Rheumatologic Institute, Cleveland Clinic, 9500 Euclid Ave, Cleveland, OH 44195, USA

G.C. Chang Chien, DO (✉)
Cleveland Clinic, Anesthesia Institute Pain Management, 9500 Euclid Ave, Dept C-25, Cleveland, OH 44195, USA
e-mail: gchangchien@gmail.com

J.E. Pope, T.R. Deer (eds.), *Treatment of Chronic Pain Conditions*, DOI 10.1007/978-1-4939-6976-0_11

Table 11.1 Differential diagnosis of lower extremity pathology

Differential diagnosis	
Primary hip pathology	Sacroiliitis
	Femoroacetabular arthritis
	Femoroacetabular impingement
	Gluteus medius bursitis
	Piriformis syndrome
Primary leg and foot pathology	Knee joint arthritis
	ACL/PCL Tears
	Knee bursitis
	Achilles tendinopathy
	Plantar fasciitis
Neurologic disorders	Lumbar plexopathy\
	Lumbar radiculopathy
	Peripheral mononeuropathy
	Neurogenic claudication
Muscle and connective tissue disorders	Myofascial pain syndrome
	Fibromyalgia
Non-neuromusculoskeletal Disorders	Peripheral vascular disease
	Gout

Table 11.2 Muscle strength grading

Strength grade	Description
0	No movement
1	Trace movement, muscle twitch only
2	Full range of motion with gravity eliminated
3	Full range of motion Against gravity
4	Full range of motion with partial resistance or asymmetric to contralateral side
5	Full strength (appropriate for age/body build)

Table 11.3 Muscle stretch reflex grading

Reflex grade	Description
0	Absent
1+	Diminished
2+	Normal
3+	Increased
4	Sustained clonus

talofibular, posterior talofibular, and calcaneofibular and deltoid ligaments. The anterior talofibular ligament is the primary lateral ankle ligament stabilizer and is also the most commonly injured ligament of the ankle.

Innervation

The innervation of the pelvis and lower extremity are derived from the lumbosacral plexus. A thorough anatomical understanding of these nerve roots and how they course the lower extremity is important. Specifically, the clinician must familiarize themselves with courses of the sciatic, common peroneal, tibial, and obturator nerves as they are often culprits of lower extremity neuromuscular pathology. The clinician should also be familiar with the lateral femoral cutaneous nerve, which provides sensation to the anterior/lateral aspect of the thigh, and pathology to this nerve may result in paresthesias.

Physical Examination

A comprehensive physical examination begins with close observation of the patient's posture and gait. This is followed by inspection of the lower limbs for signs of inflammation, infection, and anatomical discrepancies (length, alignment, and asymmetry). Neuromuscular testing follows palpation of the hip, knee, and ankle joints. Pain and tenderness along a dermatomal distribution should be noted (refer to Fig. 10.1). Quantification of the clinical motor strength and reflexes are provided in Tables 11.2 and 11.3.

Hip Physical Examination Maneuvers

The examination of the pelvic/hip should include observation for hip symmetry. Palpation of the SI and hip joints may help localize the pathology. An evaluation for full range of motion includes hip flexion, extension, abduction, adduction, and internal/external rotation. Refer to Table 11.4 for interpretation of motor strength.

Knee Physical Examination Maneuvers

The examination of the knee should include inspection of symmetry paying attention to any valgus or varus deformities. Next, palpation of the joint and surrounding tissue may reveal tenderness and effusion (Table 11.5). Evaluation for full range of motion at the joint includes knee flexion and extension. An abnormal reflex at the patellar tendon may be indicative of an L4 radiculopathy (see Fig. 10.1). Refer to Tables 11.2 and 11.3 for an interpretation of motor strength and reflexes.

Foot and Ankle Physical Examination Maneuvers

First the patient should be evaluated standing, and one must note any abnormality in stance. The arch should also be examined for pes planus or pes cavus. Palpation along all aspects of the foot can reveal common pathologies such as Achilles tendinopathy and plantar fasciitis. An evaluation for full range of motion includes foot inversion/eversion, plantar flexion, and dorsiflexion. An abnormal Achilles tendon reflex can be an indicative of a S1 neuropathy (Table 11.6).

Table 11.4 Interpretation of motor strength

Examination name	Description
Femoroacetabular Arthropathy	
Hip Scour Test	Patient in supine position with the knee and hip flexed. Apply a downward pressure at the knee along the shaft of the femur to the hip joint. With the hip adducted, rotate the hip alternatively in the internal and external direction. Presence of pain at the hip joint is a positive test
Sacroiliac arthropathy	
FABER test	Patient in supine position with one foot crossed over the opposite thigh in a figure four position with the leg in external rotation. With one hand stabilizing the opposite ASIS, apply gentle pressure on the medial aspect of the flexed knee. Presence of pain at the SI joint is a positive test
Piriformis syndrome	
FAIR test	Patient in a sitting position with 90° flexion of the hip and knee. Provide resistance at the lateral side of the knee while the patient abduct at the hip joint. Presence of pain in the piriformis muscle is a positive test

Table 11.5 Knee physical examination maneuvers

Examination name	Description
Medial capsule/medial collateral ligament tear	
Valgus stress test	With the knee extended, place one hand as pivot against the knee while using the other hand to push against the foot in the opposite direction in a valgus maneuver. Positive test is pain and laxity
Lateral capsule/lateral collateral ligament tear	
Varus stress test	With the knee extended, place one hand as pivot against the knee while using the other hand to push against the foot in the opposite direction in a varus maneuver. Positive test is pain and laxity
Anterior cruciate ligament tear	
Anterior drawer test	The patient is in supine position with hips flexed to 45° and knee flexed to 90°. The examiner should grasp the knee with both hands with thumbs resting along the joint line and index fingers on the hamstring tendons. The tibia is then drawn anteriorly. Positive test is pain and laxity
Posterior cruciate ligament tear	
Posterior Drawer Test	The patient is in supine position with hips flexed to 45° and knee flexed to 90°. The examiner should grasp the knee with both hands with thumbs resting along the joint line and index fingers on the hamstring tendons. The tibia is then pushed posteriorly. Positive test is pain and laxity
Meniscus tear	
McMurray test	The patient is in supine position with knee completely flexed. Provide external rotation while extending the knee. Repeat with internal rotation while extending the knee. Positive test is pain and clicking from the joint

Table 11.6 Foot and ankle physical examination maneuvers

Examination name	Description
Anterior talofibular ligament tear	
Anterior drawer test	Stabilize the leg with one hand and pull the heel forward with the opposite hand. Positive test is pain and laxity
Calcaneofibular and anterior talofibular ligament tear	
Talar tilt test	Stabilize the leg with one hand and invert the foot with the opposite hand. Positive test is pain and laxity
Achilles tendon tear	
Thompson test	The patient is in prone position with knees flexed 90°. Squeeze the calf to induce passive plantar flexion of the foot. Positive test is absence of foot plantar flexion
High ankle sprain	
Squeeze test	Gently squeeze the tibia and fibular together. Positive test is pain in the high ankle

Imaging Studies

Imaging studies in combination with the history and physical examination can further help the clinician decipher the diagnosis for the patient. X-ray imaging can assist in the diagnosis of lumbar facet arthropathy, hip osteoarthritis, and knee osteoarthritis. Magnetic resonance imaging can help the clinician delineate between a lumbar radiculopathy/myelopathy versus a lumbar muscle strain/sprain. Musculoskeletal ultrasound can be used as an adjunct imaging modality to assess for tendinopathy and bursitis.

Additional Studies

Electromyography/nerve conduction studies (EMG/NCSs): NCSs assess the ability of the peripheral nerve to conduct electrical impulses. Needle EMG assesses nerve and muscle function. EMG/NCSs may help the clinician elucidate and localize the neurological lesion.

Suggested Reading

1. http://www.hss.edu/musculoskeletal-exam-videos.asp.
2. Malanga GA, Andrus S, Nadler SF, McLean J. Physical examination of the knee: a review of the original test description and scientific validity of common orthopedic tests. Arch Phys Med Rehabil. 2003;84(4):592–603.
3. Reiman MP, Goode AP, Cook CE, Hölmich P, Thorborg K. Diagnostic accuracy of clinical tests for the diagnosis of hip femoroacetabular impingement/labral tear: a systematic review with meta-analysis. Br J Sports Med. 2014. pii: bjsports-2014-094302.
4. Solomon DH, Simel DL, Bates DW, Katz JN, Schaffer JL. The rational clinical examination. Does this patient have a torn meniscus or ligament of the knee? Value of the physical examination. JAMA. 2001;286(13):1610–20.

History and Physical Examination for Neuropathy

12

Reda Tolba

Key Concepts

- Thorough history taking is an essential first step for identifying the etiology and obtaining a proper diagnosis and treatment of peripheral neuropathic conditions.
- Physical examination, including a focused neurological examination, follows history taking and could help the clinician to identify the severity of the condition.
- Electrodiagnostic studies like electromyography (EMG) and nerve conduction studies can serve as tool to confirm the nature and degree of pathology.

History and Pain Assessment

Detailed history is obtained from the patients suffering from neuropathy. Neuropathic pain is usually characterized by being spontaneous, burning, shooting, and lancinating. It can be associated with paresthesia, frequently described as "pins and needles." The patients could describe other abnormal sensations such as hyperalgesia, allodynia, hyperpathia, and dysesthesia. The patient is asked about the onset of pain, duration of the pain, character of the pain, precipitating factors, relieving factors, and intensity of the pain. Asking about the presence of any red flags such as significant motor or sensory deficits, urine or bowel incontinence, fever, and night sweats is essential to rule out any emergent condition that requires immediate attention and intervention.

Ask about previous treatment tried including oral and topical medications, physical therapy, chiropractor treatment, and interventional pain procedures. Ask about medication dose, frequency, side effects, and tolerance.

Patient is asked about various conditions that could lead to peripheral neuropathies. Metabolic causes, most importantly diabetes mellitus (DM), will be on top of the list. Pain associated with diabetic neuropathy is usually worse at night time. Patient is asked about how long he has been having DM and how well controlled is his condition. Labs should be reviewed including HbA1C. Thyroid functions should be reviewed to rule out hypothyroidism. History of cancer (multiple myeloma) or treatment with chemotherapy is asked. Toxic causes like chemotherapy-induced neuropathy are not uncommon (such as isoniazid, cisplatin, and others). A history of alcohol abuse is asked. Infectious causes like HIV or Guillain-Barré syndrome can lead to painful neuropathy. Nutritional causes such as beriberi (thiamine deficiency) or pellagra (niacin deficiency) should be ruled out and promptly treated. Peripheral neuropathy could be idiopathic with no identifiable cause.

Distribution and location of the painNeuropathy:history and pain assessment, whether it involves all limbs (polyneuropathy) or rather one limb (mononeuropathy). Entrapment neuropathies follow a specific nerve distribution when these nerves are vulnerable to compression in certain anatomical locations. Common examples are carpal tunnel syndrome, ulnar neuropathy, and thoracic outlet syndrome. EMG can help confirm the diagnosis of such conditions.

Review of other systems should be performed. Associated comorbidities are not uncommon with patients with diabetic neuropathy. It is important to keep that in mind and coordinate care with the patient's primary care physician to optimize his health and treat comorbid conditions. Dose adjustment for instance is important in diabetic patients with renal insufficiency.

Physical Examination

Focused and detailed neurological examination should be performed for patients with neuropathy. This should include complete sensory and motor evaluation.

Sensory evaluation includes light touch, pressure, temperature, vibration, and proprioception, particularly in your feet and legs. This can be done by several methods. To test

R. Tolba, MD (✉)
200 west Esplanade Avenue, Kenner, LA 70005, USA
e-mail: redatolba@hotmail.com

J.E. Pope, T.R. Deer (eds.), *Treatment of Chronic Pain Conditions*, DOI 10.1007/978-1-4939-6976-0_12

temperature, ice or cold tuning fork can be used and held to the patient's leg. To test light touch and pressure, a cotton swab or thin plastic fiber can be applied by touching the end of the toe. A vibrating tuning fork can be used to test the sense of vibration. Simply applying light touch such as rubbing to the affected extremity can test for allodynia (pain produced by non-noxious stimuli). Single pinprick test can test for integrity of the sensations and rule out sensory deficit or some abnormal sensations such as hyperalgesia (increase response to a stimulus that is normally painful). Repeated pinprick testing can elicit a phenomenon called "summation" (pain growing more intense with subsequent stimulation).

Complete motor examination including muscle tone, deep tendon reflexes, and muscle strength should be performed. Although motor exam can be normal in many patients with polyneuropathy, abnormalities should be detected.

Complete examination including general, heart, lung, musculoskeletal, abdomen, skin, and other systems should be performed. Inspection of the legs and feet for diabetic ulcers, skin blisters, and joint deformities can be seen in patients with diabetic neuropathy. Decreased or absent peripheral pulses can be seen in diabetic patients due to associated peripheral vascular disease.

Important Tests

Electromyography (EMG) and nerve conduction studies can be used for confirmation of the type of neuropathy (axonal or demyelinating). It can also detect the severity of the pathology and the site of the pathology whether it is proximal or distal. Those studies can be specifically useful for ambiguous cases, when it is difficult to localize the source of the neuropathic pain. EMG and NVC only detect large fiber neuropathy and cannot detect small fiber neuropathy. Small fiber neuropathy is considered a diagnosis of exclusion. It usually presents with painful neuropathic pain in the feet in older patients. When EMG is WNL, other tests can be used to confirm small fiber neuropathy such as skin biopsy or quantitative sensory testing.

Suggested Reading

1. Benzon H, Raja SN, Fishman SM, Liu S, Cohen SP. Essentials of pain medicine. 3rd ed. Saunders Title. ISBN: 978-1-4377-2242-0. 2011
2. Fishman SM, Ballantyne JC, Rathmell JP, editors. Bonica's management of pain. 4th ed. Philadelphia, Wolters Kluwer/Lippincott, Williams and Wilkins, 2010

History and Physical Exam: Systemic Rheumatologic Disorders

13

John Hau

Key Concepts

- Patients typically present with diffuse symmetric joint or muscle pain.
- Look for systemic manifestations, which may occur in many different organ systems, including the skin, heart, lungs, liver, kidneys, and eyes.
- Morning stiffness is a common finding in systemic rheumatologic disorders.
- In addition to a thorough musculoskeletal examination, a directed examination of other involved organ system should be carried out.

Introduction

Systemic rheumatologic disorders are a diverse group of disorders that typically cause chronic pain and inflammation of joints and muscles. They may include other systemic manifestations that can affect almost any organ system. Many of the systemic rheumatologic disorders are due to an autoimmune process. Patients with systemic rheumatologic disorders often present with a complex clinical picture, making their diagnosis difficult. One of the most useful tools at a physician's disposal is a thorough history and physical examination, which oftentimes alone can lead to a correct diagnosis.

History

It is imperative to take a thorough history. One should focus on the location of pain, duration, quality of the pain, exacerbating/relieving factors, presence of morning stiffness, and any underlying family history. A thorough history and review of systems to determine extra-articular manifestations will be helpful in determining the possibility of a systemic rheumatologic disorder.

Physical Examination

A thorough physical examination should utilize all the examination skills discussed in the previous chapters. Due to the diffuse and variable organ involvement of the systemic rheumatologic disorders, the clinician should not only employ a thorough musculoskeletal examination but should be attentive to examine other organ systems that may be involved.

Some of the most common systemic rheumatologic disorders are presented in Table 13.1 with their typical presenting history and physical examination findings.

Suggested Reading

1. Gill JM, Quisel AM, Rocca PV, Walters DT. Diagnosis of systemic lupus erythematosus. Am Fam Physician. 2003;68(11):2179–86.
2. Salvarani C, Cantini F, Boiardi L, Hunder GG. Polymagia rheumatica and giant-cell arteritis. N Engl J Med. 2002;347:261–71.
3. Sieper J, Braun J, Rudwaleit M, et al. Ankylosing spondylitis: an overview. Ann Rheum Dis. 2002;61(Suppl III):iii8–iii18.
4. Waldman, S. Pain review. Philadelphia: Saunders Elsevier; 2009. Print.
5. Wasserman AM. Diagnosis and management of rheumatoid arthritis. Am Fam Physician. 2011;84(11):1245–52.

J. Hau, MD (✉)
Summit Pain Alliance, 392 Tesconi Court, Santa Rosa, CA 95401, USA
e-mail: summitpainalliance@gmail.com

J.E. Pope, T.R. Deer (eds.), *Treatment of Chronic Pain Conditions*, DOI 10.1007/978-1-4939-6976-0_13

Table 13.1 Some of the most common systemic rheumatologic disorders with their typical presenting history and physical examination findings

Rheumatologic disorder	History	Physical examination
Ankylosing spondylitis	Typically presents in the third decade of life Men are three times more likely to be affected Pain in the axial spine and sacroiliac joints Associated with uveitis	Tenderness to palpation axial spine, sacroiliac joints, iliac crests, trochanteric bursas Lumbar lordosis and thoracic kyphosis as disease progresses with loss of spinal mobility Photophobia, decreased visual acuity
Polymyalgia rheumatica	Typically presents after the age of 50 Women are twice as likely to be affected Patients present with polyarthralgias and pain involving the shoulders, neck, and hip Patients typically complain of fatigues and generalized weakness	Shoulder and hip stiffness Synovitis and bursitis of peripheral joints Decreased range of motion of the shoulders, neck, and hips
Polymyositis	Typically presents between the age of 40–60 Women are twice as likely to be affected Inflammation of muscles leading to muscle degeneration and atrophy Cutaneous manifestations common High correlation with underlying malignancy Proximal muscles affected initially followed by the distal muscle groups	Profound muscle weakness on examination Patients may demonstrate difficulty rising from sitting position or raising arms above head Periorbital heliotrope rash is pathognomonic Small muscles of the hands and feet are typically spared
Rheumatoid arthritis	Typically presents between the age of 30–50 Women are two to three times more likely to be affected Symmetric involvement of three or more joints, typically PIP, MCP, MTP, wrist, ankles, or knees Extra-articular manifestations include rheumatoid nodules, ocular involvement, vasculitis, and pericarditis	Tenosynovitis and joint effusions are a characteristic finding leading to joint destruction Swan neck deformity
Scleroderma	Typically presents between the age of 30–50 Women are four times more likely to be affected Polyarthritis, diffuse skin fibrosis, vascular damage Extra-articular manifestations may affect the esophagus, GI tract, kidneys, lungs, and heart	Polyarthralgias Sclerodactyly Raynaud's phenomenon Dysphagia Shiny and atrophic looking skin Patients may have masklike facies Ulcerations of affected skin
Systemic lupus Erythematosus	90% affected are women More common in African Americans and Asians Diffuse polyarthritis Variable presentation that can affect many different organ systems	Polyarthritis but typically less destructive compared to rheumatoid arthritis Butterfly rash Extra-articular manifestations can affect the heart, lungs, liver, or kidneys

Part IV

Evaluation and Assessment: IV. Imaging and EMG/NCV

Indications/Interpretation for Advanced Imaging: MRI and CT

14

Nomen Azeem

Key Points

- Magnetic resonance imaging (MRI) uses a magnet to form a strong magnetic field around the area to be imaged.
- MRI is the preferred diagnostic imaging technique for persistent axial spine pain with radicular symptoms if they are potential candidates for surgery or epidural steroid injection.
- The presence of some types of metal in your body is a contraindication for MRI scan as it may be a safety hazard.
- Computed axial tomography (CT) scan uses x-rays at different angles to generate cross-sectional images of structures in the body based on their ability to block the x-ray beam.
- Computed axial tomography (CT) imaging for the spine may be preferred for bony abnormalities as well as in those patients that cannot tolerate MRI or have a contraindication for MRI scan.
- Poor correlation between magnitude of pain symptoms and morphologic changes seen on spinal imaging.

Introduction

Magnetic resonance imaging was invented by Paul C. Lauterbur of the University of Illinois Urbana-Champaign in September 1971 who published the theory behind it in March 1973. In 2003 Lauterbur along with Sir Peter Mansfield of the University of Nottingham was awarded a Nobel Prize in physiology or medicine for "discoveries concerning magnetic resonance imaging." Most of the early research that involved MRI revolved around the detection of cancerous tissue. In 1980, the first MRI scanner was built by professor John Mallard at the University of Aberdeen which obtained the first clinically useful image of a patient's internal tissues using magnetic resonance imaging (MRI), which identified a primary tumor in the patient's chest, an abnormal liver, and secondary cancer in his bones. An MRI scanner uses a magnet to form a strong magnetic field around the area to be imaged. Hydrogen atoms in tissues containing water molecules are used to create a signal that is processed to form an image of the body. When you lie inside an MRI machine, the magnetic field temporarily realigns hydrogen atoms in your body, which then emit radio waves, which are measured by a receiver coil that is used to create MRI images. In time the use of MRI has spread beyond detection of tumors and now can help assess a multitude of medical pathologies and disease processes.

Determining the cause of back pain, with or without radicular symptoms, is undertaken by incorporating a good history and physical examination, provocative testing, and diagnostic imaging. Per guidelines established by the American College of Physicians and American Pain Society, it is recommended that diagnostic imaging be reserved for patients with low back pain that present with serious or progressive neurologic deficits. The most common diagnostic imaging modalities for assessment of spinal pathology are MRI and CT scan.

Magnetic resonance imaging (MRI) is the preferred diagnostic imaging technique for persistent axial spine pain with radicular symptoms if they are potential candidates for surgery or epidural steroid injection. The high resolution of MRI for soft tissues allows elucidation of the morphology and potential pathology of the intervertebral disc, the nerve roots, the central spinal canal, neural foramina, and facet joints without radiation exposure. Image contrast is weighted in two categories, T1-weighted images and T2-weighted images. In T1-weighted images, fatty tissue appears lighter which allows for greater anatomic visualization and the appreciation of mass effect on adjacent structures. In T2-weighted images, fluid appears lighter which allows

N. Azeem, MD (✉)
Sarasota Orthopedic Associates,
2750 Bahia Vista St, Ste 100, Sarasota, FL 34239, USA
e-mail: azeemnx@gmail.com

J.E. Pope, T.R. Deer (eds.), *Treatment of Chronic Pain Conditions*, DOI 10.1007/978-1-4939-6976-0_14

Table 14.1 MRI findings of common spinal pathologies

Spinal pathology	T1 weighted	T2 weighted	T1 contrast +
Annular tear		High intensity zone in annulus	Focally enhancing liner nidus in posterior disc margin
Facet arthropathy		Hyperintense fluid in facet joint	Enhancing inflammatory soft tissue changes surrounding facet joint
Spinal metastasis		Focal hyperintensity (intramedullary, extramedullary, intradural, or extradural)	Focal enhancing lesion(s) within spinal canal
Degenerative disc disease		Hypointensity within NP of dis, decreased disc height, appreciation of potential disc bulge vs. focal herniation vs. extrusion	Possible linear enhancement within disc, enhancement within Schmorl nodes
Discitis	Hypointensity of the disc and potential destruction of the vertebral endplate	Hyperintensity of disc	Enhancement of disc, adjacent vertebrae, paravertebral soft tissue, epidural abscess
Osteomyelitis	Hypointensity within the two contiguous vertebral bodies	Hyperintensity within vertebral bodies 2/2 associated edema	Enhancement of vertebral body
Arachnoiditis	Hypointensity surrounding spinal nerves		
Epidural scarring	Hypointensity in proximity to previous surgical site		
Spondylolysis		Hyperintensity in region of pars interarticularis	
Myelopathy		Intramedullary hyperintensity	Variable depending on etiology
Modic type I	Hypointensity along end plate	Hyperintensity along end plate	May show prominent enhancement along end plate
Modic type II	Hyperintensity along end plate	Hyperintensity or isointensity	
Modic type III	Hypointensity along end plate	Hypointensity along end plate	
Spondylolisthesis	Anterior or posterior shifting of one vertebral body appreciated relative to adjacent vertebral body	Anterior or posterior shifting of one vertebral body appreciated relative to adjacent vertebral body	
Spinal stenosis	Decreased AP diameter 2/2 disc encroachment, ligamentum flavum hypertrophy, facet joint hypertrophy	Decreased AP diameter 2/2 disc encroachment, ligamentum flavum hypertrophy, facet joint hypertrophy	Enhancing and crowded nerve roots

greater appreciation of disease processes including degenerative changes of intervertebral discs, inflammation, infection, and neoplasm. Van Goethem et al. stress the importance of MRI in patients following lumbar discectomy and intervertebral fusion in achieving the most beneficial and timely outcome in patients with failed back surgery syndrome. Gadolinium, a non-nephrotoxic contrast agent, can be used to enhance visualization and help identify structures with increased vascularity on T1-weighted images. Spinal MRI images are presented in three orientations, sagittal, axial, and coronal views, which allow for a three-dimensional interpretation of spinal pathology. Further having the ability to compare and contrast T1- and T2-weighted images allows the visualization of most spinal pathology (Table 14.1).

The presence of some types of metal in your body is a contraindication for MRI scan as it may be a safety hazard. This includes artificial heart valves, brain aneurysm clips, heart defibrillator or pacemaker, inner ear (cochlear) implants, older metallic artificial joints, metallic vascular stents, spinal cord stimulator, metallic foreign bodies in the orbits, or metallic surgical hardware including rods, plates, screws, pins, staples, and wiring. There are some metallic implants used for spinal fusion surgery that are no longer a contraindication for MRI. Generally an MRI scan is conducted with the patient lying supine within a closed bore magnet which can cause patient anxiety and claustrophobia leading to movement during the exam or aborting the exam altogether. Although there are now magnets, which allow for upright, sitting, or standing spine imaging to ease feelings of anxiety, the resolution leaves much to be desired.

Although a sensitive imaging test, MRI may not be very specific in determining the cause of back pain. There is a poor correlation between magnitude of pain symptoms and morphologic changes seen on MRI scan. Boden demonstrated that one-third of 67 asymptomatic patients were found to have a substantial abnormality on MRI of the lumbar spine. Per a publication by Jarvik JG and Deyo RA, high intensity zones representing annular disc tears are equivocal due to the high prevalence of these zones in asymptomatic patients, and further disc bulges and protrusions are common in asymptomatic persons. It is thus vital to correlate clinical findings with imaging in order to appropriately determine the source of pain. Further with the emphasis on cost control in medicine, it is important to limit the utilization of MRI to those patients that will most likely benefit long term from this diagnostic imaging modality.

In 1974, Robert Ledley, a professor of physiology, biophysics, and radiology at Georgetown University School of Medicine, is known to have developed, what we know today as, the computed axial tomography scanner. Computed axial tomography scan also known as CAT scan or CT scan is a type of imaging that uses x-rays at different angles to generate cross-sectional images of structures in the body based on their ability to block the x-ray beam.

CT images of the spine can be obtained in the axial, sagittal, and coronal planes. A CT scan of the spine can be useful to appreciate the alignment of the spine, herniated discs, central canal, and foraminal stenosis. A CT scan may be preferred over MRI for evaluation of fractures of the posterior elements, ossification spinal ligaments, or in post-surgical patients with hardware for better visualization without artifact. A CT scan is also an excellent option for patients in which MRI is contraindicated or those that cannot tolerate the MRI exam (i.e., claustrophobia). A study by Thornbury and colleagues compared CT with MRI for herniated discs by establishing an expert panel to review all initial radiographic and clinical data and 6-month follow-up data that served as a reference standard. It revealed CT had a sensitivity of up to 94% and specificity up to 64%, which was similar to that of MRI. CT can accurately depict the foraminal and extraforaminal nerve root because surrounding fat provides natural contrast that allows for direct visualization of nerve root displacement or compression. Although the cost of CT is favorable when compared to MRI, there should be consideration of radiation exposure during a CT scan. As with MRI, abnormalities found with CT may be found in normal, asymptomatic persons and may result in unnecessary procedures or surgery; thus, CT of the spine should only be used alongside a strong history and physical exam.

Suggested Reading

1. Boden SD, Davis DO, Dina TS, et al. Abnormal magnetic-resonance scans of the lumbar spine in asymptomatic subjects. A prospective investigation. J Bone Joint Surg Am. 1990;72(3):403–8.
2. Chou R, Qaseem A, Snow V, Casey D, Cross T, Shekelle P, Owens D; Clinical Efficacy Assessment Subcommittee of the American College of Physicians and the American College of Physicians/American Pain Society Low Back Pain Guidelines Panel*. Diagnosis and treatment of low back pain: a joint clinical practice guideline from the American College of Physicians and the American Pain Society. Ann Intern Med. 2007;147(7):478–91. doi:10.7326/0003-4819-147-7-200710020-00006.
3. Jarvik JG, Deyo RA. Diagnostic evaluation of low back pain with emphasis on imaging. Ann Intern Med. 2002;137:586–97.
4. Rinck P. Magnetic resonance in medicine. The basic textbook of the European Magnetic Resonance Forum. 8th ed. 2014. E-version 8.9 (April 2015).
5. Thornbury JR, Fryback DG, Turski PA, Javid MJ, McDonald JV, Beinlich BR, et al. Disc-caused nerve compression in patients with acute low-back pain: diagnosis with MR, CT myelography, and plain CT. Radiology. 1993;186:731–8.
6. Van Goethem J, Parizel P, Jinkins J. Review article: MRI of the postoperative lumbar spine. Neuroradiology. 2002;44(9):723–39.

Indications for/Interpretation of Electrodiagnostic Testing

15

Prin X. Amorapanth and George C. Chang Chien

Key Concepts

- Electrodiagnostic testing is an extension of the physical exam and is dynamic, assessing the real-time function of nerves and muscles.
- Electrodiagnostic testing can help diagnose multiple treatable causes of acute and chronic pain.
- Electrodiagnostic testing requires a patient who is able to both tolerate a moderate level of pain and recruit their musculature under painful conditions.
- Electrodiagnostic testing is an operator-dependent test.

Introduction

Electrodiagnostic testing (EDX) is used to answer questions regarding the physiologic status of nerves and muscles, as well as to help localize pathology and provide prognostic information about that pathology. EDX typically refers to two types of testing, nerve conduction velocity (NCV) studies and electromyographic (EMG) studies, though, colloquially, "EMG" is often used to refer to both of these studies.

NCV bypasses the normal activation of sensory and motor nerves by using an externally applied burst of current to activate a peripheral nerve. This burst then propagates throughout the nerve and is detected by an electrode applied at specific distance, which allows the measurement of latency, the amplitude, and the calculation of velocity. The sensory response is recorded as the sensory nerve action potential (SNAP) and the motor response as the compound muscle action potential (CMAP).This information is a sensitive indicator of axonal injury (e.g., abnormally low action potential amplitude), as well as the integrity of nerve myelination (e.g., abnormally reduced conduction velocity). By stimulating the nerve at different sites, a trained practitioner can localize the site of injury to a peripheral nerve. Common pathologies identified by NCS include an array of neuropathies, ranging from entrapment neuropathies to peripheral neuropathies (Chart 1). The particular pattern of NCS findings can also help identify the specific site of injury in mononeuropathies, plexopathies, and radiculopathies. One important caveat is that NCV only tests relatively large-diameter nerves (Ia) and does not provide information about smaller fibers (IIb, II, III) and thus cannot help diagnose small fiber neuropathies.

In contrast to NCV, EMG does not involve passing electrical current, but rather "listens" to muscle activity by way of passing a thin needle electrode into specific muscles in order to assess the response of motor units within these muscles in different stages of activity: rest, minimal contraction, and maximal activity. Abnormal activity as a result of pathology can result in characteristic changes to these stages in specific ways. At rest, motor units should be quiet, and so the presence of any activity is abnormal and indicates damaged muscle tissue. Abnormal resting activity includes positive waves, fibrillation potentials, complex repetitive discharges, myokymia, etc. After assessment of resting activity, voluntary activation is induced, with the examiner assessing the quality and quantity of both individual and aggregate motor unit action potentials (MUAPs). Characteristics of individual MUAPs that are noted include amplitude, frequency, and waveform complexity. Increased amplitudes and complex waveforms can reflect complex reinnervation of formerly denervated muscles, with the particular amplitude and morphology findings also lending information about the time course of the process in question. When activating muscles, individual muscle fibers fire in a progressive and sequential pattern. Changes in recruitment patterns can help identify

P.X. Amorapanth, MD, PhD
Brain Injury Medicine, Rusk Rehabilitation, NYU Langone Medical Center, Department of Physical Medicine and Rehabilitation, New York, NY, USA

G.C. Chang Chien, DO (✉)
Cleveland Clinic, Anesthesia Institute Pain Management, 9500 Euclid Ave, Dept C-25, Cleveland, OH 44195, USA
e-mail: gchangchien@gmail.com

J.E. Pope, T.R. Deer (eds.), *Treatment of Chronic Pain Conditions*, DOI 10.1007/978-1-4939-6976-0_15

Table 15.1 Common entrapment neuropathies

Affected nerve	Clinical presentation	Site of lesion
Median nerve "Carpal tunnel syndrome"	Dysesthesia in digits 1 and 2 and radial 1/2 of 3 Weakness in median-innervated hand muscles Atrophy of median-innervated muscles in severe cases	Carpal tunnel in the wrist Other entrapment sites: Ligament of Struthers Pronator teres
Ulnar nerve "Cubital tunnel syndrome"	Dysesthesia in digits 4 and 5 Weakness in ulnar-innervated hand muscles Atrophy of ulnar-innervated muscles in severe cases	Proximal: ulnar groove in the elbow Other entrapment sites: Guyon's canal in the wrist
Peroneal nerve	Dysesthesia along lateral foreleg and dorsum of the foot Weakness of foot dorsiflexion, "foot drop" Atrophy of common peroneal-innervated muscles in severe cases	Deep to the peroneal longus muscles at the fibular head
Cervical or lumbosacral radiculopathy	Radicular pain in a sclerodermal or dermatomal distribution. Myotomal weakness corresponding to the affected nerve roots	Impinged nerve root in the epidural or neuroforaminal space

injury and inform prognosis. However, characterizing recruitment patterns is a complex skill and can also require a certain minimum level of technical equipment.

A good EDX report will include a history and physical that sets the stage for interpretation of the EDX data. In addition to data and waveforms enumerating NCV values and EMG findings, there should be a summary statement that presents especially salient findings to be used in the overall interpretation, with disclaimers denoting any abnormalities or technical issues that may limit or influence the data that was gathered. This report is not used to make the diagnosis in and of itself, but rather to support a diagnosis that the clinician should already be considering.

Patient Selection

One unique property of EDX that is both an advantage and disadvantage is that it is a dynamic and functional test. Thus, it requires a patient who can actively participate in the diagnostic test by activating muscles when asked. With regard to timing, the typical recommendations for obtaining EDX are to check after the acute period of injury due to the idea that changes in membrane stability and innervation take weeks to months to manifest. However, there are findings that manifest acutely following complete nerve transection, including loss of motor recruitment, decrease in motor nerve amplitude, and decreases in sensory nerve amplitude. Furthermore, testing in the acute period may be pursued to assess for preexisting pathology that may complicate the diagnostic picture.

Best Practices

Electrodiagnostic studies can be performed by a number of practitioners, but as they are an operator-dependent test, studies are best performed by a physician board certified in electrodiagnostic medicine by the American Board of Electrodiagnostics or the American Board of Neurology. Subtle pathology can be easily missed, and spurious abnormal values may be overcalled as pathologic by practitioners who are inexperienced. Furthermore, lack of good clinical history and physical exam skills can lead to a suboptimally designed EDX study that is not powered to detect pathology; the testing needed to rule out carpal tunnel syndrome is different from that need to rule out a C8-T1 cervical radiculopathy or a brachial plexopathy. In patients who suffer from acute or chronic pain, designing an optimal study that addresses the most likely etiologies of the patients' complaint is especially crucial (Table 15.1).

When interpreting EDX, it is crucial to keep in mind that the normal values used for NCV are often lab specific and determined empirically from a particular population of normal subjects. There are numerous technical confounds that can throw EDX results into questions including ambient and body temperature, body habitus, and electrical interference.

Conclusion

Electrodiagnostic studies are an extension of the history and physical exam and obtain unique data regarding the function of peripheral nerves and muscles. When there is a clinical question of peripheral neuropathy, EDX is useful for characterizing the distribution, severity, time course (acute, subacute, chronic, old), and prognosis, as well as underlying pathology. EDX is useful to direct pathology-specific interventions, such as an epidural steroid injection versus carpal tunnel injection in a patient with neck and hand pain. Practitioners should consider ordering EDX studies in patients without an unequivocal diagnosis based on history and physical examination.

Suggested Reading

1. Dumitru D, Amato AA, Zwarts M. Electrodiagnostic medicine. 2nd ed. Philadelphia: Hanley & Belfus publishing; 2001.
2. Preston DC, Shapiro BE. Electromyography and neuromuscular disorders: clinical-electrophysiologic correlations. 3rd ed. Philadelphia: Saunders publishing; 2013.

Part V

Evaluation and Assessment: V. Surgical Referral

Indications for Surgery for Low Back Pain

16

Ryan Galica

Key Points

- Cauda equina syndrome (CES) is an emergent, absolute indication for operative treatment of lower back pain.
- Most patients with progressive motor deficits should be considered for surgery.
- Operative treatment in patients without CES or progressive neurologic deficits should be considered after failure of more conservative therapies.
- Surgery may provide faster relief of lower back pain, although long-term outcomes may only be slightly favorable when compared with conservative treatment.

Introduction

Patients have a wide array of options for treating low back pain including pharmacologic therapy and minimally invasive procedures. Operative management is the most invasive treatment option, has the most potential complications, and requires extensive rehabilitation. However, surgery may offer the most rapid and complete correction of symptoms in patients experiencing low back pain. In the absence of absolute indications for urgent decompression surgery (i.e., cauda equina syndrome, progressive motor deficits, etc.), risks and benefits of postponing surgery as well as alternative, less invasive therapies should be considered.

R. Galica, MD (✉)
University Hospitals Case Medical Center, Department of Anesthesiology, Pain Medicine, Cleveland Heights, OH, USA
e-mail: Ryangalica@gmail.com

Absolute Indications

Lower back pain caused by cauda equina syndrome (CES) is an absolute indication for operative treatment. CES is caused by compression of the nerve roots in the lumbosacral spine. Although relatively rare in the patient presenting with low back pain, CES is a neurosurgical emergency for which urgent decompression should be pursued. All patients with symptoms suggestive of CES (such as new onset urinary retention, fecal incontinence, new onset lower extremity weakness and sensory deficits, or saddle numbness) should undergo emergent MRI of the entire spine (the lesion may also be above the cauda equina) and neurosurgical referral.

Patients with progressively worsening motor deficits are commonly considered for operative measures. While not an acute presentation as with CES, these patients experience a gradual decline in function and motor weakness noted subjectively by the patient or seen on serial office visits. These patients may have undergone minimally invasive, conservative therapy throughout their course of treatment. Surgical correction should be pursued in an attempt to prevent further loss of function.

Other potential causes of lower back pain that must be treated operatively, such as abdominal aortic aneurysm or infection, should be considered and ruled out. This is best done through a careful history and physical exam with special attention to red flag symptoms (i.e., age greater than 50, fever, chills, etc.). Further imaging studies and surgical referral should be pursued where indicated.

Relative Indications

When patients experience minimal improvement in lower back pain despite maximum conservative treatment including pharmacologic therapy and minimally invasive procedures, surgical management is appropriate. Often, patients

J.E. Pope, T.R. Deer (eds.), *Treatment of Chronic Pain Conditions*, DOI 10.1007/978-1-4939-6976-0_16

may be referred for a trial of conservative therapy due to a desire to avoid more invasive surgical correction or because of comorbid conditions that place them at higher than average perioperative risk. If these patients fail maximum conservative therapy, surgery may be their best option. The ideal amount of time to trial conservative therapy before moving onto surgical decompression remains ambiguous and must be defined through ongoing discussions between the patient and practitioner.

Several studies have shown that when compared to more conservative measures, surgical treatment provides faster and superior control of lower back pain symptoms initially. These studies show long-term results of surgery for lower back pain in regards to patient pain level, satisfaction, and function are comparable to slightly better than those of conservative treatment. No drawback has been shown to first trialing conservative management before moving onto surgery if less invasive measures are unsuccessful. Thus, the urgency of the patient's desire for pain relief is factored against the risks inherent to surgery and challenges of rehabilitation. Patients with severe intractable pain preventing them from participating in most activities of daily living are likely to benefit from the rapid results of decompression surgery. However, the primary location of the patient's pain must also be taken into account as decompression surgery is thought to be more helpful in patients with predominant leg pain when compared to predominant low back pain.

Conclusion

In determining whether a patient's low back pain requires surgery, one must first rule out absolute indications for operative intervention such as cauda equina syndrome. If no absolute indications exist, conservative options should be presented to the patient before pursuing surgery.

Suggested Reading

1. Amundsen T, Weber H, Nordal HJ, Magnaes B, Abdelnoor M, Lilleas F. Lumbar spinal stenosis: conservative or surgical management?: a prospective 10-year study. Spine. 2000;25:1424–35. discussion 35–6.
2. Atlas SJ, Keller RB, Wu YA, Deyo RA, Singer DE. Long-term outcomes of surgical and nonsurgical management of sciatica secondary to a lumbar disc herniation: 10 year results from the maine lumbar spine study. Spine. 2005;30:927–35.
3. Benzon HT, Rathmell JP, Wu CL, Turk DC, Argoff CE, Hurley RW. Practical management of pain. 5th ed. Philadelphia: Elsevier/Mosby; 2014. Print.
4. Dagenais S, Haldeman S. Evidenced-based management of low back pain. 1st ed. St Louis: Elsevier/Mosby; 2012. Print.
5. Weber H. Lumbar disc herniation. A controlled, prospective study with ten years of observation. Spine. 1983;8:131–40.
6. Weinstein JN, Lurie JD, Tosteson TD, et al. Surgical vs nonoperative treatment for lumbar disk herniation: the Spine Patient Outcomes Research Trial (SPORT) observational cohort. JAMA. 2006;296:2451–9.

Part VI

Conservative Treatment: VI. Medical Conservative Care

17 Spectrum of Pain Care

John Hau

Key Concepts

- Conservative management as a starting treatment has been the mainstay of pain management.
- Pharmacotherapy and injection therapies should be incorporated as part of a comprehensive pain management plan.
- Interventional techniques can dramatically reduce pain and obviate the need for medications along with their potential side effects.
- Implantable therapies should be considered earlier in the pain care algorithm and not relegated as a final treatment option.
- Although the up-front costs of implantable therapies may be higher, over time, they can be more cost-effective when compared to continued conservative management.

Introduction

Pain can frequently be a challenging and complex condition to manage given the multitude of causes in addition to its overall impact on patients. Contemporary pain medicine has therefore evolved into a field, where patients receive care through a multimodal and multidisciplinary team approach. As the field of pain medicine has changed, the spectrum of pain care has broadened. Providers are tasked with increasing demands as our knowledge of the mechanisms underlying pain continues to grow with increasing treatment options at our disposal.

J. Hau, MD (✉)
Summit Pain Alliance, Inc.,
392 Tesconi Court, Santa Rosa, CA 95401, USA
e-mail: Johnhau@gmail.com

Conservative Management

The goal of pain care is to improve pain and functionality and to facilitate return to previous levels of activity. Conservative management as an initial starting treatment has been the cornerstone in treating patients who suffer from pain. Classic pain care algorithms favor starting with treatments that are overall efficacious, least invasive, and cost-effective. Conservative non-pharmacologic management options include physical therapy and psychological therapy, which comprises cognitive behavioral therapy, group therapy, biofeedback, and relaxation. Complimentary treatment options such as acupuncture, chiropractic care, and massage therapy may be beneficial in certain patients.

Pharmacologic Treatment

Pharmacologic agents have been shown to be beneficial in the management of pain. Incorporating pharmacologic treatment options alongside conservative management options should be considered as part of a comprehensive pain management plan. The World Health Organization presented the analgesic treatment ladder in 1986 as a guide to help clinicians better manage chronic cancer-related pain. This treatment ladder has important and applicable ideas that can be considered in the treatment of noncancer-related pain as well. The ladder advocates starting with non-opioid medications and stepping up the strength of medications depending on patient response. When initiating pharmacologic agents, starting with non-opioid therapies such as acetaminophen and nonsteroidal anti-inflammatories is recommended. Other adjuvant medications that can be incorporated include antidepressants, antiepileptic medications, topical agents, and muscle relaxants. Opioid therapy is a powerful tool in pain management, but judicious usage and patient selection are of paramount importance. The Center for Disease Control (CDC) published recommendations on chronic opioid use

J.E. Pope, T.R. Deer (eds.), *Treatment of Chronic Pain Conditions*, DOI 10.1007/978-1-4939-6976-0_17

for noncancer-related pain, and the recommendations suggest that opioids be given at a quantity under 90 morphine equivalents per day, with increased vigilance if patients are given more than 50 morphine equivalents per day, later than should be placed after other regional treatments. Opioid therapy for chronic nonmalignant pain must be carefully evaluated on an individual patient basis. Providers should be vigilant for side effects, tolerance, hyperalgesia, and misuse of opioids when prescribing. Guidance suggests compliance testing be performed randomly, commonly with urine testing, along with motoring of the pharmacy board for schedule II medications, typically available in most states.

Injections

Interventional pain management techniques should be considered as part of a comprehensive pain care plan. The breadth of interventional pain management modalities available is remarkable. Injections can be a relatively safe and effective means to help manage many painful conditions. Central nerve blocks, peripheral nerve blocks, sympathetic nerve blocks, epidural steroid injections, facet injections, radio-frequency lesioning, neurolysis, joint injections, bursa injections, and trigger point injections are some of the available injection techniques that can be used to treat many painful conditions. A thorough understanding of anatomy and pathophysiology is critical to safely select and perform interventional techniques for pain management. When employed appropriately, injections can improve pain and restore functionality. A key benefit to interventional techniques is a potential to reduce pain without the need for oral medications that carry potential systemic effects.

Implantable Therapies

Traditional pain management algorithms focused on starting with conservative treatment options that are typically less invasive and costly. Depending on the response to the treatment, progressing to more invasive and usually more costly interventions would then follow. Based on these older algorithms, implantable therapies were relegated as last-resort treatment options in patients who have exhausted more conservative options. This approach unfortunately can lead to worse outcomes for the patient, such as prolonged pain, disability, overall costs, countless procedures, and medication toxicity. Identifying appropriate patients and implementing advanced implantable therapies such as neuromodulation or implantable drug-delivery systems earlier in the care algorithm can lead to better pain management and overall cost-effectiveness. Although implantable therapies may carry a higher up-front cost, over the long term, they can be more cost-effective by reducing physician follow-up visits, hospitalizations, and reliance on chronic pain medications.

Surgery

Despite the available treatment options we have for pain, some patients have continued and persistent pain. Referral for surgical evaluation should be considered in patients who demonstrate anatomic abnormalities consistent with their pain which may be amenable to surgical correction. Patients with significant functional disability and unremitting pain despite undergoing multiple nonsurgical treatments may benefit from surgical consultation. In the multidisciplinary model of pain care, working closely with a surgeon to address any possible surgical options should be considered.

Suggested Reading

1. Chou R, Qaseem A, Snow V, et al. Diagnosis and treatment of low back pain: a joint clinical practice guideline from the American College of Physicians and the American Pain Society. Ann Intern Med. 2007;147:478–91.
2. Cohen SP, Bicket MC, Jamison D, et al. Epidural steroids, a comprehensive, evidence-based review. Reg Anesth Pain Med. 2013;38:175–200.
3. Coleman SD, Mackey S. Spinal cord stimulation compared with medical management for failed back surgery syndrome. Curr Pain Headache Rep. 2009;13(1):1–3.
4. Krames E, Poree L, Deer T, Levy R. Implementing the SAFE principles for the development of pain medicine therapeutic algorithms that include neuromodulation techniques. Neuromodulation. 2009;12:104–13.
5. Kumar K, Taylor RS, Jacques L, et al. Spinal cord stimulation versus conventional medical management for neuropathic pain: a multicentre randomised controlled trial in patients with failed back surgery syndrome. Pain. 2007;132:179–88.
6. Mueller-Schweffe G, Hassenbusch SJ, Reig E. Cost effective of intrathecal therapy for pain. Neuromodulation. 1999;2:77–87.
7. Taylor RS, Taylor RJ, Van Buyten JP, Buschser E, et al. The cost effectiveness of spinal cord stimulation in the treatment of pain: a systemic review of the literature. J Pain Symptom Manag. 2004; 27:370–8.
8. Van Kleef M, Barendse GA, et al. Randomized trial of radiofrequency lumbar facet denervation for chronic low back pain. Spine. 1999;24:1937–42.
9. Vargas-Schaffer G. Is the WHO analgesic ladder still valid? Can Fam Physician. 2010;56:514–7.

Chronic Pain Rehabilitative Programs

18

George C. Chang Chien, Randy L. Calisoff,
and James W. Atchison

Key Concepts

- Pain is a multidimensional phenomenon that affects an individual's mood, health, and function.
- Interdisciplinary pain rehabilitation utilizes the biopsychosocial model of care which approaches health as best understood in terms of a combination of biological, psychological, and social factors rather than purely in biological terms.
- Interdisciplinary treatment is an effective approach to pain care and has demonstrated improvements in pain, mood, and function including return to work in a chronic pain population.
- Providers should consider referral to a chronic pain rehabilitation program that offers interdisciplinary care for patients who also suffer from significant functional limitations secondary to their chronic recalcitrant pain.

Introduction

Chronic pain is a debilitating condition that affects people all over the world. In the United States, the prevalence of chronic pain is estimated at 30.7%. Spine and musculoskeletal disorders account for nearly 70 million physician office visits annually and 130 million outpatient, hospital, and emergency room visits. The multidimensional experience of chronic pain results in individualized perceptions and coping mechanisms that reflect the complex biopsychosocial aspects of a patient in chronic pain. The biopsychosocial model states that health is best understood in terms of a combination of biological, psychological, and social factors rather than purely in biological terms. Functional restoration or interdisciplinary pain management programs incorporate this model in assessing and treating pain and have demonstrated lasting results in pain reduction, improved quality of life, as well as psychosocial functioning. The key component to program success is collaborative ongoing communication among team members, the patient, and their support system.

G.C. Chang Chien, DO (✉)
Cleveland Clinic, Anesthesia Institute Pain Management, Cleveland, OH, USA
e-mail: gchangchien@gmail.com

R.L. Calisoff, MD
Rehabilitation Institute of Chicago, Center for Pain Management, Chicago, IL, USA

J.W. Atchison, DO
Rehabilitation Institute of Chicago, Chicago, IL, USA

Interdisciplinary Pain Rehabilitation Team

There is no consensus about what constitutes an interdisciplinary pain rehabilitation program. These programs typically involve multiple providers of different specialties including pain medicine specialists (physiatry, psychiatry, or anesthesiology), pain psychology, physical and occupational therapy, social work, as well as vocational rehabilitation. Dedicated functional restoration programs often have a defined duration and schedule of daily activities. More intensive programs are scheduled for 8 h a day for upward of 4 weeks and show stronger benefits and improved outcomes. Group therapies are a hallmark of some functional restoration programs and often include the goal of de-escalation and discontinuation of chronic opioid medications. Interventional pain management techniques such as sympathetic blocks for complex regional pain syndrome may be appropriate to facilitate physical and occupational therapies.

Patient Selection

Although all patients with chronic recalcitrant pain may benefit from comprehensive pain rehabilitation, patients with significant psychiatric comorbidities such as depression, anxiety, substance abuse, and history of physical or emotional abuse may require this comprehensive type of pain

J.E. Pope, T.R. Deer (eds.), *Treatment of Chronic Pain Conditions*, DOI 10.1007/978-1-4939-6976-0_18

rehabilitation in order to optimize successful treatment of their pain. Providers should consider referral to a chronic pain rehabilitation program in patients who also suffer from significant functional limitations secondary to their chronic recalcitrant pain.

History and Physical Examination

Intake to a pain rehabilitation program typically includes a detailed pain history such that the patient describes the characteristics of their pain and the circumstances in which it began. Practitioners should inquire about pain location, quality, intensity, temporal characteristics, aggravating and alleviating factors, impact of pain on function, sleep and quality of life, past treatment and response, patient expectations, and goals. Previous testing such as medical evaluation, imaging, neurophysiologic testing, and laboratory work should be reviewed. The results of prior interventional procedures, surgeries, and medications should be detailed and noted.

Past medical history including vision or hearing impairment, amputation, diabetes or other endocrine problems, cancer, or cardiovascular disease is important to note as they can affect performance and participation in therapy sessions.

Social history should include support networks, substance abuse (tobacco, drugs, medications, and alcohol), hobbies, and medicolegal confounders such as an active injury lawsuit or ongoing worker's compensation claim.

Functional history should include premorbid and current levels for daily activities, vocational status, exercise, and work history.

Psychological history should include a detailed screen for depression, anxiety, and other psychiatric illness. History of psychiatric illness and/or hospitalization, history of abuse (emotional, sexual, or physical, etc.), significant pain catastrophizing, or pain behaviors should also be noted.

Physical examination should be thorough, and identify any limitations that should be addressed in physical and occupational therapy.

Medical Management

Supervision by a physician specializing in pain medicine is not always necessary but can provide close monitoring for titration of pain medications. Rapid de-escalation of opioid medications may cause withdrawal symptoms, which can be treated with medications such as clonidine. Initiation of new medications such as tricyclic antidepressants may require medical monitoring for potential life-threatening side effects such as QT prolongation. Other groups of medications used to assist with pain and opioid reduction include the skeletal muscle relaxants, antiepileptic drugs (AEDs), and selective-norepinephrine reuptake inhibitors (SNRIs).

Physical Therapy

Physical therapy (physical therapists or PT) is a branch of rehabilitation medicine that includes prescription of or assistance with specific exercises, manual therapy, and education to promote strength, endurance, as well as increase functional capacity. There is considerable evidence to support the incorporation of physical therapy and exercise in the management of many types of chronic musculoskeletal disorders including osteoarthritis, fibromyalgia, rheumatoid arthritis, low back pain, as well as myofascial pain. Exercise or exercise therapy in patients with chronic pain has been demonstrated to improve function and reduce disability. Among the numerous benefits, physical therapy can reduce pain associated with movement by strengthening the musculoskeletal system, improve cardiac function, and boost metabolic efficiency. Weight loss may improve pain associated with the lower back or joint degeneration.

Occupational Therapy

Occupational therapy (occupational therapists or OT) is a branch of rehabilitation medicine that focuses on adapting the environment, modifying the task, teaching the skill, as well as educating the client/family in order to increase participation in and performance of daily activities including bathing, showering, toileting, and functional mobility. The role of OT in chronic pain is to identify activities and behaviors that aggravate pain and to teach methods for decreasing the frequency/duration of painful episodes. There is an emphasis on proper posture and body mechanics.

Together, PT and OT implement therapy interventions to decrease dependence on pain medications. These processes are especially important in disease processes such as complex regional pain syndrome and neuralgias which can lead to *kinesiophobia* as well as *fear avoidance behaviors.* Desensitization therapy and movement therapies are effective modalities to reduce the aforementioned disabilities.

Psychology

Pain psychology is an important aspect of pain rehabilitation and functional restoration. Up to 60% of patients with chronic pain have comorbid depression or anxiety. Additionally, patients with chronic pain may have poor cop-

Table 18.1 Sample of psychological treatment modalities in chronic pain

Treatment	Description
Relaxation Biofeedback Progressive muscle relaxation Guided imagery Altered focus	*Biofeedback* is a method of monitoring physiologic parameters including heart rate, sweating, skin temperature, muscle tension, and brain activity as part of relaxation exercises *Progressive muscle relaxation* involves tensing and then relaxing muscles to create awareness of tension and relaxation *Guided imagery* involves focusing your imagination to create calm, peaceful images in your mind, thereby providing a "mental escape" *Altered focus* involves shifting attention to any specific nonpainful part of the body (hand, foot, etc.) and alter sensation in that part of the body
Group therapy	Group therapy develops camaraderie between patients who can help each other solve a problem and impediments to relaxation techniques Positive peer pressure may exist to practice exercises between sessions
Cognitive behavioral therapy	Modality of therapy that is designed to address maladaptive behaviors, thoughts, or beliefs about the pain experience to enable the patient to change the behaviors related to it

ing strategies of dealing with their pain or pain exacerbating factors. Psychological treatment goals are designed to predict/manage pain, teach coping skills to minimize pain and pain-aggravating factors such as anger and anxiety, as well as how to maximize function and positive attitude, despite the presence of chronic pain (Table 18.1).

Partial list of university-based interdisciplinary pain rehabilitation programs:

Rehabilitation Institute of Chicago Center for Pain Management
Cleveland Clinic
Johns Hopkins University
Spaulding Rehabilitation Hospital
Kennedy Krieger Institute
Mayo Clinic
Stanford

Conclusion

The multidimensional experience of chronic pain results in individualized perceptions and coping mechanisms that reflect the complex biopsychosocial aspects of a patient in chronic pain. Comprehensive pain rehabilitation programs have been demonstrated effective in reducing the use of pharmacologic treatment, surgeries, and implantable pain devices while improving function and mood, as well as facilitating return to work. Providers should consider referral to a chronic pain rehabilitation program in patients who also suffer from significant functional limitations secondary to their chronic recalcitrant pain.

Suggested Reading

1. Flor H, Fydrich T, Turk DC. Efficacy of multidisciplinary pain treatment centers: a meta-analytic review. Pain. 1992;49:221–30.
2. Murphy JL, Clark EM, Banou E. Opioid cessation and multidimensional outcomes after interdisciplinary chronic pain treatment. Clin J Pain. 2013;29(2):109–17.
3. Stanos S. Focused review of interdisciplinary pain rehabilitation programs for chronic pain management. Curr Pain Headache Rep. 2012;16(2):147–52.
4. Theodore BR, Mayer TG, Gatchel RJ. Cost-effectiveness of early versus delayed functional restoration for chronic disabling occupational musculoskeletal disorders. J Occup Rehabil. 2015;25(2):303–15. doi:10.1007/s10926-014-9539-0

Physical Therapy in the Management of Chronic Pain

19

Justin F. Averna and George C. Chang Chien

Key Concepts

- Physical therapy is a branch of rehabilitation medicine that includes prescription of or assistance with specific exercises, manual therapy, and education to promote strength and stamina as well as increase functional capacity.
- There is considerable evidence to support the incorporation of physical therapy and exercise in the management of many types of chronic musculoskeletal disorders including osteoarthritis, fibromyalgia, rheumatoid arthritis, back, and myofascial pain.
- Physical therapy can reduce pain associated with movement by strengthening the musculoskeletal system, improve cardiac function, and boost metabolic efficiency. Weight loss may improve pain associated with the lower back or joint degeneration.

Introduction

Chronic pain is a multidimensional pathological process that is best understood in terms of a combination of biological, psychological, and social factors rather than purely in biological terms. Comprehensive pain management is a multifaceted approach that includes multiple modalities including physiatry, psychiatry, pain psychology, physical and occupational therapy, as well as social work. Physical and occupational medicine modalities have been demonstrated to facilitate functional restoration, decrease in pain, and improve return-to-work rates. Physical therapy (PT) is overseen by physical therapists, which are formally trained and licensed healthcare professionals that possess a skill set to help patients reduce pain, restore function, and help prevent disability. Physical therapists incorporate active and passive therapeutic exercises to address muscle strength, flexibility, neuromuscular control, functional mobility, endurance, balance, and locomotion to maximize function and maintain physical activity in an effort to ultimately decrease pain.

Physical Therapy Strategies

Formal physical therapy programs should include passive joint mobilization and range of motion exercises and address muscle function to restore joint mobility and stability. These programs should be tailored to each individuals needs and include assessment of current and premorbid functional capacity and medical conditions that may impair therapy and include objective goals.

Throughout the course of treatment, therapists will help monitor and progressively increase the level and complexity of therapeutic exercises. Ultimately, the patient should be transitioned to a daily structured home exercise program with aerobic, stretching, and strengthening exercises. Exercise prescriptions should be specifically designed to enhance physical fitness, address weight loss, and promote health by reducing risk factors for associated chronic disease processes.

Modalities commonly employed in PT include moist heat, transcutaneous electrical stimulation, cryotherapy, and ultrasound (Table 19.1).

Shoulder

The shoulder is a complex joint made up of the humerus, clavicle, and scapula and stabilized by 18 muscles, ligaments, and tendons. The muscles and joints of the shoulder allow it to move through a large range of motion. The shoulder can abduct, adduct, rotate, and be raised in front of and

J.F. Averna, DO
Temple University Hospital, Department of Physical Medicine and Rehabilitation, Philadelphia, PA, USA

G.C. Chang Chien, DO (✉)
Cleveland Clinic, Anesthesia Institute Pain Management, 9500 Euclid Ave, Dept C-25, Cleveland, OH 44195, USA
e-mail: gchangchien@gmail.com

J.E. Pope, T.R. Deer (eds.), *Treatment of Chronic Pain Conditions*, DOI 10.1007/978-1-4939-6976-0_19

Table 19.1 Goals of physical therapy

To educate patients on the principles of stretching and strengthening
To educate patients on proper posture and ergonomic principles
To accelerate the stages of healing by reducing pain and the inflammatory cycle
To restore muscular flexibility, joint mobility, and proper biomechanics
To strengthen the involved muscles
To prevent future occurrence and manage exacerbations of pain
To facilitate return to normal activities

behind the torso and move through a full 360° in the sagittal plane. The consequence of this range of motion is instability, and the shoulder joint is prone to dislocation. One of the most common pathologies is a rotator cuff injury. Pathologic changes in the rotator cuff extend across a spectrum of disease including tendinopathy, impingement, and tearing. Medical management and physical therapy protocols depend on the cause and severity of disease.

In general, strengthening of the rotator cuff should initially incorporate closed chain exercises and progress to open chain exercises for correction of strength imbalance. In the acute rehabilitation stage, strengthening exercises for the scapular stabilizing muscles rather than the rotator cuff should be emphasized. The serratus anterior and inferior trapezius, which retract and depress the scapula, should be strengthened. The pectoralis minor and upper trapezius should be stretched to reduce impingement. Additionally, posterior glenohumeral joint capsular tightness and scapulothoracic kinematics should be corrected. See Table 19.2 for post shoulder surgery rehabilitation protocol.

Table 19.2 Post shoulder surgery rehabilitation protocol

Phase 1 (0–6 weeks) Passive range of motion phase	
Goals	Protect healing tendon Restore passive ROM of the shoulder
Recommended exercises	Pendulums Standing scapular mobility (no resistance) Supine or standing passive external rotation Passive shoulder flexion
Phase 2 (6–12 weeks) Active range of motion phase	
Goals	Continue to improve passive ROM Initiate progression of active ROM Initiate gentle submaximal rotator cuff isometrics
Recommended exercises	Continue exercises from phase 1 until each can be progressed to active assisted or active motion Supine passive external rotation in scapular plane progressing to 90 deg. of abduction Table slides in flexion with progression to wall slides
Phase 3 (12–24 weeks) Strengthening phase	
Goals	Continue to focus on restoration of ROM, biomechanics, and strength Initiate progressive strengthening of rotator cuff and periscapular muscle groups Begin to use arm for daily activities
Recommended exercises	Scapular retraction Prone horizontal abduction Manual resistance patterns Dynamic strengthening Push up progression Progress to diagonal patterns and multi-planar and Functional planes of motion

Hip

The femoral-acetabular joint translates forces from the pelvis and axial skeleton into the ground. As a large weight-bearing joint, it is prone to degenerative forces that may lead to painful conditions. In patients with hip pain from osteoarthritis, strengthening of the pelvis and lower extremity may improve function and reduce pain. Strengthening should address the hip abductors, external hip rotators, and knee flexors and extensors. Patients should be evaluated for gait abnormality, which should be corrected when appropriate. In general, strengthening exercises should initially incorporate closed chain exercises and progress to open chain exercises for correction of strength imbalance. Postoperative total hip arthroplasty patients should have weight-bearing status maintained according to surgical recommendations. Posterior hip precautions, which include no hip flexion greater than 90 degrees, no hip adduction or internal rotation beyond neutral, and none of the motions combined, will be initially instituted. Anterior hip precautions include avoiding lying supine or prone, and there should be no external rotation of the hip. In these patients, it is crucial that the treating physical therapist addresses hip range of motion and isometric strength training of the hip flexors and quadriceps, hamstrings, as well as the hip abductors, adductors, and gluteal muscles. Resistive exercises for the quadriceps and hamstrings are commonly initiated within 2 months postoperatively.

Knee

Common conditions that cause pain in the knee include osteoarthritis, meniscal injury, anterior or posterior cruciate ligament injury, disorders of the patella, and quadriceps or patella tendinopathy. After an injury and once weight-bearing restrictions are reestablished, patients can begin exercises to stretch and strengthen the knee. In general, strengthening exercises should initially incorporate closed chain exercises and progress to open chain exercises for correction of strength imbalance. This includes strengthening and range of motion exercises of the hip abductors, adductors, flexors, and extensors. Active and passive range of motion of the knee and proprioception training of the lower limb should be emphasized. Postoperative total knee arthroplasty patients should be ambulatory as soon as deemed appropriate and maintain range of motion exercises with appropriate soft tissue balance to ensure proper biomechanics.

Ankle

Achilles tendinopathy is relatively common and is characterized by pain in the posterior part of the heel most commonly in the midportion of the Achilles tendon. Alfredson's model of eccentric training should be instituted by the treating physical therapist. It is a 12-week program that is successful in approximately 90% of patients with pain in the midportion of the Achilles tendon. The protocol involves no concentric loading but eccentric training in which patients undertake painful heel-drop exercises (180 repetitions/day) (Table 19.3). It should be noted that the exercise protocol should elicit pain in the tendon. If a patient does not experience pain in the tendon, the load should be increased until pain is provoked.

Spine

Chronic cervical and lumbar spine pains are common indications for physical therapy. Therapies should address range of motion, soft tissue mobilization, strengthening and stretching of postural muscular, the hip girdle and abdominal core. A thorough posture and ergonomic assessment should be performed to assess for aggravating factors for chronic pain. A progressive therapeutic exercise program with an extension bias for stretching and strengthening of the lower limb and core musculature is commonly implemented for the lumbar spine. Gait training, safety awareness, proper use of assistive devices, modification of activities, and proper body mechanics should also be addressed by the treating physical therapist.

Table 19.3 Summary of Alfredson's heel-drop exercise program

Exercise	The patient should stand on the edge of a step and rise up on their toes first lifting the non-painful leg and then slowly lowering their weight through the painful leg The heel should drop below the step Exercises are performed with both straight and bent knee Pain should be elicited when performing exercises
Repetition	3 sets of 15 repetitions with a straight knee 3 sets of 15 repetitions with a bent knee
Frequency	Twice daily
Progression	A weighted backpack can be utilized as exercises become more comfortable

Conclusion

Chronic pain can be reduced by properly addressing common musculoskeletal complaints with comprehensive physical therapy programs that promote conditioning of musculature, flexibility, and range motion with improved overall fitness and weight loss. A multifaceted and interdisciplinary approach utilizing conservative modalities has been shown to help facilitate functional restoration and decrease pain. Addressing mobility and preventing and correcting deformity can not only slow the progression of disease and decrease pain but can also substantially improve quality of life. Individualized therapy programs should be designed and overseen by medical providers and implemented by physical therapists. It is paramount to properly monitor a patient's progression in a physical therapy program for proper adjustment in therapeutic exercises and modalities. By specifically addressing muscle strength, flexibility, neuromuscular control, myofascial dysfunction, functional mobility, endurance, balance, and locomotion, patients can maximize function and ultimately better manage their chronic pain.

Suggested Reading

1. Alfredson H, Cook J. A treatment algorithm for managing Achilles tendinopathy: new treatment options. Br J Sports Med. 2007; 41(4):211–6.
2. Alfredson H, Lorentzon R. Chronic Achilles tendinosis: recommendations for treatment and prevention. Sports Med. 2000; 29:135–46.
3. Bang M, Deyle G. Comparison of supervised exercise with and without manual physical therapy for patients with shoulder impingement syndrome. J Orthop Sports Phys Ther. 2000;30(3):126–37.
4. Bhave A, Mont M, Tennis S, et al. Functional problems and treatment solutions after total hip and knee arthroplasty. J Bone Joint Surg. 2005;87(2):9–21.
5. Faas A. Exercises: which ones are worth trying, for which patients, and when? Spine (Phila Pa 1976). 1996;21:2874.
6. Hayden JA, van Tulder MW, Malmivaara A, Koes BW. Exercise therapy for treatment of non-specific low back pain. Cochrane Database Syst Rev. 2005;20(3):CD000335.
7. Hayden JA, van Tulder MW, Tomlinson G. Systematic review: strategies for using exercise therapy to improve outcomes in chronic low back pain. Ann Intern Med. 2005;142:776.
8. Liddle SD, Baxter GD, Gracey JH. Exercise and chronic low back pain: what works? Pain. 2004;107:176.
9. Machado LA, de Mv S, Ferreira PH, Ferreira ML. The McKenzie method for low back pain: a systematic review of the literature with a meta-analysis approach. Spine (Phila Pa 1976). 2006;31:E254.
10. vanTulder MW, Malmivaara A, Esmail R, Koes BW. Exercise therapy for low back pain. Cochrane Database Syst Rev. 2000:CD000335.

Opioid Medications for Chronic Noncancer Pain

20

Jonathan D. Carlson and Joshua Peloquin

Key Concepts

- Prescribing opioids for chronic pain
- Tailoring opioid doses for patient-specific needs
- Proper rotation and conversions of opioid treatments
- Risks and side effects associated with opioid medications

Introduction

Opioid medications have grown in popularity in recent years and are seen as an effective and essential medication in managing many forms of severe painful pathology. However, the benefits opioids provide to patients are accompanied by significant risks which must be addressed and mitigated by physicians and patients alike. This chapter outlines the appropriate protocol for implementing opioids as a form of pain management in patients with confirmed pathology.

Prescribing Opioids for Chronic Pain

If and when opioids are deemed necessary for the treatment of a patient's chronic pain, the prescribing physician should adhere to the following protocol before writing any opioid prescriptions (Table 20.1):

1. Confirmation of pathology by a thorough history and physical and appropriate diagnostic testing.
2. Exhaust non-opioid-based medications.
3. Review of medical records to rule out contraindications.
4. Implement patient/physician opioid agreement.
5. Screen for opioid diversion.

Once the decision has been made to prescribe opioids, the screen for diversion should be conducted at every touch point that involves prescribing opioids to the patient. This is often considered standard of care and essential to optimize patient safety. As stated, the physician should require the patient to sign an opioid agreement. It should include compliance to obtain pain medications from a single doctor/practice and to only fill pain medication prescriptions at one pharmacy. Many states and pharmacies participate in controlled prescription monitoring programs. These programs have become a vital tool that may be used to track the origination of controlled prescriptions as well to monitor where prescriptions are being filled.

When treatment is initiated, it should be required by the physician that the patient agree to not consume any alcohol, marijuana, or other illegal substances. Patients must also agree to undergo periodic and unscheduled urine drug screens (UDS) to test for illegal substance abuse as well as to monitor if the prescribed medication is being utilized. Random pill counts are another means to rule out diversion.

Clinic Pearl

Patients who use heroin in conjunction with prescribed opioids will have a UDS test positive for 6-monoacytlmorphine (6-MAM) for approximately 12 h after substance abuse occurs. Beyond this 12-h window, only morphine will be present in the patient's UDS. Figure 20.1 illustrates the metabolites of heroin and its eventual metabolism to morphine in the body.

On the onset of treatment, the total daily pill amount and dose prescribed should be at the lowest possible dosage that is estimated to adequately control the patient's pain. The dose may then be incrementally increased until adequate pain relief is achieved or the risks of increasing the opioid

J.D. Carlson, MD (✉)
Arizona Pain/Pain Doctor, Glendale, AZ, USA
e-mail: jcarlsonmd@gmail.com

J. Peloquin, DO
Midwestern Medica School, Placentia, CA, USA

J.E. Pope, T.R. Deer (eds.), *Treatment of Chronic Pain Conditions*, DOI 10.1007/978-1-4939-6976-0_20

dosage outweigh the benefits. Titration increases must be done at a slow interval. Most iatrogenic overdoses/deaths are related to too high of an initial dose and/or escalating the opioid medication too quickly over a short period of time without proper monitoring. When the dosage is incrementally increased, the risks associated with opioid medications also increase in tandem. The adverse effects of opioids increase significantly when a patient's daily equivalent dose of morphine exceeds 50–100 mg per day. There is a threefold increase in deaths related to opioid overdose when the daily oral morphine equivalent exceeds 200 mg.

When prescribing opioids, the physician should attempt to never provide more than 30 days worth of medication. This will mitigate the possibility of abuse and promote frequent interaction between the physician and patient for better monitoring of the patient's current pain levels and current opioid safety compliance. The prescribing physician must inform patients to not share their prescribed medications with other individuals. Such abuses are illegal and dangerous. Physicians should also instruct patients to store their medications in a secure location where they cannot be accessed by anyone other than themselves. Four out of five patients who overdose on opioids did not have the medication prescribed to them. Lost or stolen medications should not be replaced, unless under rare and extenuating circumstances. It is always the patient's or their assigned caretaker's responsibility to monitor the safety of the opioid medications.

Again, opioid medications should be used for the treatment of pain only when the severity of the pain warrants such use, and non-opioid pain medications have previously been tried but failed to adequately control the patient's pain. Each patient's reaction to opioid treatments will be different, and a tailored approach should be implemented to reduce the possibility of over-medicating.

Table 20.1 Contraindications for opioids

Lack of appropriate pathology
Severe respiratory instability
Severe psychiatric instability or suicide risk
Unaddressed or recent substance use disorder
Severe opioid allergy/side effects
Coadministration of drugs capable of inducing life-threatening interactions
Inappropriate use of medication (providing medication to others, concurrent alcohol use, concurrent or illegal substance use)

Tailoring Opioid Doses for Patient-Specific Needs

A tailored approach requires the potency and dose of opioids to be increased incrementally as pain and patient comorbidities dictate. For cases of mild pain, the initial regimen should be a nonsteroidal anti-inflammatory drug (NSAIDs) or acetaminophen. For moderate levels of pain, an opioid receptor agonist such as tramadol or hydrocodone can be paired

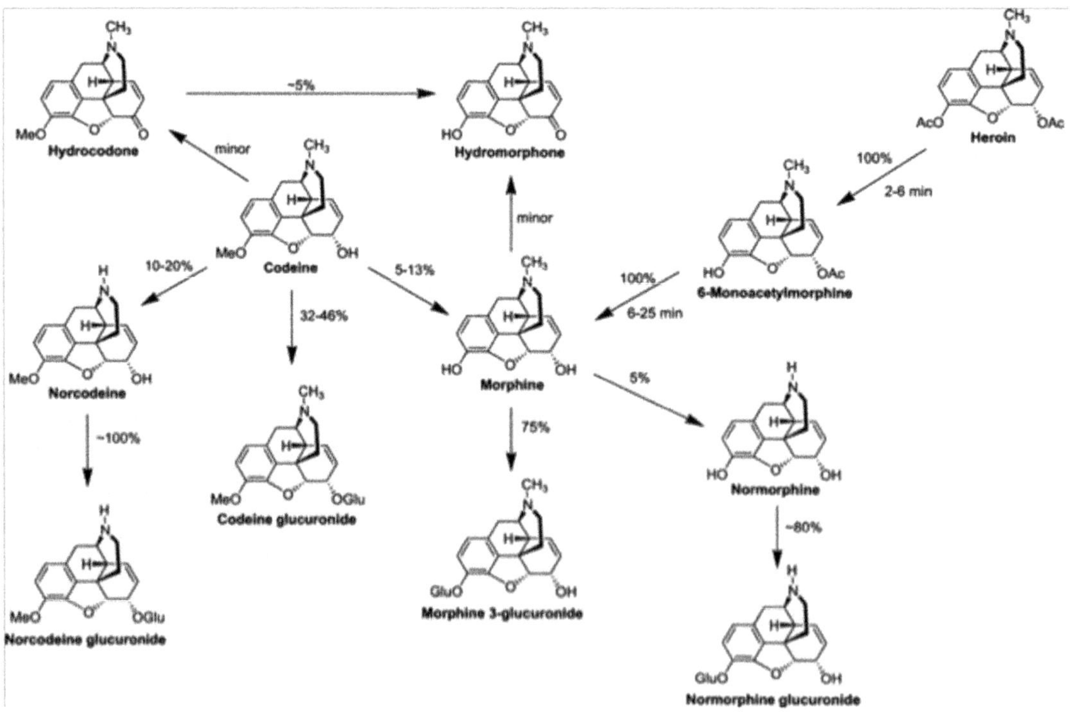

Fig. 20.1 Opioid-based metabolites

alongside with NSAIDs or acetaminophen when deemed appropriate. In cases of severe pain, a higher potency opioid receptor agonist such as oxycodone, morphine, oxymorphone, hydromorphone, methadone, or fentanyl may be considered for use.

Many of the opioids listed above can be modified to increase the duration of their effectiveness. These modified opioids are typically found in forms such as extended-release tablets. These longer-lasting opioid treatments should only be given to patients who are considered to have high opioid tolerance, and other short-acting opioids are less effective. Patients who fall into this category of treatment must be treated in a controlled environment where monitoring and assessment for adverse effects can be routinely performed. Extended-release tablets should never be used as first-line therapy to treat acute or postoperative pain. Patients should be warned to never split extended-release pills into partial doses or be crushed. Such actions can cause an unreliable amount of drug to be released, which could lead to overdose.

When physicians are developing a tailored approach for patient care, it is important to note opioid medications are only one variable in the treatment of a patient's pain. They do not encompass the entirety of a patient's pain symptoms. The use of opioids should not hinder or delay early implementation of other therapies and modalities such as exercise and physical therapy. A multifaceted approach paired with supplementation of opioids to alleviate pain is the hallmark of best practices.

Table 20.2 Opioid conversions

1. Calculate total mg dose taken in the past 24 h
2. Determine equianalgesic dose
3. If pain is controlled on current opioid, reduce the new opioid daily dose by 30–50% to account for cross-tolerance
4. If inpatient with proper monitoring, methodically titrate to achieve analgesic effect during first 24 h and/or consider patient-controlled analgesia (PCA)
5. Monitor for adverse events and effectiveness

Buprenorphine (IM/IV): 0.4 mg	Meperidine (IV/IM/SC): 75 mg
Butorphanol (IM/IV): 2.0 mg	Meperidine (PO): 300 mg
Codeine (IM/IV): 120 mg	Methadone (acute IV): 5.0 mg
Codeine (PO): 200 mg	Methadone (acute PO): 10 mg
Fentanyl (IM/IV): 0.1 mg	Morphine (IV/IM/SC): 10 mg
Fentanyl (Transdermal): 0.2 mg	Morphine (acute PO): 60 mg
Hydrocodone (PO): 30 mg	Morphine (chronic PO): 30 mg
Hydromorphone (IV/IM/SC): 1.5 mg	Oxycodone (PO): 20 mg
Hydromorphone (PO): 7.5 mg	Oxymorphone (IV/IM/SC): 1.0 mg
	Oxymorphone (PO): 10 mg

Disclaimer: It should be noted that these conversions are not definitive and should only be used as a guide. Vigilance with individual patient application of opioids conversions is still at the sole discretion of the prescribing provider

Proper Rotation and Conversion of Opioids for Ongoing Pain Management

As treatment continues, chronic pain patients may develop a tolerance to the opioid medications they are currently prescribed. It maybe necessary for opioid medications to be rotated periodically. The proper conversion dosages for opioid rotation can be calculated as shown in Table 20.2.

Risks and Side Effects Associated with Opioid Medications

The addictive nature of opioids paired with their growing availability from physicians has advanced their popularity for abuse. In the USA, death related to opioid overdose has risen significantly. Consequently, physicians must continually be aware of the dangers of prescribing opioids. To decrease the chance of addiction, overdose, and death, physicians should adhere to opioid prescribing guidelines. It is important to remember risks should be identified and assessed before treatment commences. Side effects and non-abuse-related risks may also manifest. Examples are as follows: increased falls, traffic, and work-related accidents; impaired decision-making, depressed breathing, sleep disorders, endocrine dysfunction, cognitive deficits, increased cancer risk, and opioid-induced hyperalgesia. These risks and side effects paired with the high abuse potential of opioid medications require the prescribing physician to be vigilant. Discernment between patients who require these medications to function in daily life and those who seek out opioids for abuse or secondary gain should constantly be exercised. Following established guidelines for prescribing these medications will help physicians mitigate the pitfalls associated with opioid prescribing (Box 20.1).

Box 20.1 States that participate in prescription monitoring programs

Alabama, Arizona, California, Colorado, Connecticut, Florida, Hawaii, Idaho, Illinois, Indiana, Iowa, Kansas, Kentucky, Louisiana, Maine, Massachusetts, Michigan, Minnesota, Mississippi, Nevada, New Mexico, New York, North Carolina, North Dakota, Ohio, Oklahoma, Oregon, Pennsylvania, Rhode Island, South Carolina, Tennessee, Texas, Utah, Vermont, Virginia, West Virginia, and Wyoming

Suggested Reading

1. Katz N. The impact of opioids on the endocrine system. Pain Manag Rounds. 2005;1(9):1–6.
2. Kissin I. Long-term opioid treatment of chronic nonmalignant pain: unproven efficacy and neglected safety? J Pain Res. 2013;6:513–29.
3. Lennon F, Mirzapoiazova T, Mambetsariev B, Salgia R, Moss J, Singleton P. Overexpression of the μ-opioid receptor in human non-small cell lung cancer promotes Akt and mTOR activation, tumor growth, and metastasis. Anesthesiology. 2012;116:857–67.
4. Manchikanti L, Abdi S, Atluri S, et al. American Society of Interventional Pain Physicians (ASIPP) guidelines for responsible opioid prescribing in chronic non-cancer pain: part 1 – evidence assessment. Pain Physician. 2012;15(3 Suppl):S1–65.
5. Mardian A, Patel T,Derksen D, Carlson J, Thompson IV W, St. Mars T, Sjolander S. Arizona opioid prescribing guidelines: www.azdhs.gov/clinicians/documents/clinical-guidelines-recommendations/prescribing-guidelines/141121-opiod.pdf.
6. Opioid conversion: www.globalrph.com/narcoticonv.htm.

Nonsteroidal Anti-inflammatory Drugs (NSAIDs)

21

Reda Tolba

Key Concepts

- NSAIDs have analgesic, anti-inflammatory, and antipyretic properties by inhibiting prostaglandin synthesis through cyclooxygenase COX pathway.
- NSAIDs can have adverse effects on different systems including the gastrointestinal, renal, and cardiovascular systems. Patient's medical history should be reviewed prior to treatment.
- NSAIDs can be used alone or in conjunction with other pain medications in treatment of varieties of nociceptive pain conditions.

Background

NSAID class of medications has been used by millions of patients worldwide for many years. They have analgesic, anti-inflammatory, and antipyretic properties. They are commonly used to treat nociceptive pain conditions such as osteoarthritis, low back pain, rheumatoid arthritis, inflammatory arthropathies (e.g., gout, lupus, ankylosing spondylitis), dysmenorrhea, renal colic, and headaches, to mention a few. They have been used alone or in conjunction with opioid medications in acute pain settings such in the perioperative period. Their use for neuropathic pain has been less effective.

R. Tolba, MD (✉)
200 west Esplanade Avenue, Kenner, LA 70005, USA
e-mail: redatolba@hotmail.com

Mechanism of Action

- NSAIDs inhibit prostaglandin synthesis by inhibiting cyclooxygenase COX enzyme leading to inhibition of prostaglandins synthesis. After tissue damage, cell membrane phospholipids form substances called eicosanoids (such as arachidonic acid) by the action of phospholipase A2. Arachidonic acid then is converted into prostaglandin G2 and H2 by the action of cyclooxygenase COX enzyme. NSAID analgesic action is thought to be both centrally in the CNS and peripherally at the nociceptive nerve endings.
- There are two isoforms of cyclooxygenase enzyme: COX1 is responsible for the production of prostaglandins involved in GI protection and enhancing platelet aggregation, while COX2 is only created when there is inflammation and tissue damage. It produces prostaglandins responsible for pain and inflammation. NSAIDs inhibit both COX1 and COX2 and, thereby, the synthesis of prostaglandins and thromboxanes. Selective COX2 inhibitors such as celecoxib have less adverse effects on the GI system.

Classification

- NSAIDs can be classified by their chemical structure into:
  - Salicylates (e.g., aspirin)
  - Propionic acid derivatives (e.g., ibuprofen, naproxen, ketoprofen)
  - Acetic acid derivatives (e.g., indomethacin, etodolac, diclofenac, ketorolac, nabumetone)
  - Enolic acid derivatives (e.g., meloxicam, piroxicam)
  - Anthranilic acid derivatives (e.g., mefenamic acid, meclofenamate)
  - Selective COX2 inhibitors (e.g., celecoxib, rofecoxib, valdecoxib, etoricoxib)

J.E. Pope, T.R. Deer (eds.), *Treatment of Chronic Pain Conditions*, DOI 10.1007/978-1-4939-6976-0_21

Side Effects and Contraindications

Gastrointestinal GI

Peptic ulcers/bleeding, dyspepsia, gastropathy, nausea, and vomiting and diarrhea. Formulations combining NSAIDs with proton pump inhibitors or prostaglandin analogue are available to reduce GI side effects. Avoid use with patients with history of peptic ulcer or stomach bleeding.

Renal

Constriction of the afferent arteriole and decrease in renal perfusion pressure due to inhibition of prostaglandin formation leading to renal toxicity including acute renal failure and acute tubular necrosis, hypertension, sodium, and fluid retention. Other less common renal effects can occur including nephrotic syndrome and interstitial nephritis. Avoid use in patients with renal disease.

Cardiovascular

Aside from aspirin, NSAIDs increase risk of acute coronary syndrome and stroke. That includes nonselective NSAIDs and COX 2 inhibitors. This is due to inhibition of platelet activation by inhibiting formation of thromboxane A2. Nonaspirin NSAIDs can increase the risk of heart failure in patients with preexisting heart disease. Avoid use (excluding Aspirin) in patients with history of stroke, history of myocardial infarction, or hear failure. Avoid use of NSAIDs in patients taking daily aspirin to reduce cardiovascular risk as NSAIDs can inhibit cardioprotective effects of aspirin.

Hepatic

On rare occasions, long-tern NSAID therapy can cause minor increase in liver functions and hepatocellular injury. It is advisable to follow liver functions in those patients.

NSAID-Induced Asthma

Due to increase leukotrienes, which can trigger bronchospasm.

Others

Impaired bone healing after lumbar fusion (short duration of treatment or use of fewer doses postoperatively is advised), allergic reactions, and possible erectile dysfunction. NSAID use can produce adverse effects during pregnancy (premature closure of the ductus arteriosus, miscarriage, and premature birth). Avoid use of NSAIDs during third trimester of pregnancy.

Rofecoxib (Vioxx) is a selective COX2 inhibitor that was withdrawn from the market due to increased risk of heart attacks and stroke with long-term use.

Drug Interactions

- NSAIDs should be used with caution with patients taking warfarin due to increased risk of bleeding.
- NSAIDs can antagonize the antihypertensive effects of ACE inhibitors in patients with hypertension.
- By reducing renal blood flow, NSAIDs can decrease elimination of renal excreted drugs such as lithium. Lithium level should be cautiously monitored. It also can decreases efficacy of diuretics.

Uses and Role in Perioperative Period

As mentioned above, NSAIDs can be used in a variety of acute and chronic nociceptive pain conditions but less effectively for neuropathic pain conditions. There is now an emerging role for use of NSAIDs in combination with opioid medications for treatment of acute pain in the perioperative setting. NSAIDs can be used in a multimodal approach due to its synergic effect with opioid medications. This allows for dose reduction of the opioid medications and better analgesia in the postoperative period with fewer side effects. It also can improve quality of analgesia provided. Caution should be taken when using NSAIDs in the postoperative period. Avoid use for patients with preexisting heart disease, renal, or hepatic disease. The postoperative use of NSAIDs in certain patient populations can be based on clinician judgment. One patient population for instance is patients who underwent spinal fusion. For those patients the risks of impairing bone healing are weighted against the analgesic benefits that NSAIDs can provide. Proper dosing, timing, and monitoring of toxicity are essential to avoid complications.

Conclusion

NSAIDs play an essential role in the treatment of a variety of acute and chronic nociceptive pain conditions. Their role in neuropathic pain has been less effective. There is an emerging role for NSAIDs in the treatment of acute pain in the perioperative period. Side effects of NSAIDs can limit their use despite their analgesic benefits. There is hope in the future to developing more COX isoforms that can lead to more selective action of NSAIDs, with isolated central analgesic effects and without peripheral toxic side effects.

Suggested Reading

1. Benzon H, Raja SN, Fishman SM, Liu S, Cohen SP. Essentials of pain medicine. 3rd ed.
2. Fishman SM, Ballantyne JC, Rathmell JP. Bonica's management of pain. 4th ed.
3. Katzung B, Masters S, Trevor A. Basic and clinical pharmacology. 12th ed. Lange Basic Science. McGraw Hill Companies; 2012. ISBN-13: 978-0071764018; ISBN-10: 0071764011

22 Anticonvulsants

Radhika P. Grandhe and George C. Chang Chien

Key Concepts

- Anticonvulsants have been used in pain management since the 1960s, very soon after they were first used for treatment of epilepsy.
- Anticonvulsants are effective in the treatment of neuropathic and mixed pain conditions.
- Dizziness and somnolence are the most common side effects reported with use of anticonvulsant medications in the treatment of pain.
- Titrate the dose of these medications to effect and tolerability. Gradual titration may improve treatment adherence by minimizing initial adverse effects.

Introduction

Neuropathic pain arises from dysfunction or a lesion in the central or peripheral nervous system or both. Following nerve injury, alteration in the expression, distribution, and voltage dependence of ion channels leads to enhanced excitability and ectopic firing that in turn leads to increased perception of pain. Anticonvulsant medications with unique channel blocking and membrane-stabilizing properties have been used in neuropathic and mixed pain since the 1960s.

Anticonvulsants have demonstrated efficacy for several chronic pain conditions including painful diabetic neuropathy, postherpetic neuralgia, trigeminal neuralgia, phantom limb pain, postoperative or traumatic neuropathic pain, complex regional pain syndrome, cancer-related neuropathy, HIV neuropathy, spinal cord injury, multiple sclerosis, and fibromyalgia.

Mechanism of Action

Anticonvulsant medications inhibit transmission of electrical signals within the nervous system. This can occur via many mechanisms, at unique points within signal transmission, with the overall effect of preventing neuronal membrane depolarization. This effect is one reason why the term anticonvulsants has now fell off in favor of the term "membrane stabilizers" and explains why the use of antiseizure medication is useful in the treatment of neuropathic pain.

Gabapentin and pregabalin bind to the alpha 2-delta subunit of voltage-gated calcium channels in the dorsal horn, reducing opening of these channels. Subsequently calcium influx and thus depolarization is reduced leading to an inhibition of the ascending pain signal. Anticonvulsants like carbamazepine and topiramate predominantly exert their action via blockade of voltage-gated sodium channels. Other drugs such as valproic acid have additional actions via GABA and glutamate pathways (Table 22.1).

Scientific Evidence

The Neuropathic Pain Special Interest Group (NeuPSIG) of the International Association for the Study of Pain has recommended gabapentin or pregabalin as one of the three first-line medications for treatment of neuropathic pain other than trigeminal neuralgia. Pregabalin in doses of 300–600 mg daily has been found effective in patients with postherpetic neuralgia, painful diabetic neuropathy, central neuropathic pain, or fibromyalgia. Gabapentin in doses greater than 1200 mg daily was associated with moderate or substantial benefit in 43% or 31% of patients, respectively, in a Cochrane overview (Table 22.2).

R.P. Grandhe, MBBS, MD
Cleveland Clinic, Department of Pain Management, Cleveland, OH, USA

G.C. Chang Chien, DO (✉)
Cleveland Clinic, Anesthesia Institute Pain Management, 9500 Euclid Ave, Dept C-25, Cleveland, OH 44195, USA
e-mail: gchangchien@gmail.com

J.E. Pope, T.R. Deer (eds.), *Treatment of Chronic Pain Conditions*, DOI 10.1007/978-1-4939-6976-0_22

Table 22.1 Mechanism of action for common membrane stabilizers

Drug	Na channel blockade	Ca channel blockade	Glutamate mechanism	GABA mechanism
Gabapentin pregabalin		Binds voltage-gated or L type		
Topiramate	Yes		Inhibits AMPA- type glutamate receptor	Potentiates GABA inhibition
Carbamazepine Oxcarbazepine	Yes			
Lamotrigine	Stabilizes slow Na+ channel		Prevents release of glutamate	
Valproic acid	Yes			Acts on GABA A receptor
Phenytoin	Yes			

Table 22.2 Common membrane stabilizer medications

Drug	Dose titration	Common side effects	Clinical tips
Gabapentin	Start at 300 mg (100 mg in elderly) increase over 2–4 weeks to a dose of 1200–3600 mg/day as tolerated	CNS depression including somnolence and dizziness, edema, and gait disturbances	Dose reduction in renal impairment
Pregabalin	Start at 100 mg (75 mg in elderly) increase over 2–4 weeks to 300–600 mg/day	Peripheral edema, dizziness, somnolence, ataxia, headache, fatigue, weight gain, xerostomia, blurred vision, diplopia	Dose reduction in renal impairment Possible angioedema in some patients
Carbamazepine	Start at 100–200 mg BID increase by 200 mg/week to a max dose of 1200 mg a day	Drowsiness, dizziness, nausea, vomiting Leukopenia and agranulocytosis	Monitor Na+ levels and CBC Dose reduction in hepatic impairment Possible Stevens- Johnson syndrome and TEN in patients of Asian descent
Oxcarbazepine	1200–1800 mg/day	Similar to carbamazepine except for lower risk of agranulocytosis and leukopenia. Risk of hyponatremia	Monitor Na+ levels
Topiramate	Start with 50 mg/ day and titrate to 200–400 mg/day	Sedation, cognitive impairment. Risk for kidney stones, glaucoma, and weight loss	
Lamotrigine	Start at 25–50 mg and titrate over 4–6 weeks to 300–500 mg/day	Sedation, rash	Has been used in HIV-associated neuropathy
Valproic acid	800 mg/day	Somnolence, dizziness, gastrointestinal upset	May be effective for migraine headaches
Phenytoin	200–300 mg/day	Dizziness, sedation, ataxia, bleeding gums, anemia	Potential for drug interactions due to enzyme induction

A growing volume of evidence suggests moderate-to-large reduction in the development of chronic postsurgical pain (CPSP) with gabapentin and a very large reduction in the development of CPSP with pregabalin. Carbamazepine has been demonstrated in crossover, placebo-controlled, double-blind studies to be an effective medication in the treatment of trigeminal neuralgia with a low number needed to treat of less than 2.

Conclusion

Anticonvulsants (membrane stabilizers) are an important tool in the armamentarium of a pain physician. Common side effects of anticonvulsant medications include dizziness and somnolence. The pain physician should be apprised of how to monitor and treat the unique and potentially fatal adverse effects associated with medications such as lamotrigine, oxcarbazepine, and carbamazepine. Anticonvulsant medications require gradual upward titration of dosage until clinical effects are perceived or side effects are intolerable or the maximum dose is reached.

Suggested Reading

1. Andrew Moore R, Wiffen PJ, Derry S, McQuay HJ. Gabapentin for chronic neuropathic pain and fibromyalgia in adults. Cochrane Database Syst Rev. 2011;3:CD007938.
2. Benzon HT. Essentials of pain medicine. 3rd ed. 2011. Ch 16, p. 123–29.
3. Dworkin RH, O'Connor AB, et al. Recommendations for the pharmacological management of neuropathic pain: an overview and literature update. Mayo Clin Proc. 2010;85(3 Suppl):S3–14.

Antidepressants

23

Alexander Bautista and George C. Chang Chien

Key Concepts

- Antidepressants have shown proven efficacy in the treatment of chronic pain syndromes and neuropathic pain.
- The analgesic effect of antidepressants is of a much lower dose in comparison to the dose used to treat depression.
- It has a diverse range of pharmacologic actions but primarily inhibition of serotonin, norepinephrine, and epinephrine reuptake.
- Newer antidepressants have increased receptor specificity resulting in analgesia with minimal side effect profile.
- Weight gain and cholinergic symptoms are the usual adverse effects reported by patients.
- Dosing of antidepressants should always start at a lower dose and slowly titrated until adequate pain relief is achieved or side effects limit dose escalation.

Background

The management of chronic pain is complex and requires multimodal approach as well as "polypharmacy" to provide pain relief, to increase functionality, and to improve quality of life. Also, the concept between the causal relationship between chronic pain state and depression exists, and patients would manifest features of both.

Antidepressants have shown efficacy in the treatment of many chronic pain syndromes and regarded as one of the first-line treatment in neuropathic pain. Data supports its effectiveness in patients experiencing brief, lancinating pain and constant burning pain. Its analgesic effect is independent of the presence of depression or mood improvement, which is usually achieved at lower doses.

Pharmacologic Mechanism

The analgesic effect of antidepressants is primarily due to the inhibition of reuptake of serotonin, epinephrine, and norepinephrine. The presence of a higher level of these neurotransmitters modulates the activation of the descending inhibitory pathway in the pain pathway (pain mechanisms chapter). Its diverse range of antinociceptive action includes monoamine modulation, inhibition of ion channel activity (i.e., sodium and calcium), N-methyl-D-aspartate (NMDA), histamine, and cholinergic receptors. It has also shown interaction with opioid receptors and stimulation of endogenous opioid release.

Clinical Application

Classification of antidepressants is typically based on their specificity on the neurotransmitter reuptake (Table 23.1).

The potential efficacy of each drug in terms of providing analgesia has been inconsistent in comparative studies. However, a significant body of evidence suggests its use in neuropathic pain conditions such as postherpetic neuralgia, painful diabetic neuropathy, painful mononeuropathy and polyneuropathy, spinal cord injury, fibromyalgia, osteoarthritis, low back pain, cancer-related neuropathic pain, and *Human immunodeficiency virus* sensory neuropathy.

Tricyclic Antidepressants (TCA)

- TCAs have been shown to be efficacious in the treatment of neuropathic pain and headache syndromes.
- TCAs also have anti-inflammatory effect by inhibiting prostaglandin and substance P as shown in animal studies.

A. Bautista, MD
Cleveland Clinic, Anesthesia Institute Pain Management, Cleveland, OH, USA

G.C. Chang Chien, DO (✉)
Cleveland Clinic, Anesthesia Institute Pain Management, 9500 Euclid Ave, Dept C-25, Cleveland, OH 44195, USA
e-mail: gchangchien@gmail.com

J.E. Pope, T.R. Deer (eds.), *Treatment of Chronic Pain Conditions*, DOI 10.1007/978-1-4939-6976-0_23

Table 23.1 Common antidepressant and neuropathic pain medications

Class of antidepressants	Antidepressant	5-HT	NE	DA	H	Anticholinergic side effects
Tricyclic antidepressants (TCA)	Amitriptyline	++	+	++++	+	+
	Clomipramine	+++++	+	++	++	+
	Desipramine	+++++	+	++++	+++	++
	Imipramine	+++++	+	++	+	+
	Nortriptyline	++	+	++++	+	+
Selective serotonin reuptake inhibitors (SSRIs)	Citalopram	+++++	++++	?	+	+++
	Fluoxetine	++++	+++	++++	++++	++++
	Fluvoxamine	+++++	+++++	+++++	+++++	+++++
	Paroxetine	+++++	++	+++++	+++++	++
	Sertraline	+++++	+++	+++++	+++++	++
Selective norepinephrine reuptake inhibitors (SNRIs)	Duloxetine	+++	+	+++++	+++	+++
	Milnacipran	?	++	?	?	?
	Nefazodone	++	+++	++	+++++	+++++
	Venlafaxine	+++++	++++	+++++	+++++	+++++
Monoamine oxidase inhibitors	Isocarboxazid Selegiline Tranylcypromine					
Dopamine reuptake inhibitors	Bupropion	++++	++++	+++++	+++++	+++++
Tetracyclic antidepressants	Mirtazapine	+	++++	++++	+	++
Selective serotonin reuptake enhancer	Tianeptine	+	–	++	?	+

5HT serotonin, *NE* norepinephrine, *DA* dopamine, *H* histamine

- Added benefit of TCAs besides elevation of mood includes normalization of sleep pattern and muscle relaxation.
- These are generally prescribed due to its affordability in comparison with other antidepressants.
- There are no clear guidelines that support optimum dosage to achieve pain relief; however, some data suggest that higher dosage may potentially provide additional pain relief.
- Secondary amine TCAs such as nortriptyline and desipramine have better side effect profiles and less toxicity than tertiary amine TCA drugs.

Selective Serotonin Reuptake Inhibitors (SSRI)

- Clinical trials have demonstrated variability and inconsistencies for the treatment of chronic pain syndrome.
- Reduction of pain was seen in patients with peripheral diabetic neuropathy, fibromyalgia, and headache.

Serotonin-Norepinephrine Reuptake Inhibitors (SNRI)

- The degree of serotonin selectivity across the specific drugs on this class varies with venlafaxine having the 30-fold selectivity for 5-hydroxytryptamine (5-HT)/serotonin receptors.
- Duloxetine is the first prototype drug that has been approved by the FDA for the treatment of painful diabetic neuropathy.

Tetracyclic Antidepressants

- Studies have shown limited analgesic property exists with its use and showed inferior analgesia when compared to other antidepressants.
- May consider its use if patients are not tolerant to other agents.

Monoamine Oxidase Inhibitors

- There is limited evidence that its analgesic effect exists for chronic pain condition.
- Its use is limited due to multiple side effects and drug-to-drug interaction.

Dopamine Reuptake Inhibitors

- Its prototype bupropion also has noradrenergic activity, but the evidence of analgesic effect is limited.

Side Effects

The use of antidepressants has its potential dangers for abuse and overdose. Careful considerations should always be given to patients who show signs of overt depression and suicidal tendencies. It is advocated to start on a lower dose with slow titration to achieve maximum pain relief and/or side effects are not tolerated.

- Weight gain is the most common complaint of patients taking antidepressants. The mood alteration effect may have an effect on appetite and general well-being.
- Anticholinergic-type side effects are the usual complaints of patients that include dry mouth; sedation and urinary retention may limit its use.
- Its use in pregnancy is not advocated due to the risk of fetal malformation.
- Cardiac toxicity has been reported in patients taking TCA, manifested as, but not limited to, myocardial infarction, sinus tachycardia, and increased ventricular ectopy. Some authors suggest screening EKG in patients over the age of 40 and starting a new TCA.

Conclusion

Antidepressants can be used to treat chronic pain states especially if there is a component of depression. It is also vital to know that its use may be associated with untoward side effects inherent to the drug.

Suggested Reading

1. Benzon HT. Raj's practical management of pain. 4th ed. Mosby 2008: Mosby; 2002. p. 643–57. ISBN: 9780323041843.
2. Dwrokin RH, O'Connor AB, et al. Pharmacologic management of neuropathic pain: evidence-based recommendations. Pain. 2007;132: 237–51.
3. Leon AC, Fiedorowicz JG, et al. Risk of suicidal behavior with antidepressants in bipolar and unipolar disorders. J Clin Psychiatry. 2014;75(7):720–7.

Antispasmodics

24

Andrew M. Hall

Key Concepts

- Skeletal muscle relaxants are thought to help break the acute "pain-spasm-pain" cycle by either depressing central or spinal reflexes (antispasmodics) or reducing skeletal muscle hypertonicity and involuntary contractions (antispasticity agents).
- Muscle relaxants may also exert their effect by causing general CNS depression.
- Acetaminophen and NSAIDs are considered first-line therapies for nonspecific low back pain. There is no indication for muscle relaxants in chronic low back pain.
- Due to their sedating nature, as well as potential for misuse, abuse, and concomitant use of alcohol, opioids, benzodiazepines, or other sedatives, use extreme caution when prescribing.

Introduction

Antispasmodics and antispasticity agents, often called "skeletal muscle relaxants," are often used to treat low back pain and generalized muscle spasms. They are frequently used in the setting of acute musculoskeletal, soft tissue, or ligamentous injury or strain. The exact cause of muscle spasms is controversial. A commonly accepted theory is that they are thought to be part of a "pain-spasm-pain" cycle in which (1) part of the body is injured, (2) muscle contracts or "spasms" involuntarily to protect the area from injury, (3) muscle contracture contributes to local tissue ischemia, (4) ischemia causes release of additional nociceptive chemical mediators, and (5) the cycle continues.

A.M. Hall, MD (✉)
Department of Anesthesiology and Perioperative Care, Division of Pain Medicine, University of California, San Francisco, CA, USA
e-mail: andrew.hall@ucsf.edu

Background

Antispasmodics (carisoprodol, chlorzoxazone, cyclobenzaprine, metaxalone, methocarbamol, and orphenadrine) are FDA-approved for relief of acute (1–3 weeks) musculoskeletal discomfort. Although frequently prescribed long-term, none are indicated in the treatment of chronic back pain. Definitive mechanisms of action of antispasmodics are less understood. These agents are thought to primarily act by inhibiting spinal interneurons, depressing polysynaptic reflexes within the dorsal horn of the spinal cord and the descending reticular formation in the brain. It is unclear, however, whether antispasmodics may exert their effect via sedation, as other sedatives also decrease these polysynaptic reflexes. Benzodiazepines (i.e., diazepam) are sedatives commonly used as skeletal muscle relaxants. Benzodiazepines act on postsynaptic γ-aminobutyric acid ($GABA_A$) neuronal receptors to decrease neuronal nociceptive transmission. These decreases in spinal reflexes from benzodiazepines and nonbenzodiazepine antispasmodics are thought to indirectly relax skeletal muscle.

Antispasticity agents work at the level of the spinal cord or skeletal muscle to reduce skeletal muscle hypertonicity and involuntary contractions. Oral baclofen and possibly tizanidine are antispasticity agents and are FDA-approved for muscle spasticity due to upper motor neuron conditions, i.e., multiple sclerosis and spinal cord lesions. Baclofen is a $GABA_B$ agonist, whereas tizanidine is a central α_2 agonist similar to clonidine. Tizanidine is thought to have antispasmodic properties as well. Although antispasmodics and antispasticity agents are not technically interchangeable, clinicians often use the antispasticity agents to treat muscle spasm.

Application

For initial treatment of nonspecific low back pain, acetaminophen and nonsteroidal anti-inflammatory drugs (NSAIDs) are relatively safe and thus recommended as

J.E. Pope, T.R. Deer (eds.), *Treatment of Chronic Pain Conditions*, DOI 10.1007/978-1-4939-6976-0_24

first-line therapy by the American Pain Society and American College of Physicians based on their 2007 guidelines. Comparatively, there are no quality data that support the use of skeletal muscle relaxants over NSAIDs. However, muscle relaxants may be an acceptable alternative in patients with contraindication to NSAID use or when NSAID therapy has failed. There is no clear evidence that one muscle relaxant agent is more effective than others for treatment of muscle spasm and low back pain. Understanding the differences among the muscle relaxant classes in terms of use, mechanism of action, and side effects will aid in tailoring therapy to patient needs.

Prolonged use of benzodiazepines and carisoprodol may result in physical and psychological dependence and thus should not be used as first-line agents. Caution should be used when prescribing any muscle relaxant/antispasmodic agent given its sedative effects and potential for abuse or misuse, especially concomitant use with alcohol, opioids, benzodiazepines, or other sedative.

Specific Drugs (Table 24.1)

Antispasmodics: metaxalone, methocarbamol, orphenadrine, chlorzoxazone, carisoprodol, cyclobenzaprine

Antispasticity agents: baclofen, dantrolene (not discussed here)

Both: tizanidine, benzodiazepines (diazepam)

Table 24.1 Antispasticity agents and antispasmodics

Drug and class	Onset	Duration (h)	Mechanism of action	Side effects	Important considerations[a]
Sedatives/CNS depressants					
Carisoprodol (Soma)	30 min	4–6	Decreased communication at reticular formation and spinal cord	Dizziness, drowsiness, HA, N/V, seizures, withdrawal	Converts to meprobamate in liver; may result in physical or psychological dependence and abuse; reduce dose in hepatic disease and elderly
Chlorzoxazone (Paraflex)	30–60 min	4–6	Inhibits multisynaptic reflex arc spinal cord and subcortical levels	Dizziness, drowsiness, HA, N/V	Rare idiosyncratic hepatocellular toxicity
Cyclobenzaprine (Flexeril)	60 min	12–24	Acts at brain stem to reduce tonic somatic motor activity, some 5-HT_2 antagonism	Blurry vision, dizziness, drowsiness, dry mouth, prolonged QTc, urinary retention	Structurally related to TCAs; reduce dose in hepatic disease and elderly; caution use with SSRIs; seizures with tramadol and MAOIs
Metaxalone (Skelaxin)	60 min	4–6	General CNS depressant	Dizziness, drowsiness, HA, N/V	Contraindicated in severe hepatic/renal disease
Methocarbamol (Robaxin)	30 min	4–6	General CNS depressant	Diplopia, dizziness, drowsiness, light-headedness	Less sedating than others in similar class; almost 100% excreted in urine
Orphenadrine (Norflex)	60 min	4–6	Analgesic and euphoric properties; central atropine-like effects	Anxiety, dizziness, light-headedness, palpitations, syncope	Anticholinergic; caution use in cardiac arrhythmias, elderly, heart failure; taper in chronic use
GABA agonists					
Baclofen (PO) (Lioresal)	3 days	Variable	Presynaptic $GABA_B$ agonist; decreases transmission at spinal cord	Drowsiness, HA, hypotension, N/V, withdrawal, urinary retention	Reduce dose in renal disease; gradually reduce dose over several weeks upon discontinuation
Diazepam (PO) (Valium)	30 min	Variable	Presynaptic $GABA_A$ agonist; decrease transmission at spinal and supraspinal sites	Fatigue, hypotension, psychiatric reactions, sedation	Controlled substance; minimize use for low back pain; avoid use in elderly
Central α2 agonists					
Tizanidine (Zanaflex)	2 weeks	Variable	Central 2 agonist; increases presynaptic inhibition of motor neurons	Dizziness, drowsiness, dry mouth, hypotension, prolonged QTc	Reduce dose in hepatic/renal disease; taper in chronic use

CNS central nervous system, *HA* headache, *GABA* gamma-aminobutyric acid, *SSRIs* selective serotonin reuptake inhibitors, *MAOIs* monoamine oxidase inhibitors, *N/V* nausea and vomiting, *TCA* tricyclic antidepressant

[a]All sedatives may have additive effects when combined with alcohol or other CNS depressants

Suggested Reading

1. Baclofen Tablet package insert. Sellersville: Teva Pharmaceuticals USA; 2010 Jun.
2. Chlorzoxazone package insert. Sayreville: Vertical Pharmaceutical; 2010 Oct.
3. Chou R, Qaseem A, Snow V, et al. Diagnosis and treatment of low back pain: a joint clinical practice guideline from the American College of Physicians and the American Pain Society. Ann Intern Med. 2007;147(7):478–91.
4. Jackson K, Argoff C, Dubin A. Skeletal muscle relaxants. In: Practical management of pain. 5th ed. Philadelphia: Elsevier; 2014. p. 569–73.
5. Metaxalone package insert. Bristol: King Pharmaceuticals, Inc.; 2008 Apr.
6. Methocarbamol package insert. Philadelphia: Lennett Co., Inc.; 2007 Jan.
7. Orphenadrine citrate package insert. Schaumburg: Sagent Pharmaceuticals; 2009 Dec.
8. Soma (carisoprodol) package insert Charlotte. North Carolina: Vintage Pharmaceuticals, Inc.; 2006 June.
9. Valium (diazepam) package insert Nutley. New Jersey: Roche Laboratories Inc.; 2008 Jan.
10. Witenko C, et al. Considerations for the appropriate use of skeletal muscle relaxants for the management of acute low back pain. Pharmacy & Therapeutics. 2014;39(6):427–35.
11. Zanaflex tablets (tizanidine hydrochloride) package insert. Hawthorne: Acorda Therapeutics Inc.; 2006 July.

Steroids

25

Christine El-Yahchouchi and Salim Hayek

Key Concepts

- Several steroid formulations available for parenteral administration are used off-label in epidural injections.
- Catastrophic complications have been reported following epidural steroid injection with particulate steroid suspensions.
- It is now recommended that non-particulate steroid solutions be used as the initial therapeutic agent for all transforaminal epidural steroid injections.
- Only non-particulate steroid solutions (e.g., dexamethasone) are recommended for use in cervical transforaminal epidural injections.

Introduction

Epidural steroid injections have gained popularity due to their minimally invasive nature, evidence of clinical effectiveness for radicular pain, and ease of reproducibility. It is usually performed for patients with radicular symptoms on the hypothesis that radicular pain is caused by leakage of inflammatory mediators from the herniated nucleus pulposus. Glucocorticoids have anti-inflammatory effects, limiting the formation of arachidonic acid by inhibiting phospholipase A2 and ultimately the formation of prostaglandins and other eicosanoids involved in the inflammatory mechanism. Multiple steroid formulations are available for parenteral administration, and although these medications have been used in the epidural space, these are considered off-label applications.

C. El-Yahchouchi, MD (✉) • S. Hayek, MD
Division of Pain Medicine, Department of Anesthesiology,
University Hospitals Case Medical Center,
11100 Euclid Avenue, Cleveland, OH 44106, USA
e-mail: Christine.ElYahchouchi@UHhospitals.org;
christine_el_yahchouchi@hotmail.com

Indications

Epidural steroid injections are best studied in patients with radicular pain due to lumbar disc herniations and have demonstrable evidence of efficacy, clinical effectiveness, and safety. It is less studied in patients with radicular symptoms due to foraminal stenosis or neurogenic claudication from central spinal canal stenosis. Epidural injection of steroids in patients with axial back pain lacks evidence of efficacy or effectiveness.

Background

There are several steroids preparations available in approximate equipotent solutions (Table 25.1). Triamcinolone, methylprednisolone, betamethasone, and dexamethasone were commonly used for epidural injections. Triamcinolone now has a label warning against epidural use.

Historically the corticosteroids used were particulate steroid suspensions. Unfortunately catastrophic complications have been reported following transforaminal epidural injections; all occurred with particulate steroids. The proposed mechanism is embolization of a medullary artery (supplying the anterior spinal artery) known as artery of Adamkiewicz. Dexamethasone, a solution, contains no particles larger than red blood cells and cannot act as an embolic agent. Although its efficacy was questioned in small trials with short-term follow-up, recent large retrospective and randomized comparative effectiveness trials have shown outcomes to be indistinguishable from steroid suspensions. It is now recommended as the initial therapeutic agent for all transforaminal epidural steroid injections in order to prevent serious neurological complications.

Steroid preparations may also vary by added preservatives, some of which may be neurotoxic. When available, a preservative-free preparation is desirable.

J.E. Pope, T.R. Deer (eds.), *Treatment of Chronic Pain Conditions*, DOI 10.1007/978-1-4939-6976-0_25

Table 25.1 Steroid preparations

		Methylprednisolone	Triamcinolone	Dexamethasone	Betamethasone
Equivalent dose (mg)		4	4	0.75	0.6
Max particle size (microns)		>500	>500	0.5	500
Concentration		Densely packed	Densely packed	Few particles	Densely packed
Aggregation		Extensive	Extensive	None	Some
Size		Densely packed	12* RBC	<RBC	12* RBC
GC potency		5	5	27	33
Half-life (hrs)		18–36	18–36	36–54	36–54
Preservatives	Benzyl alcohol	Yes	Yes	No	No
	Methylparaben	No	No	Yes	No
	Sodium bisulfite	No	No	Yes	No

Adapted from Derby et al. [2] and Benzon et al. [1] *Practical management of pain*, 5th edn, chapter 44

Suggested Reading

1. Benzon HT, Chew T-L, McCarthy RJ, Benzon HA, Walega DR. Comparison of the particle sizes of different steroids and the effect of dilution. A review of the relative neurotoxicities of the steroids. Anesthesiology. 2007;106:331–8.
2. Derby R, Lee S-H, Date ES, Lee J-H, Lee C-H. Size and aggregation of corticosteroids used for epidural injections. Pain Med. 2008;9(2):227–34.
3. El-Yahchouchi C, Geske JR, Carter RE, Diehn FE, Wald JT, Murthy NS, Kaufmann TJ, Thielen KR, Morris JM, Amrami KK, Maus TP. The noninferiority of the nonparticulate steroid dexamethasone vs the particulate steroids betamethasone and triamcinolone in lumbar transforaminal epidural steroid injections. Pain Med. 2013;14(11):1650–7.
4. El-Yahchouchi CA, Plastaras CT, Maus TP, Carr CM, McCormick ZL, Geske JR, Smuck M, Pingree MJ, Kennedy DJ. Adverse event rates associated with transforaminal and interlaminar epidural steroid injections: a multi-institutional study. Pain Med. 2015; epub PMID: 26593277.
5. Kennedy DJ, Plastaras C, Casey E, Visco CJ, Rittenberg JD, Conrad B, Sigler J, Dreyfuss P. Comparative effectiveness of lumbar transforaminal epidural steroid injections with particulate versus nonparticulate corticosteroids for lumbar radicular pain due to intervertebral disc herniation: a prospective, randomized, double-blind trial. Pain Med. 2014;15(4):548–55.
6. MacMahon PJ, Eustace SJ, Kavanagh EC. Injectable corticosteroids and local anesthetic preparations: a review for radiologists. Radiiology. 2009;252:647–61.
7. Rathmell JP, Benzon HT, Dreyfuss P, Huntoon M, Wallace M, Baker R, Daniel Riew K, Rosenquist RW, Aprill C, Rost NS, Buvanendran A, Scott Kreiner D, Bogduk N, Fourney DR, Fraifeld E, Horn S, Stone J, Vorenkamp K, Lawler G, Summers J, Kloth D, O'Brien Jr D, Tutton S. Safeguards to prevent neurologic complications after epidural steroid injections: consensus opinions from a multidisciplinary working group and national organizations. Anesthesiology. 2015;122:974–84.

Part VII

Conservative Treatment: VII. Interventional Conservative Care

Radiologic Safety in Interventional Spine and Pain Medicine

26

W. Porter McRoberts

Key Concepts

- Use of X-ray fluoroscopy remains essential for the safe completion of many pain procedures.
- Fluoroscopy yields cumulative, dose-related morbidity to patients, staff and physician.
- The physician is responsible for everyone's exposure, and staff training is essential to reduce exposure and increase expediency.

Introduction

It's ironic that such a life improving modality can also yield such morbidity. Until other modalities supersede fluoroscopy, it will remain the primary tool for pain procedure imaging. The physician, being closest to the fluoroscopy unit, is most susceptible to cumulative effects of X-ray dose because of the multipliable effects of proximity and procedure number. Hopefully, most absorption will be through cumulative scatter radiation and not direct exposure. Understanding several basic radiation principles *and then reviewing with your OR staff* will yield enormous benefit. Lastly, by reducing exposure to the patient, the physician and staff will also benefit from exposure diminution.

Background

Fluoroscopy's origins began with X-ray when Wilhelm Conrad Röntgen discovered the previously unknown radiation "X" in 1895. The first fluoroscopes were simply cardboard funnel darkened to see the fluorescence from an activated barium salt. At first X-ray was thought to be beneficial to the body, but soon first experimenters correlated skin burns and radiation exposure. Initially there was little reason to suspect the association between exposure and morbidity; however, the first warning of negative effects came from Thomas Edison, Nikola Tesla and others who reported eye irritations. Now fluoroscopy is used routinely in medical imaging.

Dose-Limiting Strategies (Distance, Time, Barriers)

Use good technique.
Increase the distance between patient (and physician) and X-ray source.
Lower the image intensifier as much as possible.
When taking lateral projections, move away from the X-ray source as much as possible.
Collimate always, especially with digital magnification. Learn to function with tight collimation.
Limit digital magnification (use leaded, prescription eye lenses to maximize visual acuity).
Stand away when high-dose situations occur.
Limit fluoroscopy usage.
Limit use of live fluoro, and if possible use pulse mode.
Anticipate needle motion thus minimizing multiple steps of confirmatory fluoro. Use when needle is close to sensitive tissues.
Use low-dose settings as a default; train staff to do so.
Use digital subtraction when indicated and tubing to distance the operator from the beam.
Use barriers.
Lead gloves work when outside the beam, and it should be obvious, but keep hands out of beam.
Wear well-fitted lead that's comfortable. The more coverage, the better.
Use 360-lead protection when the back may be exposed to the c-arm.
Use lead glasses always.
Long-term strategies.

W. Porter McRoberts, MD (✉)
Interventional Spine, Pain and Neurosurgery, Holy Cross Hospital, 3111 NE 44th St., Fort Lauderdale, FL 33308, USA
e-mail: portermcroberts@gmail.com

J.E. Pope, T.R. Deer (eds.), *Treatment of Chronic Pain Conditions*, DOI 10.1007/978-1-4939-6976-0_26

Meet with your staff and continually train on techniques to reduce.

Educate staff on position of c-arm prior to first exposure so as to increase likelihood that first fluoro shot has medical relevance other than to serve as a reference for improved targeting. Target in the mind first and then with the fluoro.

Have machine inspected regularly by medical physicist, and incorporate education for physician and staff with physicist.

Consistently wear and monitor dosimetry badges and rings. Routinely monitor and correlate strategies for dose reduction with actual reduction.

Suggested Reading

1. European Commission (radiologic protection). www.europa.eu.int/comm./environment/radprot
2. http://www.unscear.org" www.unscear.org
3. International Atomic Energy Agency. http://www.iaea.org" www.iaea.org
4. National Commission on Radiological Protection. http://www.icrp.org
5. NDT. Nondestructive testing. https://www.ndeed.org/EducationResources/CommunityCollege/Radiography/Introduction/history.htm. Accessed 24 Apr 2015.
6. Peters P. Textbook of Radiology. In: W.C. Roentgen and the discovery of x-rays. 1995. http://www.medcyclopaedia.com/library/radiology/chapter01.aspx
7. World Health Organization. http://www.who.int

Trigger Point Injections

27

Nomen Azeem

Key Points

- A trigger point is a hyperirritable spot in the muscle associated with a hypersensitive palpable nodule in a taut band which is painful on compression.
- Myofascial trigger points are a component of a larger disorder known as myofascial pain syndrome (MPS).
- Physical and emotional stress is thought to increase susceptibility to trigger points due to fatigue of the muscles.
- Diagnosis of myofascial pain syndrome is done by history and clinical exam.
- Conservative treatment options include spray and stretch, physical therapy, and massage.
- Invasive treatment options include dry needling, trigger point injection, and botulinum toxin.

Introduction

Approximately 23 million Americans have chronic disorders of the musculoskeletal system. According to Travell and Simons, a myofascial trigger point is classically defined as a hyperirritable spot in the skeletal muscle that is associated with a hypersensitive palpable nodule in a taut band which is painful on compression and can give rise to characteristic referred pain, motor dysfunction, and autonomic phenomena. Myofascial trigger points are thought to be a component of a larger disorder known as myofascial pain syndrome (MPS). MPS is defined as sensory, motor, and autonomic symptoms that are caused by myofascial trigger points. MPS is a major progenitor of nonarticular local musculoskeletal pain and tenderness that affects every age group and is commonly recognized as "muscle knots." MPS is not to be confused with fibromyalgia syndrome, which is ascribed to a collection of complaints including chronic widespread pain, accompanied by tactile allodynia, fatigue, sleep disturbance, and psychological distress.

There are many causes of trigger points theorized. However commonly accepted causes include an initial insult to the muscle fibers either due to an acute trauma or repetitive microtrauma. Physical and emotional stress is also thought to increase susceptibility to the development of trigger points due to fatigue of the muscles or muscle groups. A local twitch response is a characteristic response of myofascial trigger points elicited by palpation or needle insertion. The origin of LTR may be due to altered sensory spinal processing resulting from sensitized peripheral mechanical receptors. According to Simons et al., the site of an LTR is a "sensitive locus," and the site where there is spontaneous electrical activity is the "active locus". It is hypothesized that a myofascial trigger point locus is formed when a sensitive locus, a nociceptor, and an active locus – the motor end plate – coincide. According to Shah et al., trigger points can be categorized into "active," which elicit pain locally and referred pain without palpation and "latent" which only cause pain when palpated. Further it was determined that there is a release of biochemicals associated with pain, inflammation, and intercellular signaling which are elevated in the vicinity of "active" trigger points.

Diagnosis of myofascial pain syndrome is mainly done by history and clinical exam, specifically the painful palpation of trigger points and identification of LTRs. Travell and Simons identified eight clinical characteristics for the diagnosis of myofascial pain syndrome (Table 27.1).

There are various conservative treatment options for trigger points which include spray and stretch, physical therapy, and massage. Simons and Travell advocated passive stretching after applying vapocoolant spray over trigger point. Physical therapy programs can be contoured to include stretching, correction of improper biomechanics and posture, and modalities such as TENS unit, ultrasound, and cryotherapy. Massage techniques such as deep

N. Azeem, MD (✉)
Sarasota Orthopedic Associates,
2750 Bahia Vista St, Ste. 100, Sarasota, FL 34239, USA
e-mail: nazeem@soa.md; azeemnx@gmail.com

J.E. Pope, T.R. Deer (eds.), *Treatment of Chronic Pain Conditions*, DOI 10.1007/978-1-4939-6976-0_27

Table 27.1 Diagnosis of myofascial pain syndrome

1. Onset description and immediate cause of pain
2. Pain distribution pattern
3. Resisted ROM and increased sensitivity to stretching
4. Weakened muscle due to pain with no atrophy
5. Compression causing pain similar to patient's chief complaint
6. Palpable taut band within muscle correlating with patient's trigger point
7. LTR elicited by snapping palpation or rapid insertion of a needle
8. Reproduction of referred pain with mechanical stimulation of trigger point

stroking, stripping, and myofascial release can be utilized to improve trigger points.

Invasive treatment options for trigger points include dry needling, trigger point injection, and botulinum toxin. Dry needling is the rapid repeated insertion of a small needle directly into the trigger point. Trigger point injections utilize a similar technique to dry needling but commonly use a local anesthetic for patient comfort. Although steroids have been used for trigger point injections, there is currently no evidence to support its use, and it carries the risk of local myotoxicity, subcutaneous tissue damage, and discoloration of the skin. Botulinum toxin blocks muscle contraction by preventing acetylcholine release presynaptically, which denervates the muscle. Botulinum toxin does not discriminate between a trigger point and surrounding tissue which could lead to complications.

With the increasing incidence of myofascial pain syndrome, a comprehensive approach must be employed to effectively improve pain symptoms with specific focus on the management of trigger points. Further large scale randomized double blind clinical trials may help to establish guidelines for the efficacious treatment of trigger points both independently and within the context of myofascial pain syndrome.

Suggested Reading

1. Immamura ST, Fischer AA, Imamura M. Pain management using myofascial approach when other treatment failed. Phys Med Rehabil Clin N Am. 1997;8(1):179–96.
2. Kao MJ, Han TI, Kuan TS, Hsieh YL, Su BH, Hong CZ. Myofascial trigger points in early life. Arch Phys Med Rehabil. 2007;88(2):251–4.
3. Lavelle ED, Lavelle W, Smith H. Myofascial trigger points. Anesthesiol Clin. 2007;25:841–51.
4. Mense S, Simons DG. Muscle pain: understanding its nature, diagnosis, and treatment. Lippincott: Williams and Wilkins; 2001.
5. Shah JP, Gilliams EA. Uncovering the biochemical milieu of myofascial trigger points using in vivo microdialysis: An application of muscle pain concepts to myofascial pain syndrome. J Bodyw Mov Ther. 2008;12:371–84.
6. Simons D. Single-muscle myofascial pain syndromes. Handbook of pain management. 2nd ed. Lippincott: Williams & Wilkins; 1994. p. 539–55.
7. Travell JG, Simons DG. Myofascial pain and dysfunction: the trigger point manual. Lippincott: Williams and Wilkins; 1993.

Knee Injection

28

Alexander Bautista, George C. Chang Chien, Julie Ann Zitterkopf Larson, and Mayank Gupta

Key Concepts

- Knee pain as manifestation of osteoarthritis is the most common indication for intra-articular knee injection.
- The diagnosis of knee pain is based on history, physical examination, and imaging modalities.
- The approaches to access the retropatellar space include anterolateral, anteromedial, superolateral, and superomedial approach.
- The most common medication used for knee injection is corticosteroids, but agents such as hyaluronic acid, botulinum neurotoxin, and platelet-rich plasma (PRP) have been described.
- The use of ultrasound and fluoroscopy guidance may help improve accuracy and outcome of knee injections.
- Special care should be taken to avoid injecting into Hoffa's fat pad as atrophy can be the result if corticosteroids are placed within this structure.

Background

Intra-articular injections of the knee are usually performed in patients complaining of knee pain following failure of conservative management. Knee pain can be caused by intra-articular processes, which involved the ligaments, by meniscal tear, or may be post-traumatic in origin. It may also result from cartilage loss secondary to degenerative processes like osteoarthritis or synovitis. Also, inflammatory causes such as inflammatory arthritis or septic arthritis along with tendinopathies and bursitis may present as knee pain. Infrequently, it may be referred pain from areas involving the spine and/or the hip joint. Multiple studies have demonstrated a positive efficacy of corticosteroid injection in noninfective inflammatory conditions in the knee joint. A recent meta-analysis shows intra-articular hyaluronic acid injections are also an effective way to treat knee joint arthritis. Many painful syndromes around the knee may mimic knee joint pain, including Baker's cyst and prepatellar, suprapatellar, iliotibial band, and pes anserine bursitis.

Diagnosis

Knee pain can be diagnosed based on clinical presentation and radiographic imaging. Typically, the pain is localized to the knee and worsens with activity. Patients will report decreased in functional status and range of motion due to pain. On physical examination, patients will have a decreased passive range of motion of the knee joint. The presence of crepitus, effusion, quadriceps weakness, and medial and lateral laxity may be noted but not necessarily present.

X-ray imaging is the simplest and cost-effective to evaluate for radiographic evidence of knee osteoarthritis. Classic signs of osteoarthritis include joint space narrowing, osteophyte formation, subchondral cyst formation, and increased subchondral bone density (Fig. 28.1).

Technical Considerations

The knee is a complex articulating joint that is prone to injury. It consists of three compartments: the tibiofemoral, lateral tibiofemoral, and patellofemoral, all of which share a common synovial cavity.

A. Bautista, MD
Cleveland Clinic, Anesthesia Institute Pain Management, Cleveland, OH, USA

G.C. Chang Chien, DO (✉)
Cleveland Clinic, Anesthesia Institute Pain Management, 9500 Euclid Ave, Dept C-25, Cleveland, OH 44195, USA
e-mail: gchangchien@gmail.com

J.A.Z. Larson, MD, MPH
University of Kansas Medical Center, Physical Medicine and Rehabilitation, Kansas City, KS, USA

M. Gupta, MD
American Society of Interventional Pain, University of Kansas Medical Center, Kansas City, KS, USA

J.E. Pope, T.R. Deer (eds.), *Treatment of Chronic Pain Conditions*, DOI 10.1007/978-1-4939-6976-0_28

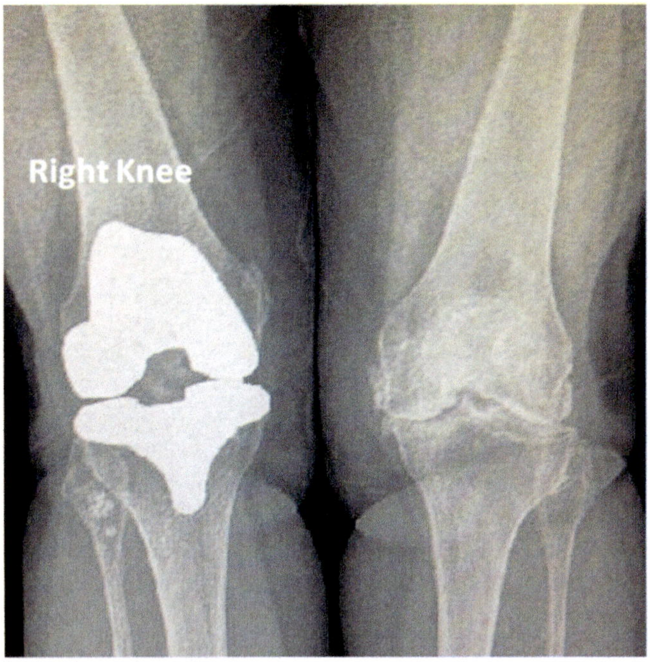

Fig. 28.1 Anterior-posterior weight-bearing radiograph. The right knee has had total knee arthroplasty. The left knee demonstrates severe medial and lateral compartment osteoarthritis. Note the decreased joint space, sclerotic bone changes, subchondral cyst formation, and osteophyte formation

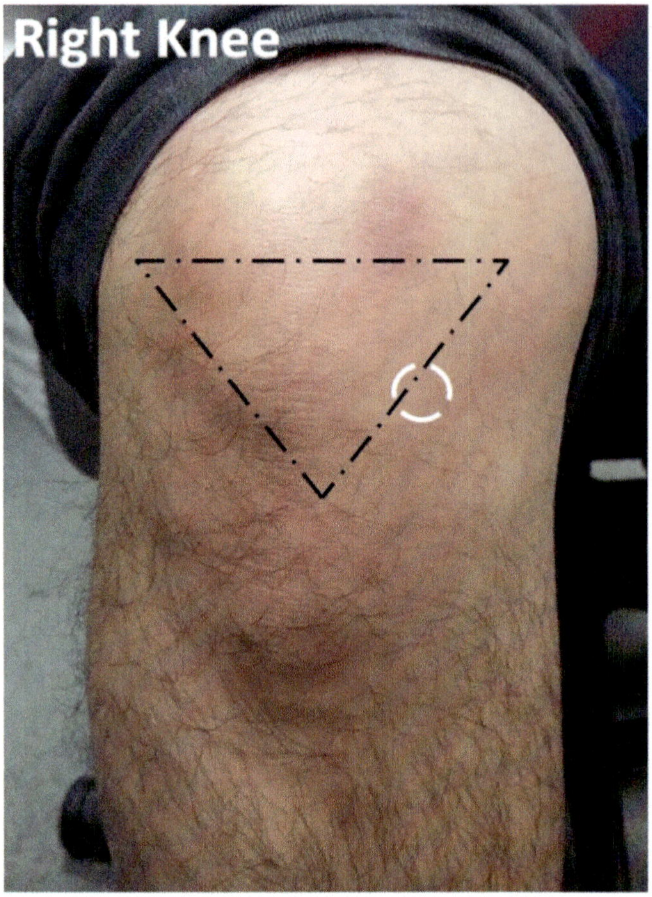

Fig. 28.2 Landmarks for knee joint injection. Insert the needle into the space between the patella and femur parallel to the middle facet of the patella. The *dashed triangle* gives/provides the technique as described by Lockman. *White dashed circle* is the medial needle insertion site, although this injection can be performed both at the medial and lateral recess

The approach to knee injection is selected based on the individual's bony anatomy and should be the path of least obstruction, with maximal access of the synovial cavity. The knee joint can be accessed by superolateral, superomedial, or anteromedial/anterolateral approaches. The patient should be sitting with the knee flexed at 90°. Locate the apex of the patella by palpation. Lockman reported the concept of the triangle technique in which one line is drawn from the apex of the patella to the lateral pole of the patella, and another line is drawn from the apex to the medial upper pole of the patella, resulting in an inverted triangle. The base of the triangle forms the upper border of the patella. The lateral line of the triangle is then marked at the midpoint, where the needle can be inserted and directed into the intra-articular knee joint (see Fig. 28.2). A 1 ½–2 inch 22-gauge needle is ideal for injections with a 5 ml syringe. However, needle sizes ranging from 22 to 25 gauges have been used depending on medication viscosity, access to arthritic joints, and if aspiration of fluid is anticipated. A higher gauge needle may increase the resistance in pushing the medication with minimal discomfort. Careful initial palpation and marking of the injection site is advocated to reduce re-palpation after preparation of the site. Maintenance of sterile technique is advised at all times. The skin can be cleansed with iodine disinfectant or chlorhexidine. Skin anesthesia can be accomplished by injection of 2–3 ml of 1% lidocaine prior to needle insertion.

If a joint effusion is noted, this should be aspirated to relieve pressure within the joint capsule. Once a needle has entered the joint space and satisfactory joint fluid has been withdrawn, the syringe can be removed and replaced with a syringe filled with medication intended for injection (Fig. 28.3).

Superolateral Knee Injection

The patient is positioned supine with the knee fully extended, with a pad to support the knee to facilitate relaxation. The physician's thumb is used to gently rock then stabilize the patella, while the needle is inserted below the superolateral surface aiming toward the center of the patella. The needle is then directed slightly posterior and inferomedially into the knee joint. The needle should not feel any resistance upon entering the skin. A hard obstruction may reflect encountering the bone or cartilage. Redirect the needle until the

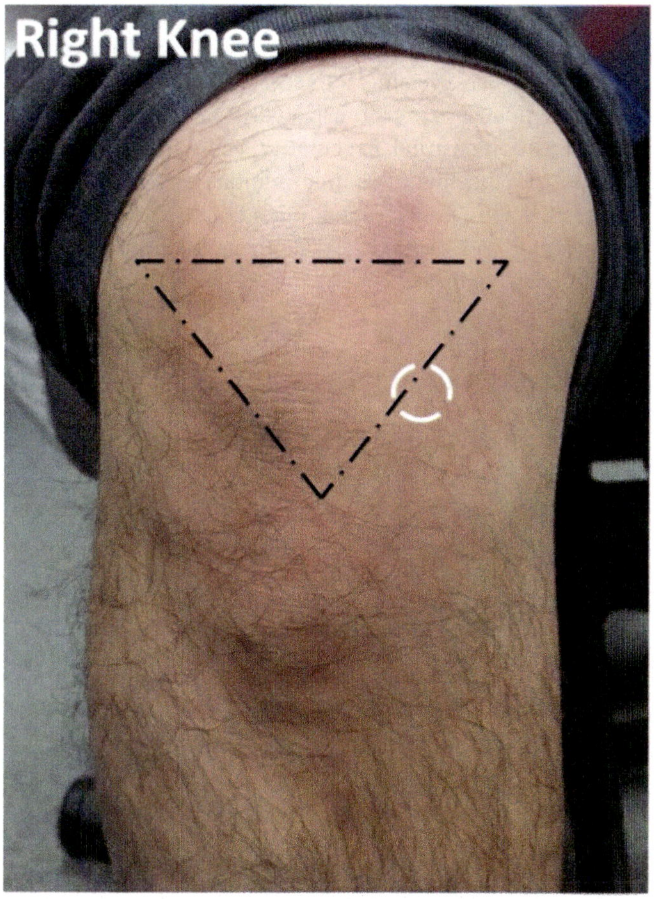

Fig. 28.3 Needle entry location described and approach

obstruction is "walked off." Injection of medication should be without any resistance.

Superomedial Knee Injection

The patient is positioned supine with the knee fully extended, with the pad support underneath the knee to facilitate relaxation. The physician's thumb is used to gently rock then stabilize the patella, while the needle is inserted below the superomedial surface aiming toward the center of the patella. The needle is then directed slightly posterior and inferolaterally into the knee joint. The needle should not feel any resistance upon entering the skin. A hard obstruction may reflect encountering the bone or cartilage. Redirect the needle until the obstruction is "walked off." Injection of medication should be without any resistance.

Anterolateral/Anteromedial Knee Injection

The patient can either sit or lie supine with the knee flexed 90° to facilitate ease of needle entry. The needle is inserted either lateral or medial to the patellar tendon approximately 1 cm above the tibial plateau and directed 15°–45° from the anterior knee surface vertical midline toward the joint space. The needle should not feel any resistance upon entering the skin. A hard obstruction may reflect encountering the bone or cartilage. Redirect the needle until the obstruction is "walked off." Injection of medication should be without any resistance.

The use of ultrasound and fluoroscopic-guided knee injections may improve accuracy and increase the likelihood of directing medication in the joint space.

Medications

A variety of medications have been used to inject the knee. The injectable amount ranges from 2 to 8 ml.

Corticosteroids

- These agents have anti-inflammatory properties which also possess varied metabolic effects and modify the body's immune response. Oftentimes, these are combined with local anesthetics depending on the physician's preference. No large trials to date have compared the value of various steroid preparations for knee injection.
- Preparation: methylprednisolone, triamcinolone, dexamethasone, hydrocortisone, prednisolone, and betamethasone.

Hyaluronic Acid

- Hyaluronic acid is an anionic, nonsulfated glycosaminoglycan which forms a viscoelastic solution in water that works as a lubricant. It plays a vital role in managing friction among adjacent tissues.
- This helps form the structural integrity of the synovium and the cartilage that helps lubricate the synovial joint. It is also a pro-inflammatory mediator that modulates cell proliferation, migration, and gene expression.
- Preparation: Synvisc, Supartz, Euflexxa, Hyalgan, Orthovisc, and Supartz.

Botulinum Toxin

- Botulinum toxin type A is an acetylcholine release inhibitor and neuromuscular-blocking agent found in the natural toxin from *Clostridium botulinum*.
- This may provide pain relief in patients with advanced knee osteoarthritis. The mechanism may be due to the neurotransmitter-mediated inhibition of sensory neurons.
- Preparation: Botox, Dysport, and Xeomin.

Platelet-Rich Plasma (PRP)

- PRP is blood plasma that has been enriched with a concentrated source of autologous platelets, growth factors, and cytokines that is known to stimulate healing of bone and soft tissues.
- The procedure is complex and requires special equipment to prepare. Its use has shown production of new hyaline/fibrocartilage formation. It also contains high levels of cytokines and growth factors.

After injection, a sterile dressing and pressure is applied at the injection site. Ice can be applied to the affected area for the first 24–48 h. The patient is also instructed to increase activity with straight leg raising exercises with avoidance of vigorous exercises and running for several days.

There are no existing guidelines for a repeat injection. However, a 4- to 6-week interval period is reasonable if symptoms persisted. Partial relief from the initial injection warrants consideration for repeat injection. Some practitioners will advocate switching between viscosupplementation and corticosteroid injections. If adequate pain relief is not achieved, consider further imaging or surgical consultation.

Complications

Complications associated with knee injections can be divided into two broad categories: infectious and noninfectious causes. With regard to infectious cause, iatrogenic septic arthritis is the most serious complication and is commonly attributed to poor sterile technique. This occurs in 1 per 2000–15,000 injections. Noninfectious complications of knee injections are usually seen as a result from steroid injection besides the inherent trauma to the surrounding structures such as soft tissue, ligaments, and nerves. Chronic steroid injections may cause tendon rupture and nerve atrophy or necrosis. Systemic effects of steroids that include impaired glucose control especially in diabetic patient, osteoporosis, menstrual irregularity, ecchymoses, and suppression of the hypothalamic-pituitary axis have been described. Though uncommon, other complications, such as skin atrophy and dystrophic calcification around the joint capsule, may occur.

Suggested Reading

1. Ahmed I, Gertner E. Safety of arthrocentesis and joint injection in patients receiving anticoagulation at therapeutic levels. Am J Med. 2012;125:265.
2. Boon AJ, Smith J, Dahm DL, Sorenson EJ, et al. Efficacy of intra-articular botulinum toxin type a in painful knee osteoarthritis: a pilot study. PM R. 2010;2(4):268–76.
3. Daley EL, Bajaj S, Bisson LJ, Cole BJ. Improving injection accuracy of the elbow, knee and shoulder: does injection site and imaging make a difference? As systematic review. Am J Sports Med. 2011;39(3):656–62.
4. Kelley SS, Erpelding JM, Kobs J, Nance CJ, Rendleman DA. Knee and lower leg. In: Snider RK, editor. Essentials of musculoskeletal care. 4th ed. Rosemont: American Academy of Orthopedic Surgeons; 1999. p. 368–489.
5. Lockman LE. Practice tips. Knee joint injections and aspirations: the triangle technique. Can Fam Physician. 2006;52(11):1403–4.
6. Neustadt DH. Osteoarthritis. In: Rakel RE, editor. Conn's current therapy. Philadelphia: W.B. Saunders; 2003. p. 1075–9.
7. Sampson S, Reed M, Silvers H, Meng M, Mandelbaum B. Injection of platelet-rich plasma in patients with primary and secondary knee osteoarthritis: a pilot study. Am J Phys Med Rehabil. 2010; 89(12):961–9.
8. Wang C, Lin J, Chang CJ, Lin YT, Hou SM. Theraputic effects of hyaluronic acid on osteoarthritis of the knee. A meta-analysis of randomized controlled trials. J Bone Joint Surg Am. 2004;86-A:538–45.
9. Weiss L, et al. Easy injections. 1st ed. Philadelphia: Butterworth-Heinemann/Elsevier; 2007. p. 43–7.

Ankle Injection

29

Nomen Azeem

Key Points

- Common indication for injecting the ankle joint is for pain secondary to arthritis.
- Diagnosing ankle joint arthritis is done by thorough history and clinical exam.
- Ankle joint injections done by palpation of anatomy, under ultrasound guidance, or under fluoroscopy for more precise placement of needle.
- Risks of ankle injections include cartilage deterioration, weakening or ruptured tendon, possible puncturing of a vein or artery, infection, or osteonecrosis.
- Tarsal tunnel injection is done by palpation of anatomy or ultrasound guidance for more precise needle and injectate placement.
- Risks of tarsal tunnel injections include nerve damage, puncturing of a vein or artery, or infection.

The articulation of the talus with the tibia and fibula forms the ankle joint and is stabilized by ligaments that attach to the medial and lateral malleoli. On the lateral ankle joint is stabilized by the anterior talofibular ligament (ATFL), posterior talofibular ligament (PTFL), and the calcaneofibular ligament (CFL). The medial ankle joint is stabilized by the deltoid ligament.

The ankle joint is one of the more commonly injected joints. The main indication for injecting the ankle is for pain secondary to arthritis that has failed conservative treatment including rest, ice, and the use of nonsteroidal anti-inflammatories. Arthritis of the ankle joint may occur in older patients with wear and tear or in athletes with a history of trauma to the area. Other indications for ankle joint injection include crystalloid deposition disease, mixed connective tissue disease, and synovitis.

Diagnosing ankle joint arthritis is done by obtaining a thorough history and clinical exam. Patients can present with pain, swelling, redness, warmth, crepitus, and gait disturbance. A plain film x-ray of the ankle joint can confirm findings consistent with ankle joint arthritis.

Ankle joint injections may be done by palpation of anatomy, under ultrasound guidance, or under fluoroscopy for more precise placement of needle and injectate. The patient is positioned in a supine position with the ankle relaxed, and space between the anterior border of the medial malleolus and the medial border of the tibialis anterior tendon is palpated to identify the space between the talus and tibia. As with any joint injection, a sterile technique must be utilized. Once proper entry point is identified, a 25-gauge 1.5 inch needle is inserted into the space and directed posterolaterally. Once in position, aspirate fluid to rule out intravascular needle placement and inject solution of 3–5 mL of local anesthetic and 1 mL of steroid. The needle is withdrawn and Band-Aid is applied.

Risks of ankle injections include cartilage deterioration, weakening or ruptured tendon, the possible puncturing of a vein or artery, an infection, or osteonecrosis.

The Achilles tendon or the lateral ligaments of the ankle joint including the ATFL, PTFL, and CFL can be injected with novel regenerative solutions such as platelet-rich plasma (PRP) for persistent pain secondary to tendonitis or ligament sprain (with ultrasound guidance). According to Taylor and colleagues, a systematic review found that PRP use in tendon and ligament injuries has several potential advantages, including faster recovery and possibly a reduction in recurrence with no adverse reactions described. However, due to the risk of weakening of the tendon or ligament leading to rupture, these structures should not be injected with a steroid solution.

The tarsal tunnel is formed by the medial malleolus and the flexor retinaculum under which the posterior tibial nerve passes. The posterior tibial nerve further divides into the medial/lateral plantar nerves and the calcaneal branches that

N. Azeem, MD (✉)
Sarasota Orthopedic Associates,
2750 Bahia Vista St, Ste 100, Sarasota, FL 34239, USA
e-mail: nazeem@soa.md; azeemnx@gmail.com

J.E. Pope, T.R. Deer (eds.), *Treatment of Chronic Pain Conditions*, DOI 10.1007/978-1-4939-6976-0_29

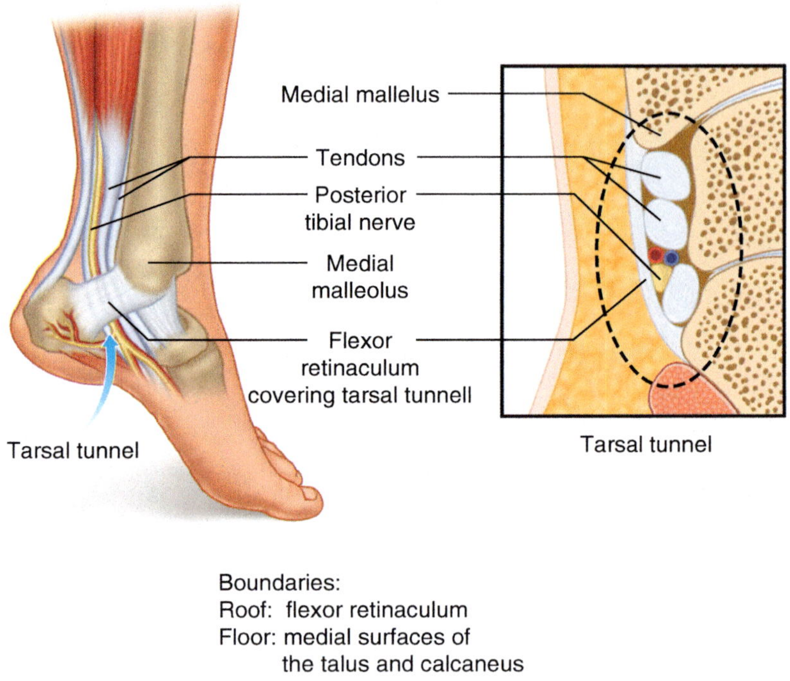

Fig. 29.1 Tarsal tunnel boundaries

innervate the base of the foot. Any compression of the posterior tibial nerve while passing through the tarsal tunnel can cause neuropathic foot pain (Fig. 29.1).

Diagnosing tarsal tunnel syndrome is done by obtaining a thorough history and clinical exam. Patients present with burning sensation, pain, and paresthesias which worsen with weight bearing. On exam, there may be a positive Tinel's test (tapping over the tarsal tunnel can exacerbate pain symptoms). EMG/NCS may also be used to detect a posterior tibial nerve compression neuropathy.

Tarsal tunnel injection may be palpation of anatomy or ultrasound guidance for more precise needle and injectate placement. The patient is positioned in a lateral decubitus position with symptomatic foot down, and the posterior tibial tendon is identified by resisted foot inversion. The posterior nerve runs posterior to posterior tibial tendon; thus, the needle entry point is behind the medial malleolus posterior to the tendon. As with any joint injection, a sterile technique must be utilized. Once proper entry point is identified, a 25-gauge 1.5 inch needle is inserted at a 30° angle and advanced a few centimeters. The needle should be repositioned if patient feels paresthesias. Once in position, aspirate fluid to rule out intravascular needle placement and inject solution of 1–2 mL of local anesthetic and 0.5–1 mL of steroid. The needle is withdrawn and Band-Aid is applied. Risks of tarsal tunnel injections include possible nerve damage, possible puncturing of a vein or artery, or an infection.

Suggested Reading

1. Braddom RL. Physical medicine and rehabilitation, vol. 2. 3rd ed. Philadelphia: Saunders/Elsevier/Mosby 2008; 2007. p. 548. ISBN: 9781416032052.
2. Khoury NJ, el-Khoury GY, Saltzman CL, Brandser EA. Intraarticular foot and ankle injections to identify source of pain before arthrodesis. AJR Am J Roentgenol. 1996;167:669–73.
3. Tallia AF, Cardone DA. Diagnostic and therapeutic injection of the ankle and foot. Am Fam Physician. 2003;68(7):1356–62.
4. Taylor DW, Petrera M, Hendry M, Theodoropoulos JS. A systematic review of the use of platelet-rich plasma in sports medicine as a new treatment for tendon and ligament injuries. Clin J Sport Med. 2011;21(4):344–52.

Hip Injections

30

Julie Ann Zitterkopf Larson and Mayank Gupta

Key Concepts

- Hip pain is a very common symptom with numerous causes. In a study of 6056 adults with ages 60 and older, 14.3% reported significant hip pain most days in the past 6 weeks.
- Injections of corticosteroid or hyaluronic acid have been shown to delay total hip replacement in patients with osteoarthritis.

Introduction

In patients with hip pain, history and physical exam are critical to diagnosis. The location and character of hip pain, along with aggravating and alleviating factors, and the impact on ambulation can all be used to distinguish conditions affecting the bursa and other soft tissues from conditions impacting the hip joint and adjacent bones. Pathology presenting from the femoroacetabular (hip) joint typically presents with pain deep within the groin. Gradual onset of groin pain with weight bearing and improvement with rest is the hallmark of osteoarthritis of the hip joint. Differential diagnosis of acute onset of groin pain with weight bearing includes occult fracture from trauma, osteonecrosis (especially in patients with a history of high glucocorticoid use), acute synovitis, or septic arthritis. By comparison, constant pain in the anterior hip region, that is, neither aggravated by direct pressure nor repetitive flexion of the hip, suggests lower abdominal/pelvic pathology, inguinal hernia, or referred pain from L2 to L3 spinal nerve roots.

J.A.Z. Larson, MD, MPH (✉)
University of Kansas Medical Center, Physical Medicine and Rehabilitation, Kansas City, KS, USA
e-mail: julie.zitterkopf@gmail.com

M. Gupta, MD
American Society of Interventional Pain, University of Kansas Medical Center, Kansas City, KS, USA

Background

The first-line treatment for most hip conditions consists of conservative management including rest of the joint and surrounding structures, ice, nonsteroidal anti-inflammatory drug (NSAID), and physical therapy. Injections are the next reasonable step for pain that is refractory to conservative measures. After ruling out a septic joint, an intra-articular injection of a 2–5 mL mixture containing corticosteroid (triamcinolone or methylprednisolone) mixed with a local anesthetic can suppress the inflammation contributing to joint pain. This can serve both as a diagnostic and therapeutic tool. It is highly suggested that image guidance with ultrasound or fluoroscopy be used for interarticular hip joint injections. When the femoroacetabular joint is injected without image guidance, the miss rate is relatively high and the femoral nerve can be injured 30% of the time. Literature supports performing about ten injections to gain proficiency at performing ultrasound guided hip injections.

With image guidance, the femoroacetabular (hip) joint can be injected successfully with either the anterior or lateral approach. The anterior approach to the hip joint is performed with the patient lying in a supine position. It is critical to mark the course of the femoral artery, with the insertion site of the needle lateral to the vascular bundle and vertical to the mid-portion of the femoral neck to avoid neurovascular injury. The needle is advanced in a straight direction until it reaches the anterior aspect of the base of the femoral neck. A small amount of iodinated contrast is injected to verify the intra-articular position of the needle before deposition of corticosteroid solution. If arterial puncture occurs, direct pressure can be applied to the injection site to prevent development of a hematoma. The joint can also be injected via the lateral approach using fluoroscopy (Fig. 30.1). Studies have demonstrated decreased rates of neurovascular injuries with the lateral approach when compared to the anterior approach because it allows visualization of the needle at all times during the insertion of the

J.E. Pope, T.R. Deer (eds.), *Treatment of Chronic Pain Conditions*, DOI 10.1007/978-1-4939-6976-0_30

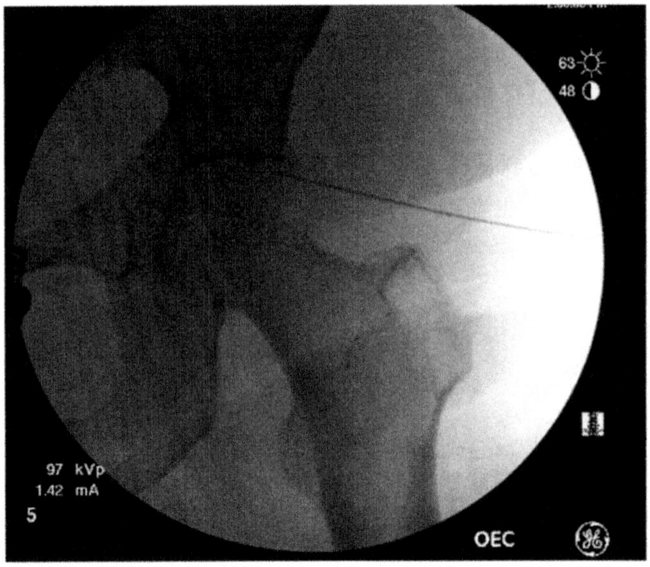

Fig. 30.1 Fluoroscopic view of intra-articular injection of the left hip via lateral approach

needle. Patients can be positioned either supine or on their side with the affected hip up. The entry site is immediately cephalad to the greater trochanter, at the mid-level of the anteroposterior dimension of the thigh. Using fluoroscopic guidance, the needle is advanced, so it enters the hip joint laterally at the junction of the femoral head and neck. Intra-articular position may be verified using iodinated contrast prior to deposition of corticosteroid solution.

Greater trochanteric bursitis is a commonly used term describing lateral hip pain with tenderness to palpation over lateral aspect of the hip. Patients often complain of pain that is made worse when lying with direct pressure on the affected side. The point of maximal tenderness is typically around 1.5 inches below the superior portion of the trochanter directly over the maximum lateral prominence. The hip range of motion is normal. Physical exam should also include analysis of gait, lower back flexibility, and sacroiliac joint dysfunction. The goals of treatment include reducing inflammation in the bursa, correcting any underlying gait disturbance, and preventing recurrent bursitis through specific hip and back stretching exercises. Initial treatments should include heat and passive stretching exercises to reduce the pressure over the bursal sac. If conservative treatment fails, the trochanteric bursa sac can be injected. With the patient lying laterally with affected hip up, the area over the greater trochanter can be palpated for the point of maximal tenderness. After the hip is prepped in a standard aseptic fashion, the needle can be directed toward this area until periosteum is contacted or fluoroscopy guided techniques. The needle is then pulled back slightly, and the medication is injected after negative aspiration. While this can be performed blindly, having experienced physicians use a fluoroscopy bursagram results in correct placement 53% of the time (Fig. 30.2).

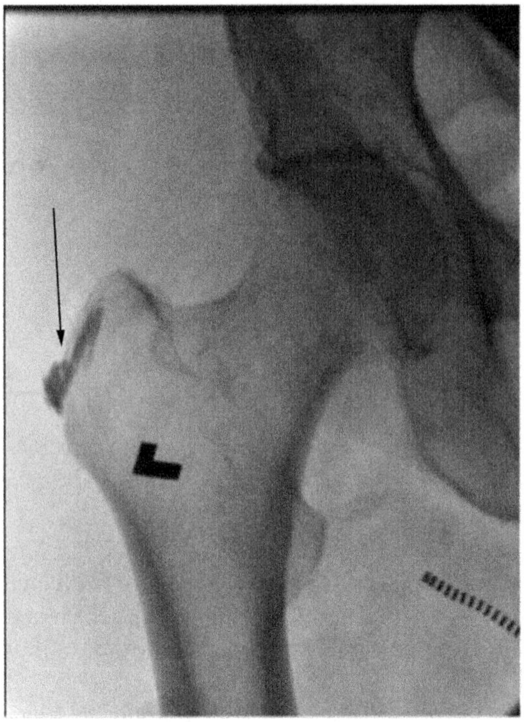

Fig. 30.2 Fluoroscopic view of the greater trochanter bursa injection with contrast

Aftercare for All Injections

The literature suggests patients rest for 3 days, avoiding direct pressure and repetitive movements of the joint. Patients are allowed to shower following injection but should avoid soaking the injection site for 3 days to decrease the risk of infection.

Candidacy

First-line treatment for hip pain includes conservative measures such as rest, ice, nonsteroidal anti-inflammatory drug (NSAID), and physical therapy. Injections are the next reasonable step for pain that is refractory to conservative measures. Contraindications to hip joint injections include patients who have an unstable or surgically implanted joint, a septic joint, and an infection of soft tissues around the joint such as cellulites, an intra-articular hip fracture, avascular necrosis, severe osteoporosis, and a clotting disorder or those who are on anticoagulants.

Suggested Reading

1. Atchia I, Birrell F, Kane D. A modular, flexible training strategy to achieve competence in diagnostic and interventional musculoskeletal ultrasound in patients with hip osteoarthritis. Rheumatology (Oxford). 2007;46(10):1583–6.
2. Christmas C, Crespo CJ, Franckowiak SC, et al. How common is hip pain among older adults? Results from the Third National Health and Nutrition Examination Survey. J Fam Pract. 2002;51:345.
3. Cohen SP, Narvaez JC, Lebovits AH, et al. Corticosteroid injections for trochanteric bursitis: is fluoroscopy necessary? A pilot study. Br J Anaesth. 2005;94(1):100–6.
4. Dobson MM. A check on the anatomical accuracy of intra-articular hip injections in relation to the therapy of coxarthritis. Ann Rheum Dis. 1950;9(3):237–40.
5. Dobson MM. A further anatomical check on the accuracy of the intra-articular steroid. J Bone Joint Surg Br. 2007;89(3):422; author reply 422.
6. Leopold SS, Battista V, Oliverio JA. Safety and efficacy of intraarticular hip injection using anatomic landmarks. Clin Orthop Relat Res. 2001;391:192–7.
7. Lovell NH. Intra-articular corticosteroid hip injections: a review of 63 consecutive patients. Eur J Orthop Surg Traumatol. 2006; 16:20–3.

Occipital Nerve Block

31

Dmitri Souzdalnitski, Syed S. Ali, Sherif Zaky, and Imanuel Lerman

Key Concepts

- Occipital nerve block (ONB) allows blockade of nociceptive afferent fibers distributed over the occipital region, vertex, sides of the head, as well as upper cervical region, which is known to interact with the trigeminal complex.
- ONB may provide acute headache relief, abort an intractable headache cycle, or serve as part of prevention strategies for occipital neuralgia, migraine, cluster headaches, and other common headache disorders; ONB typically provides rapid pain relief, lasting days to weeks and months.
- ONB can be performed blindly or with ultrasound guidance. They are technically simple and well tolerated by patients and, if accurately performed, are remarkably safe.

Introduction

Occipital nerve block (ONB) has been found effective in the treatment of occipital neuralgia, migraine headaches, cervicogenic headache, cluster headache, and some other primary and secondary headache disorders.

D. Souzdalnitski, MD, PhD (✉)
Western Reserve Hospital,
1900 23rd Street, Cuyahoga Falls, OH 44223, USA
e-mail: dsouzdalnitski@wetsrenreservehospital.org

S.S. Ali, MD
Western Reserve Hospital, Center for Pain Medicine,
Cuyahoga Falls, OH, USA

S. Zaky, MD, MSC, PhD
Pain Management Service, Firelands Regional Medical Center,
Case Western Reserve University, Sandusky, OH, USA

I. Lerman, MD, MS
University of California San Diego, Department of Anesthesiology,
Lajolla, CA, USA

Background

Occipital nerve blocks are used as a diagnostic and therapeutic instrument for management of headaches assumed to be caused by occipital neuralgia. Recently, ONB has been found to be effective in treatment of an array of acute and chronic, primary and secondary headache conditions listed below. While the number of randomized controlled studies which support the efficacy of this procedure is limited, there is an abundance of positive observational studies and case reports, in addition to a recent systemic review favoring the usefulness of this intervention. It is suggested that ONB is especially helpful in the treatment of severe headache when medications are not effective or have unfavorable or intolerable side effect profile.

Anatomy

There are three occipital nerves: the greater occipital nerve (GON), the lesser occipital nerve (LON), and the third occipital nerve (TON). The TON is a branch of the third cervical nerve and typically connects to the GON from below and medially. It is responsible for providing sensations to the back of the scalp and lower occipital region. The GON originates higher, from the dorsal primary ramus of the second cervical nerve. It is located between the *m. inferior obliquus capitis* and *m. semispinalis capitis*. As the GON travels cephalad, it penetrates the *m. semispinalis capitis* and then the *m. trapezius*. It then can be located less than 1 inch lateral to the superior nuchal line. The GON can be found lateral to the vertex and medial to the occipital artery (OA). The LON is different from TON and GON as it mainly consists of branches of the superficial cervical plexus, and it has contributions from the C2 and C3 ventral rami. The LON travels cephalad on the posterior border of the *m. sternocleidomastoid*. It provides sensory innervation of the scalp lateral to the GON distribution, up to the posterior part of the ear.

J.E. Pope, T.R. Deer (eds.), *Treatment of Chronic Pain Conditions*, DOI 10.1007/978-1-4939-6976-0_31

Candidacy

Indications for ONB include the treatment of acute or chronic headaches, which may be unresponsive to pharmacological treatment. It may also be used as abortive therapy for an intractable headache, as well as assist in weaning off of medications known to contribute to medication overuse headache. The geriatric population and expectant mothers are good candidates especially where oral analgesics/antidepressants/membrane stabilizers provide pain reduction but may cause side effects or are contraindicated. Specifically, the ONB may be utilized in treatment of migraine (with or without aura, status migrainosus, and chronic migraine), episodic or chronic tension or cluster-type headache, chronic daily headache, cervicogenic headache, posttraumatic headache, hemicrania continua, new daily persistent headache, post-dural puncture headache, trigeminal neuralgia, and occipital neuralgia.

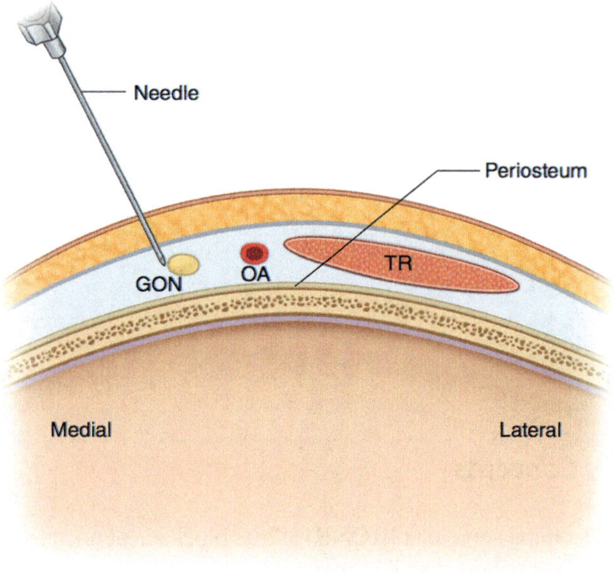

Fig. 31.1 Schematic representation of greater occipital nerve (GON) block, landmark technique. The GON is typically located medial to occipital artery (OA). TR *m. trapezius*

Techniques

The ONB uses an injectate of 3–5 ml of local anesthetic (typically 1% lidocaine or 0.5% bupivacaine) in close approximation to the GON. It can be done using 25–30-gauge ½–1-inch needle. Steroid medication, preferably, non-particulate, such as dexamethasone (1–5 mg, half-life 36–54 h) or methylprednisolone (20–125 mg, half-life 18–36 h), can be added. Adding a steroid to local anesthetic is touted as a potential adjuvant resulting in protracted therapeutic effect of the regional nerve blockade. The use of the steroids for the GON block is however controversial, with only scant evidence demonstrating improved efficacy in cluster headaches.

In the past GON blocks were performed using the landmarks technique. When using a landmark technique, a patient should be placed in a sitting or prone position. The occipital artery should be palpated on the back of the head at or slightly caudal to the superior occipital protuberance about 1.5 inch lateral to the midline. The GON is typically located medial to the artery approximately 0.5–1.5 inch lateral to the occipital protuberance (also termed inion). Palpating this will often produce occipital tenderness, or even headache, which may indicate the location for the blockade. The GON blockade can be performed on both sides depending on symptomatology. It is important to avoid injury to occipital artery during the injection. Therefore, the artery should be palpated before a skin wheal with local anesthetic is performed. The injection should be carried out *medial to pulsation* of the occipital artery (Fig. 1). The variations in the course of GON and artery may require increase in volume of local anesthetic up to 10 ml in order to achieve clinical success. The inadvertent intra-arterial injection of local anesthetic or particulate steroid (triamcinolone) can result in complications including and not limited to scalp necrosis, hair loss, and hair discoloration. The needle is typically advanced until the bony periosteum is encountered or until the patient reports paresthesia. In order to avoid injection into the periosteum, the needle should be then slightly withdrawn. The aspiration of the syringe should be performed, and if negative, the local anesthetic should be injected in the located tender point or in a fanlike manner. This technique results in a field block and improves the likelihood of successful block. In addition using this technique may result in blockade of the TON or LON, which can be in close approximation to the GON (Fig. 31.1).

Recently ultrasonographic guidance has been proven to accurately locate the GON, the surrounding muscles, soft tissues, and, most importantly, vascular structures. It also provides real-time visualization of the needle as it is advanced as well as the injectate. It has been shown that ultrasonography-

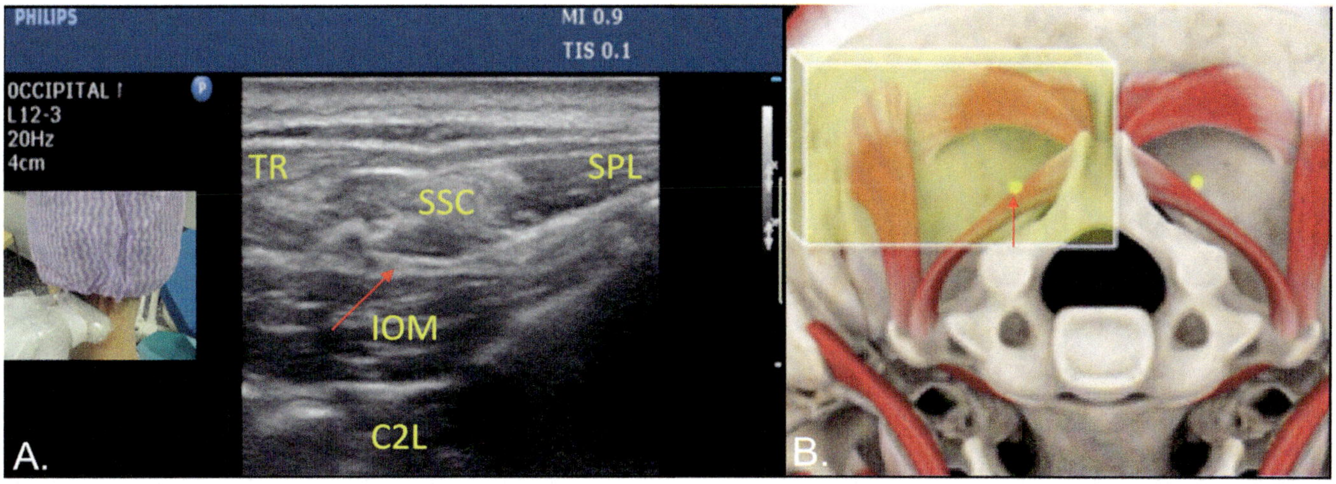

Fig. 31.2 (**a**) Ultrasonographic image of greater occipital nerve (*red arrows*), injectate spread just above the GON. M medial, L lateral, C2L Ce lamina, IOM *m. inferior obliquus capitis*, SSC *m. semispinalis capitis*, SC *m. semispinalis capitis*, *TR* m. trapezius. Inset orientation of probe tilted superolateral. Inset probe placement adapted from Greher M, Moriggl B, Curatolo M, Kirchmair L, Eichenberger U. Sonographic visualization and ultrasound-guided blockade of the greater occipital nerve: a comparison of two selective techniques confirmed by anatomical dissection. Br J Anaesth. 2010;104(5):637–42. (**b**) Transverse anatomical view of IOM and GON (*red arrow*)

guided GON blocks may have better outcomes and potentially safer interventions. Ultrasonography-guided GON block can be performed at the same location as the traditional landmark technique or lower, at the C2 level, where the GON is located just above the *m. inferior obliquus capitis* (Fig. 2). GON block typically provides rapid pain relief, within 15–30 min, lasting days to months. Patients with history of craniotomy, or if the patient has received antiplatelet or anticoagulation therapy, require detailed discussion on risk/benefits/alternative treatment options, preferably image-guided intervention and longer monitoring/special attention after the ONB (Fig. 31.2).

Suggested Reading

1. Lambru G, Abu Bakar N, Stahlhut L, et al. Greater occipital nerve blocks in chronic cluster headache: a prospective open-label study. *Eur J Neurol*. 2014;21(2):338–43.
2. Narouze S, editor. Interventional head and face pain management: nerve blocks and beyond. 1st ed. New York: Springer Science + Business Media; 2014. p. 29–34.
3. Narouze S, Souzdalnitski D. Occipital nerve entrapment within the semispinalis capitis muscle diagnosed with ultrasound. *Cephalalgia*. 2013;33(16):1358–9.
4. Tepper SJ, Stillman MJ. Cluster headache: potential options for medically refractory patients (when all else fails). *Headache*. 2013;53(7):1183–90.

32 Trigeminal Nerve Block

Eduardo Jusino and Maged Guirguis

Key Concepts

- All patients with a new diagnosis of trigeminal neuralgia should undergo brain and brainstem MRI with and without gadolinium to rule out posterior fossa or brainstem lesions and demyelinating disease.
- Skill with fluoroscopic guidance of the technique should be developed before attempting to perform this block to avoid devastating complication.
- Adequate time is needed to allow the patient to become comfortable with the approach and appropriate sedation to occur.

Anatomy

The trigeminal nerve contains sensory and motor fibers. Somatic afferent fibers transmit pain, light touch, and temperature sensation from the skin of the face, the oral and nasal mucosa, the teeth, and the anterior two thirds of the tongue. Visceral efferent fibers innervate muscles of facial expression, tensor tympani, and muscles of mastication. Also, the trigeminal nerve has multiple communications with autonomic nervous system through the ciliary, sphenopalatine, otic, and submaxillary ganglia (Fig. 32.1).

The trigeminal nerve travels as follows: brainstem, prepontine fossa, Meckel's cave (trigeminal/Gasserian ganglion location), and extracranial branch. After the Gasserian ganglion, the nerve separates into the ophthalmic, maxillary, and mandibular divisions.

E. Jusino, MD
Cleveland Clinic Foundation, Cleveland, OH, USA

M. Guirguis, MD (✉)
Ochsner Health System, Pain Management, Department of Anesthesiology & Critical Care Medicine, New Orleans, LA, USA
e-mail: magedaziz@gmail.com

The ophthalmic division carries sensory fibers to the scalp, forehead, upper eyelid, conjunctiva, cornea, nose, nasal mucosa, frontal sinus, and parts of the meninges. It divides into the nasociliary nerve, lacrimal nerve, and frontal nerve. The nasociliary nerve divides into the sensory root of ciliary ganglion, long ciliary nerve, posterior ethmoidal nerve, anterior ethmoidal nerve, and infratrochlear nerve. The frontal nerve divides into the supratrochlear nerve and supraorbital nerve.

The maxillary division provides purely sensory fibers to the lower eyelid, cheek, nares, upper lip, upper teeth, upper gums, nasal mucosa, palate, roof of the pharynx, maxillary sinus, ethmoid sinus, sphenoid sinus, and parts of the meninges. Its branches are divided into four groups, depending on the location where they branch off: the cranium, the pterygopalatine fossa, the infraorbital canal, or the face. The intracranial group includes the middle meningeal nerve. The pterygopalatine group includes the zygomatic nerve, the superior alveolar nerves, the nasopalatine nerve, the palatine nerves, and the pharyngeal nerve. The infraorbital group includes the infraorbital nerve and the anterior superior alveolar nerve. The facial group includes the inferior palpebral nerve, the superior labial nerve, and the lateral nasal nerve.

The mandibular division contains a large sensory root and a small motor root that provide innervation to the lower lip, lower teeth, gums, chin, jaw, parts of the external ear, and parts of the meninges. Its branches are divided into three groups: the main trunk, the anterior division, and the posterior division. The main trunk group includes efferent branches for the medial pterygoid, tensor tympani and tensor veli palatini muscles, and an afferent nerve for the meningeal branch. The anterior group includes the efferent masseteric, deep temporal, and lateral pterygoid nerves and the afferent buccal nerve. The posterior group includes the efferent/afferent inferior alveolar nerve and the afferent auriculotemporal and lingual nerves.

J.E. Pope, T.R. Deer (eds.), *Treatment of Chronic Pain Conditions*, DOI 10.1007/978-1-4939-6976-0_32

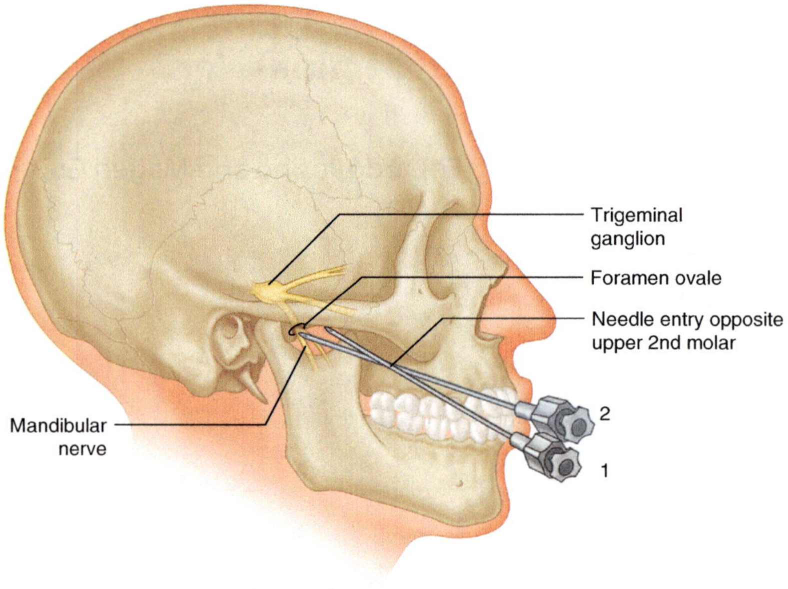

Fig. 32.1 Anatomy of trigeminal nerve block from entry site: AP and lateral views relative to mouth and pupil

Introduction

Trigeminal neuralgia is a disease characterized by distinctive, intense episodes of pain in the trigeminal nerve distribution on a unilateral side. Most cases of trigeminal neuralgia are idiopathic. Inflammatory causes (e.g., multiple sclerosis, infection, etc.) and compression of the trigeminal roots (e.g., tumors, vasculature, etc.) may be associated. Patients usually describe the pain as electric, shooting, and shock-like. The pain can be precipitated by light mechanical stimulation to the face or oral mucosa. The vast majority of cases affect either the maxillary or mandibular division (V2 or V3), alone or in combination. In approximately 5% of patients, the symptoms occur solely in the ophthalmic division (V1).

Treatment

The primary treatment for trigeminal neuralgia is pharmacologic (carbamazepine). Other anticonvulsants may also be beneficial. For patients who fail to respond to pharmacologic treatment, trigeminal nerve block is a practical next step. If this fails, more invasive options such as radiofrequency ablation, balloon compression, Gamma Knife radiosurgery, and microvascular decompression may be considered after evaluating the risk-benefit ratio.

Trigeminal Nerve Block and Neurolysis

Indications

The indications for performing a trigeminal nerve block include the following: management of trigeminal neuralgia, surgical anesthesia, anatomic differential neural blockade, prognostic nerve block before ablative procedure, alleviation of acute pain emergencies, palliation of cancer pain, management of cluster headache, and treatment of persistent ocular pain.

Contraindications

The contraindications for performing trigeminal nerve block include but are not limited to the following: patient refusal, local infection, sepsis, coagulopathy, increased intracranial pressure, behavioral abnormalities, allergy to local anesthetics, and uncooperative patient.

Technique

Injecting small, incremental doses of local anesthetic to avoid local anesthetic toxicity should be utilized for all blocks (Figs. 32.1, 32.2, 33.3, and 32.4).

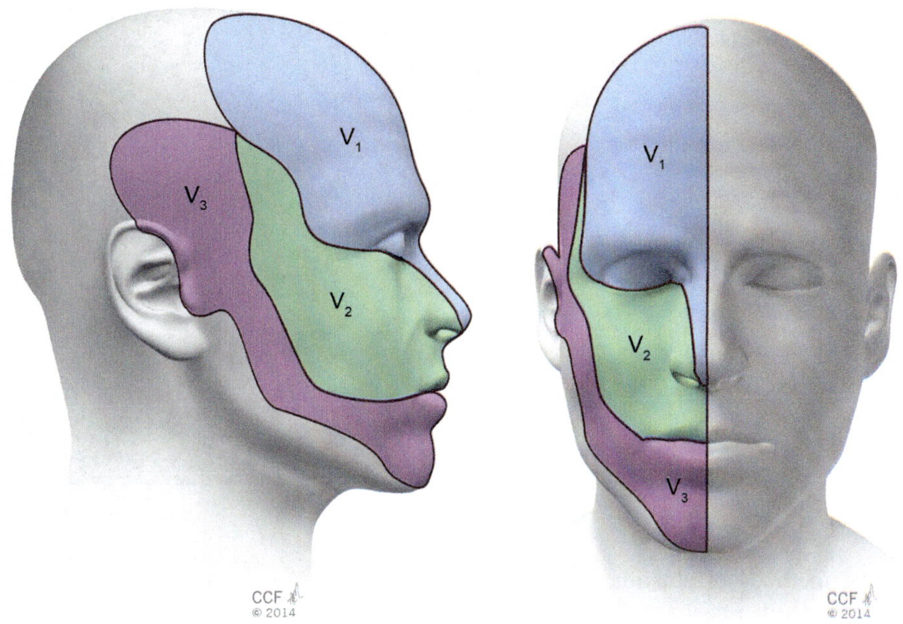

Fig. 32.2 Dermatomes: trigeminal nerve (Reprinted with permission, Cleveland Clinic Center for Medical Art & Photography © 2014. All Rights Reserved)

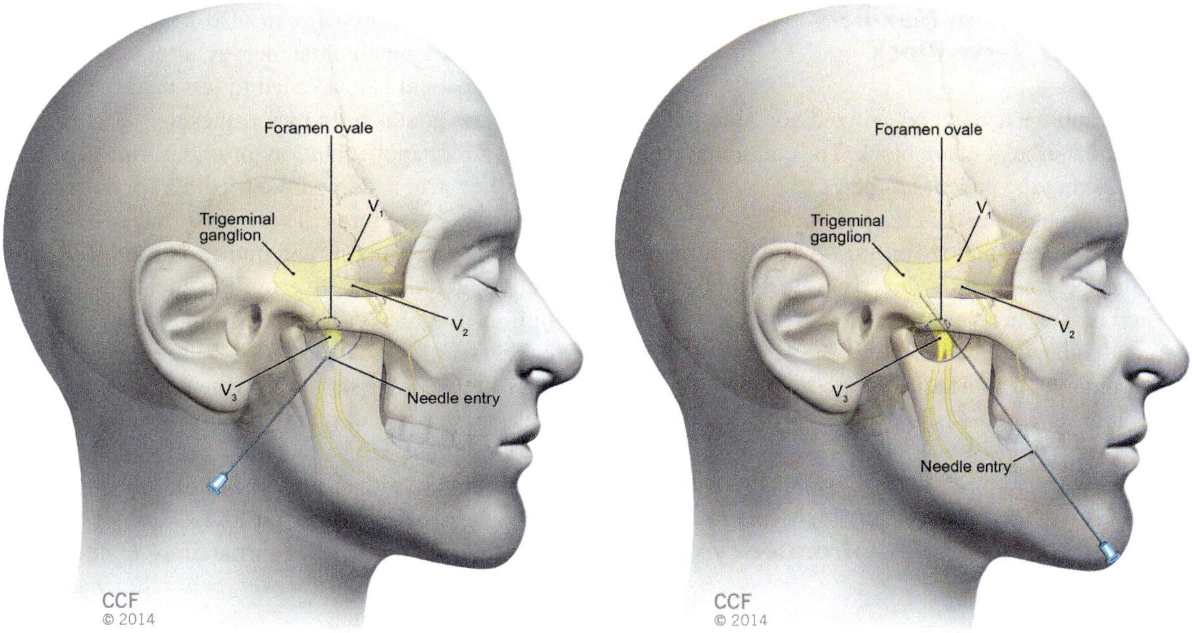

Figs. 32.3 and 32.4 Lateral trigeminal nerve block of the face (Reprinted with permission, Cleveland Clinic Center for Medical Art & Photography © 2014. All Rights Reserved)

Gasserian Ganglion Block

The patient is positioned supine with the cervical spine extended. Under fluoroscopic guidance, submental and oblique views are obtained to identify the foramen ovale. Approximately 2.5 cm lateral to the corner of the mouth, a needle is advanced perpendicular to the pupil of the eye in a cephalad direction toward the auditory meatus. After contact is made with the base of the skull, the needle tip is withdrawn slightly and walked posteriorly into the foramen ovale. Carefully aspirate for blood/CSF. After needle position is confirmed and aspiration is negative, the therapeutic solution may be injected. An average volume of 0.4 mL of neurolytic solution is usually adequate to provide long-lasting pain

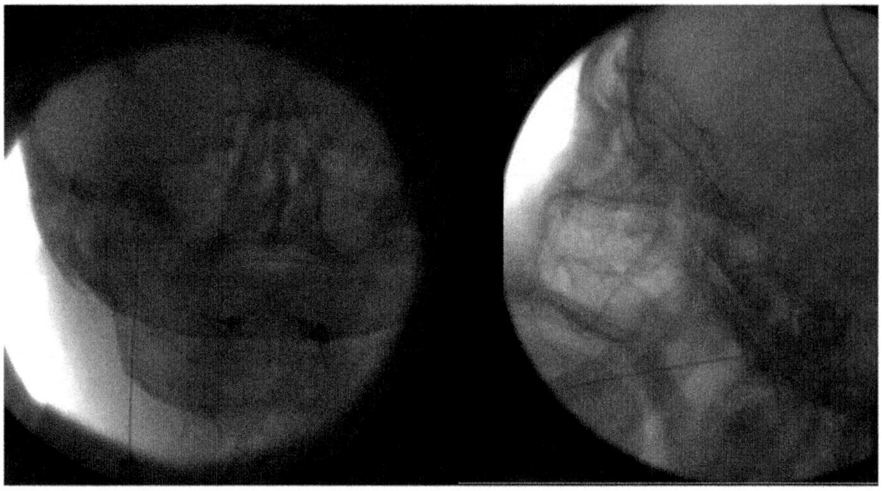

Fig. 32.5 Radiographic image: trigeminal nerve block

relief. The methods of ablation include thermal injury by radiofrequency, chemical injury by glycerol/phenol/alcohol injection, and mechanical compression by balloon inflation.

Coronoid Approach for Maxillary and Mandibular Nerve Block

The coronoid approach may be utilized for simultaneous maxillary and mandibular nerve block. The coronoid notch is identified by asking the patient to open and close the mouth several times and palpating the area just anterior and slightly inferior to the acoustic auditory meatus. A needle is inserted just below the zygomatic arch directly in the middle of the coronoid notch. The needle is advanced 1.5–2 inches in a plane perpendicular to the skull until the lateral pterygoid plate is encountered. The needle is withdrawn slightly, and 7–15 mL of local anesthetic is injected.

Gasserian Ganglion, Ophthalmic, Maxillary, and Mandibular Nerves Radiofrequency Ablation

The patient is positioned supine with the cervical spine extended. A nasal cannula and/or nasal trumpet may be utilized to maintain the airway patent. Sedation is commenced. The needle is directed as stated above in the Gasserian ganglion block section. After the needle is engaged in the foramen ovale, lateral view fluoroscopy is used to advance the needle to a point just superior to the intersection of the petrous bone and the clivus. Sedation is stopped. The stylet of the needle is removed and replaced with the radiofrequency electrode. Once the patient is adequately awake, test stimulation is started with 0.05–0.15 volts at 50 Hz to evoke paresthesia in the area desired. When the electrode location is confirmed, the patient is anesthetized again. Afterward, the electrode is heated up to 75–80 °C for 90 s.

A coronoid approach can also be used for RFA of the maxillary and mandibular nerves after neurolysis is complete; the patient is awakened to test the efficacy of the procedure. The goal is mild hypoesthesia.

Radiofrequency ablation provides the highest rate of pain relief when compared to other percutaneous nerve destructive procedures. The two forms of radiofrequency ablation are continuous and pulsed. Pulsed RFA is a nondestructive method of delivering RF energy to the trigeminal ganglion. In contrast to conventional RF described above, short bursts of RF current at 42 °C are generated with long pauses between bursts to allow heat to dissipate in the target tissue. In a recent randomized controlled study comparing both, it has been shown that continuous radiofrequency is more effective than pulsed radiofrequency. Although in recent study, patient received PRFA did not have paresthesia, which clinically shows that it is nondestructive and may be an advantage. However, pain relief was not satisfactory as it was expected.

Complications

Potential complications include but are not limited to the following: bleeding, infection, nerve injury, intravascular injection, intrathecal injection, cardiac and respiratory arrest, seizure, stroke, dysesthesia, motor weakness, and pain exacerbation.

Suggested Reading

1. Erdine S, Ozyalcin NS, Cimen A, Celik M, Talu GK, Disci R. Comparison of pulsed radiofrequency with conventional radiofrequency in the treatment of idiopathic trigeminal neuralgia. Eur J Pain. 2007;11:309–13.
2. Gulur P, Wainger BJ, Young A. Head and facial trigeminal neuralgia. In: Pain procedures in clinical practice. 3rd ed. Philadelphia: Elsevier; 2011. p. 297–304.
3. Narouze SN. Trigeminal (Gasserian) ganglion, maxillary nerve, and mandibular nerve blocks. In: Interventional management of head and face pain: nerve blocks and beyond. New York: Springer; 2014. p. 53–9.
4. Singla A. Trigeminal neuralgia. In: Essentials of physical medicine and rehabilitation. 2nd ed. Philadelphia: Saunders; 2008. p. 491–6.
5. Waldman SD. Gasserian ganglion block. In: Pain management. 2nd ed. Philadelphia: Elsevier; 2011. Expert Consult. Web 1 Aug. 2014.
6. Waldman SD. Trigeminal nerve block. In: Atlas of pain management injection techniques. 3rd ed. Philadelphia: Saunders; 2013. p. 44–6.

33 Sphenopalatine Ganglion

Robert Bolash and Reda Tolba

Key Concepts

- The sphenopalatine ganglion serves as a major intersection point for sympathetic and parasympathetic nerve fibers innervating the face.
- Application of local anesthetic to the ganglion has proven efficacy in the treatment of head and facial pain disorders including cluster headaches, herpes zoster, trigeminal neuralgia, atypical facial pain, and migraine.
- The sphenopalatine ganglion can be blocked via a percutaneous infrazygomatic approach by application of local anesthetic or by applying radiofrequency ablation of the ganglion.

Introduction

Historically, sphenopalatine ganglion blocks have been used for the treatment of a wide variety of conditions including asthma, angina, singultus, epilepsy, glaucoma, headaches, neck pain, vascular spasm, facial neuralgia, blindness, low back pain, sciatica, earache, temporomandibular joint dysfunction, hyperthyroidism, dysmenorrhea, fibromyalgia, and myofascial pain. It is uncertain if these early "successes" were due to the application of local anesthetic to the sphenopalatine ganglion or the fact that intranasal cocaine was the most commonly utilized local anesthetic.

R. Bolash, MD
Cleveland Clinic, Anesthesia Institute Pain Management, 9500 Euclid Ave, Dept C-25, Cleveland, OH 44195, USA

R. Tolba, MD (✉)
200 west Esplanade Avenue, Kenner, LA 70005, USA
e-mail: redatolba@hotmail.com

Indications

Today, the sphenopalatine ganglion block is employed for the treatment of sphenopalatine neuralgia, trigeminal neuralgia, atypical facial pain, acute migraine, cluster headaches, and herpes zoster. Most successes have been demonstrated in the treatment of chronic and episodic cluster headache likely by interrupting the parasympathetic outflow from the superior salivary nucleus. Clinical success has demonstrated improvement among patients with atypical facial pain, trigeminal neuralgia, and migraine, including refractory cases in patients who have failed numerous noninvasive modalities.

Treatment

Historically, a *transnasal approach* utilizing local anesthetic-soaked pledgets containing lidocaine, tetracaine, or cocaine has been used. The nare is anesthetized by inserting the local anesthetic-soaked pledget along the superior aspect of the middle turbinate overlying the sphenopalatine ganglion. A *percutaneous fluoroscopically guided infrazygomatic approach* to the sphenopalatine ganglion for both diagnostic blocks and radiofrequency ablation is used by interventional pain physicians. A lateral fluoroscopic view of the face is obtained with the c-arm by superimposing the two rami atop each other. A skin wheal is created inferior to the zygomatic arch and anterior to the mandible. A 22 or 25-gauge 3.5-inch spinal needle is then inserted coaxially with lateral fluoroscopic guidance. The needle is then advanced superiorly and medially toward the pterygopalatine fossa utilizing AP fluoroscopic guidance. The needle tip will terminate just lateral to the ipsilateral nasal wall. Following final needle positioning, 0.2 mL of contrast material is injected under live fluoroscopic imaging to rule out intravascular spread (Fig. 33.1).

The percutaneous technique can be modified to perform *radiofrequency ablation*. A 22-gauge 10-cm curved, blunt radiofrequency needle with a 5-mm active tip is substituted and is advanced in same manner as described above. Upon

J.E. Pope, T.R. Deer (eds.), *Treatment of Chronic Pain Conditions*, DOI 10.1007/978-1-4939-6976-0_33

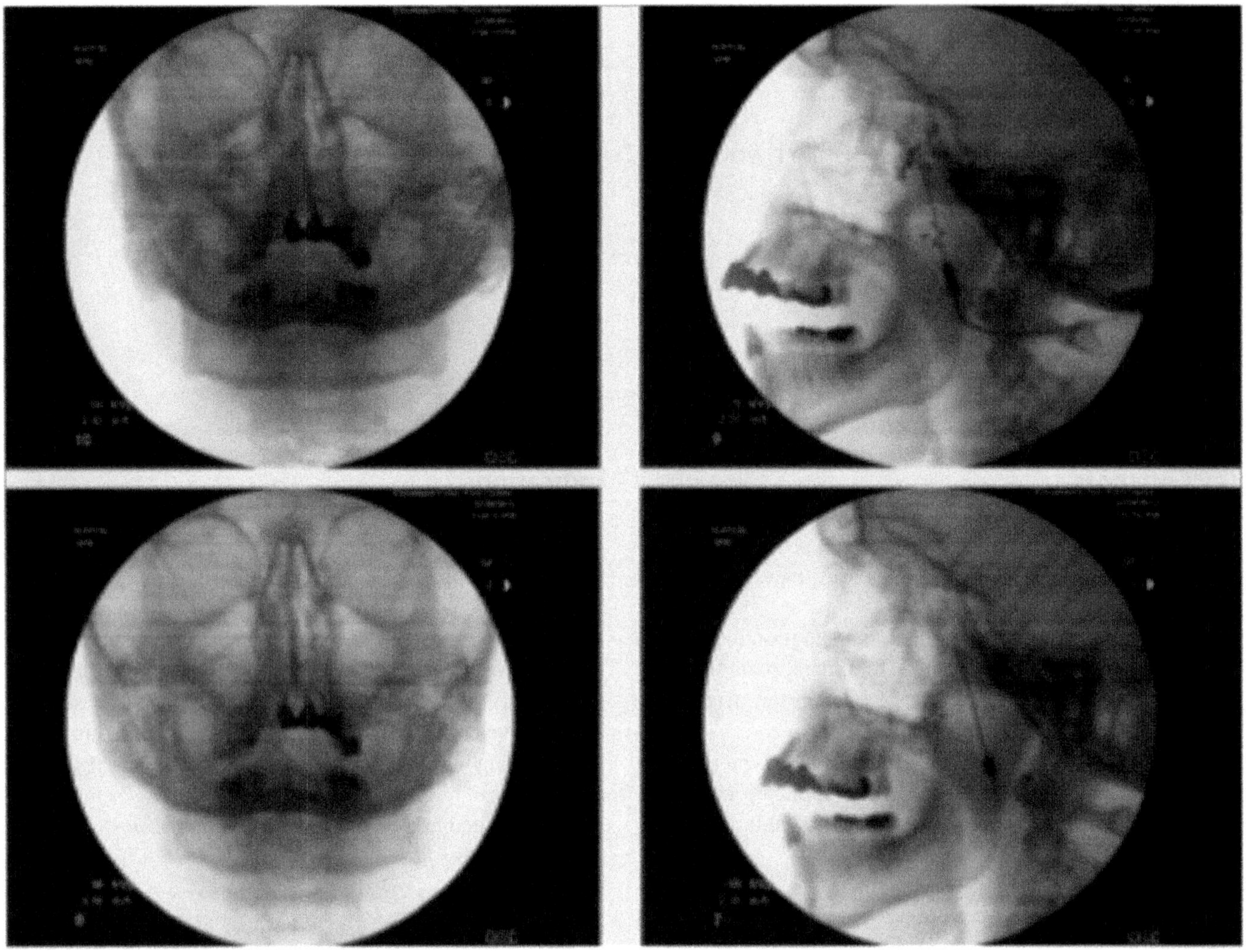

Fig. 33.1 Percutaneous fluoroscopic views: Needle courses medially toward the ipsilateral nasal wall

proper needle position, and confirmation of negative intravascular spread, sensory stimulation is carried out at 50 Hz with a 1-ms pulse duration. A favorable needle position will result in deep perinasal and maxillary paresthesias at <0.5 V. After stimulation is confirmed, local anesthetic is injected and radiofrequency neurotomy is performed at 80 °C for 90 s.

Suggested Reading

1. Day M. Neurolysis of the trigeminal and sphenopalatine ganglions. Pain Pract. 2001;1(2):171–82.
2. Narouze S. Complications of head and neck procedures. Tech Reg Anesth Pain Manag. 2007;11(3):171–7.
3. Narouze SN. Role of sphenopalatine ganglion neuroablation in the management of cluster headache. Curr Pain Headache Rep. 2010;14(2):160–3.
4. Narouze S, Kapural L, Casanova J, Mekhail N. Sphenopalatine ganglion radiofrequency ablation for the management of chronic cluster headache. Headache. 2009;49(4):571–7.
5. Sanders M, Zuurmond WW. Efficacy of sphenopalatine ganglion blockade in 66 patients suffering from cluster headache: a 12- to 70-month follow-up evaluation. J Neurosurg. 1997;87(6):876–80.
6. Spencer RF. Technique for sphenopalatine ganglion block. Reg Anesth. 1997;22(5):483–4.
7. Waldman SD. Sphenopalatine ganglion block – 80 years later. Reg Anesth. 1993;18(5):274–6.
8. Windsor RE, Jahnke S. Sphenopalatine ganglion blockade: a review and proposed modification of the transnasal technique. Pain Physician. 2004;7(2):283–6.

Auriculotemporal Nerve Block

34

Reda Tolba

Key Concepts

- Auriculotemporal nerve is a peripheral branch of the mandibular nerve and lies in close proximity to parotid gland, neck of the mandible, and temporal vessels.
- Auriculotemporal nerve is at risk of injury during surgical intervention of the parotid gland or mandibular condyle.
- "Frey's syndrome" may be a consequence of injury to the branches of the auriculotemporal nerve and is also seen as a consequence of fractures of the temporomandibular joint (TMJ).

Anatomy

The auriculotemporal nerve arises as two roots from the posterior division of the mandibular nerve. These roots encircle the middle meningeal artery then converge to form a single nerve. The auriculotemporal nerve passes between the neck of the mandible and the sphenomandibular ligament, gives off branches to parotid gland posteriorly, and gives branches to the auricle anteriorly. It then goes across the root of the zygomatic process of the temporal bone, deep to the superficial temporal artery (Fig. 34.1).

Innervation

The *somatosensory root* (*superior*) gives somatosensory fibers, which rise up to the superficial temporal area. It gives sensory supply to the skin of the auricle, external acoustic meatus, outer side of the tympanic membrane, and the skin in the temporal region (superficial temporal branches). It also gives articular branches to supply the temporomandibular joint (TMJ).

The *parasympathetic root* (*inferior*) carries postganglionic fibers to the parotid gland which serve as secretomotor fibers for the parotid gland.

Clinical Significance

The nerve as it courses posteriorly to the condylar head is frequently injured in temporomandibular joint (TMJ) surgery, causing an ipsilateral paresthesia of the auricle and skin surrounding the ear. Auriculotemporal nerve is the main nerve that supplies the temporomandibular joint (TMJ), along with branches of the masseteric nerve and the deep temporal.

"Frey's syndrome" merits consideration. Anatomically, the auriculotemporal nerve (ATN) is in close relation to the parotid gland, neck of the mandible, temporal vessels, and sphenomandibular ligament. Fine branches of the ATN are at risk of division during surgical intervention of the parotid gland or condyle of the mandible. "Frey's syndrome" or abnormal gustatory sweating can develop. This syndrome is characterized by occurrence of hyperesthesia, flushing, and warmth or sweating over the distribution of the auriculotemporal nerve and/or greater auricular nerve while eating foods that produce a strong salivary stimulus.

Auriculotemporal neuralgia (AN) is characterized by crises of strictly unilateral lancinating pain that may be perceived in the temporal region, TMJ, and in the parotid, auricular, and retro-orbital regions. The main clinical characteristic of AN is moderate to severe pain, associated with exacerbations, perceived as stabbing pain. The pain may worsen or be triggered by pressure on the periauricular region at the level of the tragus. Case reports have described about refractory facial pain after TMJ surgery attributed to AN. Pain from parotitis, a condition that can be caused by mumps, is carried by the auriculotemporal nerve to the brain.

R. Tolba, MD (✉)
200 west Esplanade Avenue, Kenner, LA 70005, USA
e-mail: redatolba@hotmail.com

J.E. Pope, T.R. Deer (eds.), *Treatment of Chronic Pain Conditions*, DOI 10.1007/978-1-4939-6976-0_34

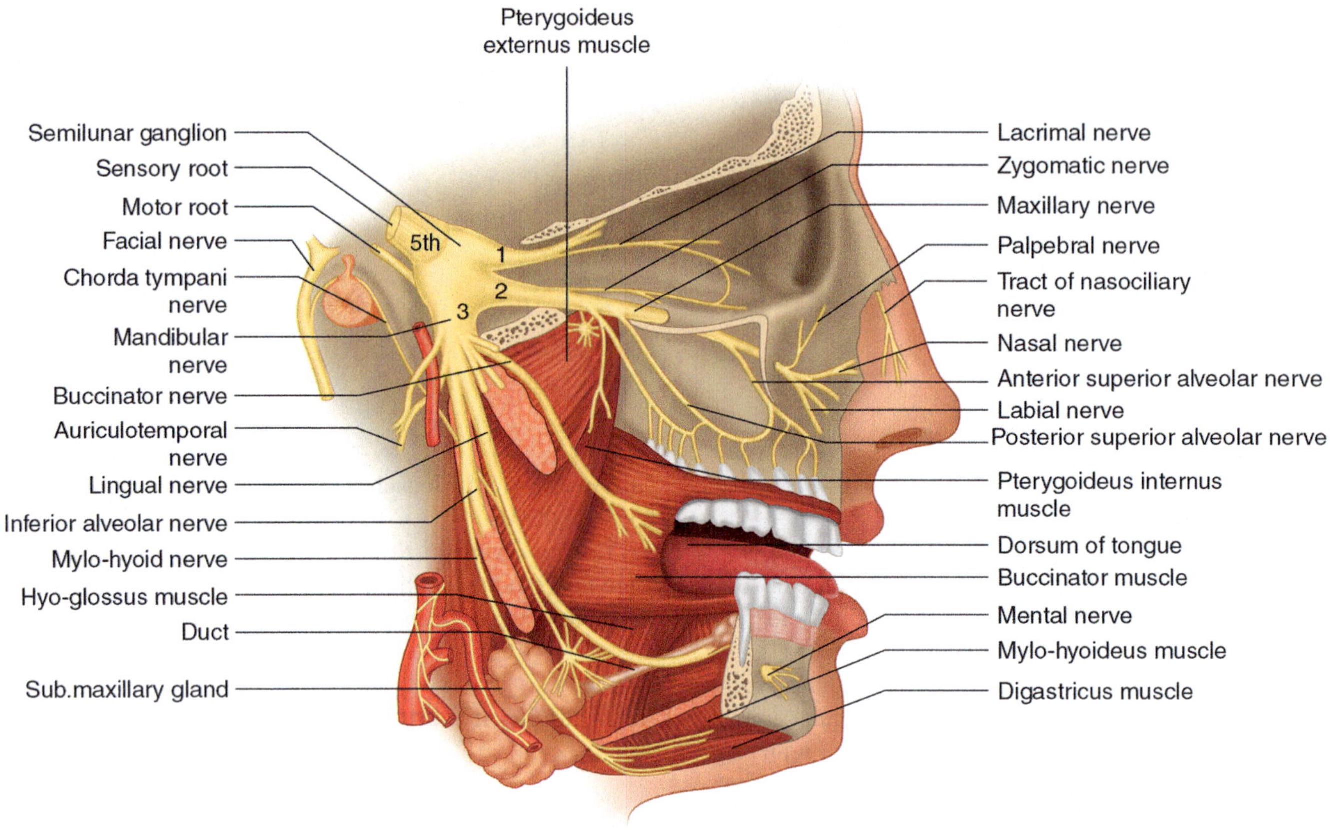

Fig. 34.1 Auriculotemporal nerve anatomy

Auriculotemporal Nerve Block

This block can be performed to relieve refractory pain attributed to auriculotemporal neuralgia. Block technique is described as follows: the needle is inserted below the TMJ, in the posterior margin of the head of the mandible, just in front of the tragus, to a depth of 1–1.2 cm, at a horizontal 45° angle in the direction of the nose, with care taken to first perform aspiration in order to avoid intravascular injection. Subsequently 0.5 cc of lidocaine 2% mixed with 0.5 cc of dexamethasone (8 mg/ml) can be injected to block the nerve. Simopoulos et al. have described a case of successful auriculotemporal nerve stimulation for treatment of chronic refractory migraine.

Suggested Reading

1. Du Toit DF. Auriculo-temporal nerve. Clinicopathological relevance to facial-maxillary practice. SADJ. 2003;58(2):62–3.
2. Kamath RAD, Bharani S, Prabhakar S. Frey's syndrome consequent to an unsual pattern of temporoMandibular joint dislocation: case report with review of its incidence and etiology. Craniomaxillofac Trauma Reconstr. 2013;6(1):1–8. Published online 2013 January 23. doi: 10.1055/s-0032-1332210.
3. Shankar H, Brethauer J. Ultrasound guided steroid injection for auriculo-temporalneuralgia. Anesthesiology. 2007;107:A903.
4. Simopoulos T, Bajwa Z, Lantz G, Lee S, Burstein R. Implanted auriculotemporal nerve stimulator for the treatment of refractory chronic migraine. Headache. 2010;50(6):1064–9.
5. Speciali JG, Gonçalves DA. Auriculotemporal neuralgia. Curr Pain Headache Rep. 2005;9(4):277–80.
6. Standring S. Gray's anatomy: the anatomical basis of clinical practice, Expert Consult. 40th ed. Churchill Livingstone; 2008. ISBN-10: 0443066841, ISBN-13: 978- 0443066849.
7. Stuginski-Barbosa J, Murayama RA. Refractory facial pain attributed to auriculo-temporal neuralgia. J Headache Pain. 2012;12(5):415–7.

35 Glossopharyngeal Neuralgia

George C. Chang Chien and Zachary McCormick

Key Concepts

- Glossopharyngeal neuralgia is characterized by unilateral paroxysmal pain in the oropharynx, nasopharynx, larynx, base of the tongue, lower jaw, and ear. These attacks are typically excruciating and described as sharp, stabbing, "shocks of electricity" that can last from seconds to minutes.
- Antiepileptic drugs and tricyclic antidepressants may be used to ameliorate the pain of glossopharyngeal neuralgia.
- Blocks with a local anesthetic with or without a corticosteroid, chemical neurolysis, and radiofrequency ablation are all options in the management of glossopharyngeal neuralgia.
- An obtunded gag reflex is one way to test for a successful glossopharyngeal nerve block.

Introduction

Glossopharyngeal neuralgia is characterized by unilateral paroxysmal pain in the oropharynx, nasopharynx, larynx, base of the tongue, lower jaw, and ear. These attacks are typically excruciating and described as sharp, stabbing, "shocks of electricity" that can last from seconds to minutes. The diagnosis is primarily based on the description of the location and pattern of the pain. A block of the glossopharyngeal nerve is a useful tool to confirm the diagnosis. MRI is routinely performed to rule out a tumor or other mass lesion, or blood vessels that may be compressing the glossopharyngeal nerve. Antiepileptic drugs and tricyclic antidepressants may be used to ameliorate the pain of glossopharyngeal neuralgia. Blocks with a local anesthetic with or without a corticosteroid, chemical neurolysis, and radiofrequency ablation are all options in the management of glossopharyngeal neuralgia. In severe cases that are refractory to other treatments, surgery that severs the glossopharyngeal nerve may be the only treatment to relieve the pain.

Background

Glossopharyngeal neuralgia is characterized by unilateral paroxysmal attacks triggered by stimulation to the oropharynx, such as mechanical swallowing, yawning, coughing, laughing, and chewing, and sensory stimulation such as cold, salty, acidic, or bitter foods.

The incidence of GPN increases with age and most often affects persons older than 50 years; however, in patients with multiple sclerosis, GPN tends to occur at a younger age. In 217 cases of glossopharyngeal neuralgia seen at the Mayo Clinic, 57% of the cases were in patients greater than 50 years old, while 43% were between the ages of 18 and 50. Twelve percent of these patients had bilateral involvement, but a frequency as high as 25% has been reported. Additionally, 12% of the patients exhibited both glossopharyngeal and trigeminal neuralgia. A greater prevalence in males has also been reported by some authors, while others have reported no difference in prevalence by gender.

Cardiovascular symptoms such as bradycardia, hypotension, and even cardiac arrest may accompany the attacks in 1–2% of the cases. The close association between the glossopharyngeal nerve and the vagus nerve (CN X) may underlie, in part, the etiology between glossopharyngeal neuralgia and the cardiac symptoms.

Glossopharyngeal neuralgia may mimic trigeminal neuralgia. Both may present with facial/jaw pain elicited by the same mechanical and sensory mechanisms. Cases may be difficult

G.C. Chang Chien, DO (✉)
Cleveland Clinic, Anesthesia Institute Pain Management, 9500 Euclid Ave, Dept C-25, Cleveland, OH 44195, USA
e-mail: gchangchien@gmail.com

Z. McCormick, MD
Northwestern University, The Rehabilitation Institute of Chicago, Chicago, IL, USA

J.E. Pope, T.R. Deer (eds.), *Treatment of Chronic Pain Conditions*, DOI 10.1007/978-1-4939-6976-0_35

to differentiate in patients with pain in the region of the tragus or deep to the angle of the jaw. However, compared to trigeminal neuralgia, glossopharyngeal neuralgia is relatively rare although dual diagnosis has been reported. A diagnostic interventional block may be useful in differentiating the two etiologies and indeed may be the only way to definitively establish the diagnosis of glossopharyngeal neuralgia.

Diagnosis

Diagnosis is based on clinical presentation, physical examination, imaging studies, and diagnostic blocks.

High-resolution MRI or CT scan of the head may reveal tumor, bony erosion, multiple sclerosis plaques, abscess, or infection. 3D visualizations of the brain stem or MRA may identify neurovascular compression or arteriovenous malformation. Visualization of the offending vessel was better in cases of compression from the posterior inferior cerebellar artery (PICA) compared to the anterior inferior cerebellar artery (AICA).

Medical Treatment

Medical treatment of GPN is similar to treatment for other forms of neuropathic pain, including trigeminal neuralgia. Antiepileptic drugs (AEDs) and tricyclic antidepressants alone or in combination have been studied with variable efficacy. AEDs that have been used include carbamazepine, lamotrigine, diazepam, and gabapentin; tricyclic antidepressants such as amitriptyline and nortriptyline have been used.

Glossopharyngeal Nerve Block

Patients that are not well managed on medication alone may benefit from a glossopharyngeal nerve block (Table 35.1).

Techniques for extraoral, intraoral, fluoroscopic, or ultrasound-assisted procedures have been described. The use of fluoroscopy allows real-time imaging of the contrast media and may help minimize intravascular injection in case the needle tip has penetrated either the carotid or jugular vessels. Injections of local anesthetic and/or steroids or chemical neurolysis and radiofrequency ablation are all options in management of glossopharyngeal nerve dysfunction. We describe the classic nonimage-guided intraoral approach to perform the glossopharyngeal nerve block.

Table 35.1 Indications for GPN block or neurolysis

Glossopharyngeal neuralgia (GPN)
Post-tonsillectomy pain control
Cancer pain
To reduce gag reflex for awake endotracheal intubation
Singultus (hiccups)
Carotid sinus syndrome
Patients that are poor candidates for microvascular decompression

Intraoral Technique

Anterior Tonsillar Pillar Method

The patient is asked to open the mouth widely (Fig. 35.1). The tongue is swept to the opposite side with a tongue depressor, laryngoscope blade, or gloved fingers. A 25-gauge, 3.5 inch spinal needle is inserted 0.5 cm deep, just lateral to the base of the anterior tonsillar pillar (ATP). The use of a spinal needle is advantageous for visualization of the tonsillar pillars by keeping the syringe out of the patient's mouth. After careful aspiration for blood or cerebrospinal fluid, 2 mL of local anesthetic (LA) plus non-particulate steroid is injected. The advantages of this method are that the ATP is easily identified and exposed, and the tongue movement does not trigger the gag reflex.

The patient is asked to open the mouth widely. The tongue is depressed down with a laryngoscope blade or a tongue blade. A 22–25 gauge, 3.5 inch spinal needle bent 1 cm from the distal end is directed laterally into the submucosa along the caudal aspect of the PTP (palatopharyngeal fold). After careful aspiration for blood and cerebrospinal fluid, 2 mL of local anesthetic and/or steroid is injected. The PTP method becomes more difficult in patients with large tongues or small oral opening and may cause greater gag reflex.

Conclusion

Pain from glossopharyngeal neuralgia can be challenging to diagnose and treat. Current best evidence supports the use of a multimodal approach to treatment including medication management and interventional techniques such as nerve blocks, radiofrequency neurolysis, and surgical decompression when indicated.

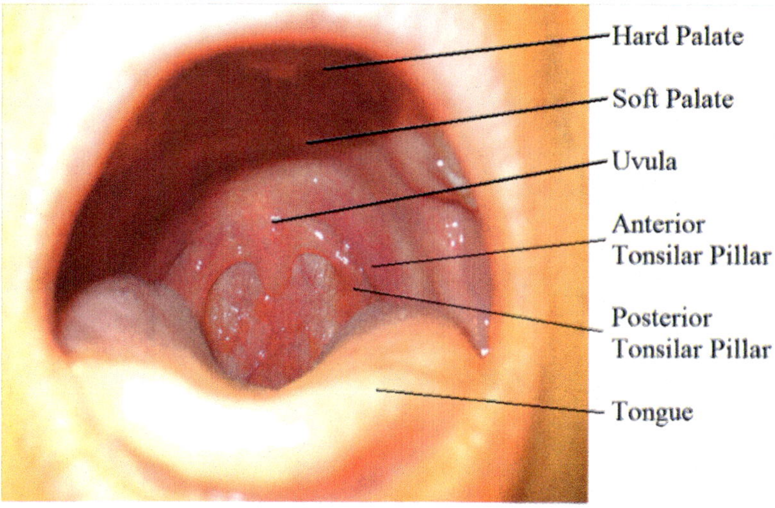

Fig. 35.1 Anatomy for intraoral glossopharyngeal nerve block. *Posterior tonsillar pillar method*

Suggested Reading

1. Gaitour E, Nick ST, Roberts C, Gonzalez-Toledo E, Munjampalli S, Minagar A, Vrooman B, Souzdalnitski D, Zamnifekri B. Glossopharyngeal neuralgia secondary to vascular compression in a patient with multiple sclerosis: a case report. J Med Case Rep. 2012;6:213.
2. Isbir CA. Treatment of a patient with glossopharyngeal neuralgia by the anterior tonsillar pillar method. Case Rep Neurol. 2011; 21(3):27–31.
3. Park HP. The effects of glossopharyngeal nerve block on postoperative pain relief after tonsillectomy: the importance of the extent of obtunded gag reflex as a clinical indicator. Anesth Analg. 2007;105:267–71.
4. Rushton JG, Stevens JC, Miller RH. Glossopharyngeal (vagoglossopharyngeal) neuralgia: a study of 217 cases. Arch Neurol. 1981;38:201–5.
5. Soh KB. The glossopharyngeal nerve, glossopharyngeal neuralgia and the Eagle's syndrome – current concepts and management. Singap Med J. 1999;40:659–65.
6. Waldman SD. The role of neural blockade in the management of headaches and facial pain. Headache Dig. 1991;4:286–92.

Atlanto-Occipital and Atlantoaxial Joint Injections

36

George C. Chang Chien and Jianguo Cheng

Key Concepts

- The atlanto-occipital (AO) and atlantoaxial (AA) joints are common causes of neck pain due to arthritic change and whiplash injury, among other causes.
- Patients typically present with both headache and neck pain aggravated by lateral rotation of the cervical spine and/or flexion or extension of the cervical spine.
- Anesthetic or corticosteroid injection into the AO/AA joints can be diagnostic and therapeutic for pain arising from these structures.
- The proximity of many vital structures necessitates complete mastery of the relevant anatomy, fluoroscopic image interpretation, and expert interventional technique.
- Injection of contrast under fluoroscopy with or without ultrasound is recommended to assure safe needle placement prior to injection of medication.
- Major complications associated with AO/AA injection are related to the close proximity of the target structures to the foramen magnum and the vertebral arteries.
- Potentially catastrophic outcomes include direct injury to the brain stem and spinal cord and intravascular injection of medication causing seizure of brain infarction.
- These injections are contraindicated in patients with cervical joint hypermobility or joint instability.

G.C. Chang Chien, DO (✉)
Cleveland Clinic, Anesthesia Institute Pain Management, Cleveland, OH 44195, USA
e-mail: gchangchien@gmail.com

J. Cheng, MD, PhD
Cleveland Clinic, Department of Pain Management, Cleveland, OH, USA

Introduction

The diagnosis of cervicogenic headache (CH) should be considered in patients with headache and concomitant history of neck pain, cervical trauma, or whiplash injury. Patients with CH pain commonly report symptoms in the back of the head and around or over the top of the head, sometimes up to the eyebrow or behind the eyes. These symptoms may be referred pain from cervical structures innervated by the upper three cervical spinal nerves including the muscles, joints and ligaments, the dura mater of the spinal cord and posterior cranial fossa, and the vertebral artery. Not surprisingly, patients with other types of head and facial pain may also report neck, shoulder, and myofascial symptoms. Thus, CH is often misdiagnosed as tension or migraine headaches leading to treatment failure. Diagnostic criteria for cervicogenic headaches have been established by the International Headache Society's International Classification of Headache Disorders (Headache chapter). Nonetheless, the great overlap in symptomatology between CH and other headache types often requires a diagnostic block.

The atlanto-occipital (AO) and atlantoaxial (AA) joints are susceptible to arthritis and can be injured during acceleration/deceleration ("whiplash") injuries. Pain following such injuries is often initially attributed to soft tissue injury such as muscle strain. AO and AA injections can be valuable during the workup for headaches. Local anesthetic infiltration of the joints has been demonstrated to provide good short-term relief of cervicogenic headaches. Due to the invasive nature and risk for injury, the criteria for a positive response to anesthetic blockade are stringent: pain must be reduced by 90% or more, ideally with a dual block paradigm. According to one retrospective study, pulsed radiofrequency treatment within the AA joint led up to 12 months of pain relief.

J.E. Pope, T.R. Deer (eds.), *Treatment of Chronic Pain Conditions*, DOI 10.1007/978-1-4939-6976-0_36

Anatomy

Occiput The occipital bone is part of the cranium at the posterior/inferior part of the skull. A prominent feature of the occipital bone is the foramen magnum, through which the cranial cavity communicates with the vertebral canal. The foramen magnum is a large oval aperture with its long diameter anteroposterior. It is wider behind than in front where the condyles that articulate with the atlas (C1) preside. Critical structures that enter the foramen magnum include the medulla oblongata, the vertebral arteries, and the anterior/posterior spinal arteries.

C1 (atlas) The *atlas* (C1) is the most superior cervical vertebra of the spine. The atlanto-occipital joint allows the head to nod up and down on the vertebral column. The atlas has a ring shape, consisting of an anterior and a posterior arch and two lateral masses (Chap. 7).

C2 (axis) The second cervical vertebrae allow for the head to rotate. The odontoid process rises perpendicularly from the surface of the anterior body and makes articulation with the atlas. It is positioned in between the anterior part of the atlas and the transverse ligament. The latter separates the odontoid process in the front and the thecal sac and the spinal cord in the back. The odontoid process acts as a pivot that allows the atlas and attached head to rotate on the axis. The processes contain the transverse foramen which gives passage to the vertebral artery, vertebral vein, and a sympathetic nerve plexus.

Nerves

The C1 nerve root (suboccipital nerve) exits between the skull and the C1 vertebrae. It provides motor innervation to the suboccipital muscles and interconnects with fibers of the C2 and C3 nerves. The greater and lesser occipital nerves (GON and LON) exit from between the first and second vertebra. The GON is the medial branch of the dorsal primary ramus of cervical spinal nerve 2. Its course often covers a large portion of the posteromedial aspect of the AA joint. The GON innervates the skin along the posterior part of the scalp to the vertex, over the ear. The LON typically arises from the lateral branch of the ventral ramus of the second and sometimes also the third cervical nerve and can sometimes be derived from the GON. The LON innervates the lateral portion of the posterior scalp and the medial surface of the pinna of the ear. The third occipital nerve (TON) is the medial branch of the posterior division of the third cervical nerve. It innervates the inferior portion of the posterior scalp. Third occipital nerve headache is common in patients with chronic neck pain and headache after whiplash (Chap. 7).

The Vertebral Artery

The vertebral arteries arise from the subclavian arteries, then typically enter the transverse process of sixth cervical vertebrae (C6), and less common at C7 (Fig. 36.1). They then proceed superiorly, in the transverse foramen. The vertebral artery lays immediately posterolateral to the atlanto-axial joint as it courses through the C2 and C1 foramina. Once they have passed through the transverse foramen of C1, the vertebral arteries travel across the posterior arch of C1 crossing the medial posterior aspect of the atlanto-occipital joint and through the suboccipital triangle before entering the foramen magnum. This diagonal course across the posteromedial aspect of the AO joint provides an important landmark for performing AO injections. Of note, the vertebral artery is covered during its entire course with a large plexus of veins.

Clinical Diagnosis

Patients often report neck pain, "stiffness," with decreased cervical range of motion and difficulty in head turning. Patients may report posterior headaches (occipital headaches) aggravated by rotation, side bending, and/or flexion or extension of the cervical spine. Additionally, some patients may report posterior or preauricular pain symptoms. CH refer into the posterior scalp but can also manifest as shoulder pain and occasionally arm pain on the side of the headache. Symptoms can be unilateral or bilateral. On physical examination, pressure on the base of the head and upper cervical spine may reproduce pain or trigger headaches. Diagnosis is made according to the criteria for cervicogenic headaches established by the International Headache Society's International Classification of Headache Disorders (Table 6.5).

Atlanto-Occipital Injection Under Fluoroscopic Guidance

The patient is placed in the prone position with a small roll or towel placed under the chin to accentuate cervical flexion. Although both AO and AA injection can be performed under ultrasound guidance, fluoroscopic guidance is most commonly utilized to identify the vertebral bodies of C1 and C2 by identifying the characteristic odontoid process of C2 (Fig. 36.2). Additionally, C2 spinous process is the first and most superior cervical vertebrae with a bifid spinous process. It is important to visualize the vertebrae of C1 and C2 midline, accounting for any rotation. The skin is prepped and draped in a sterile fashion. The skin overlying the target is anesthetized

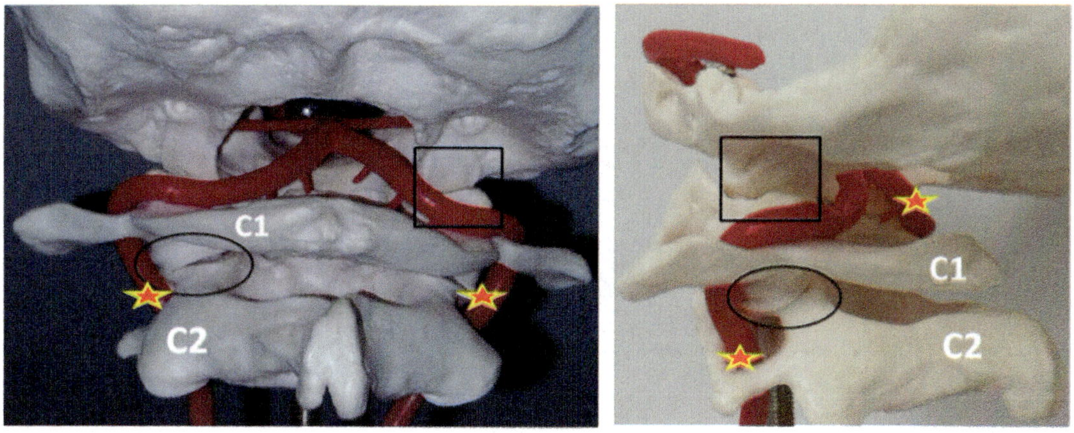

Fig. 36.1 Model of occiput, atlas, and axis. *Red star*: Vertebral artery. *Oval*: Atlantoaxial joint. *Square*: Atlanto-occipital joint

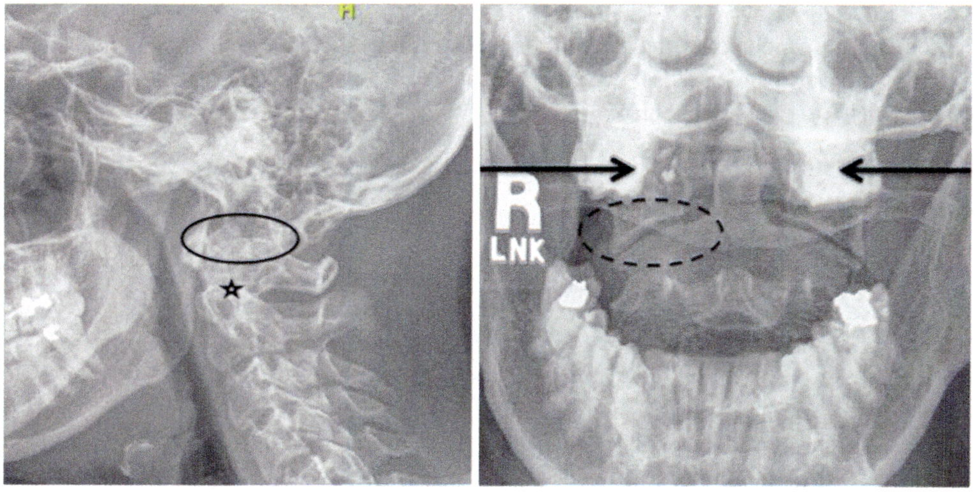

Fig. 36.2 Lateral cervical radiograph demonstrating the atlanto-occipital, atlantoaxial, and cervical facet joints. *Left*: *Oval* outlining the atlanto-occipital joint line. *Star* denotes atlantoaxial joint. *Right*: Open mouth radiograph demonstrating occiput, the ring of the atlas, and the body of the axis. *Black arrows* depict the atlanto-occipital joint line. *Dashed line oval* surrounds the right atlantoaxial joint line

with 2–3 ml of local anesthetic. Care is made not to penetrate too deeply, as many critical structures may be within 1–2 cm of the skin.

To perform an AO joint injection, the needle should be directed toward the superior posterolateral aspect of the joint to avoid the vertebral artery medially. After negative aspiration, injection of contrast under fluoroscopy is recommended to assure correct placement of the needle. If the needle is too medial, it may cause inadvertent puncture of the vertebral artery or the dural sleeve. Barring intravascular spread of contrast, medication can be incrementally injected with intermittent aspiration via extension tubing under close scrutiny for neurovascular compromise or change in neurologic status.

Atlantoaxial Injection Under Fluoroscopic Guidance

The patient is similarly positioned and prepared as above. It is critically important to adjust the C-arm and clearly visualize the AA joint (Fig. 36.2). The target for AA joint injection is the space between the exiting C2 root and the vertebral artery. A needle should be directed toward the junction of the middle and lateral thirds of the posterior aspect of the joint to avoid the C2 nerve root medially or the vertebral artery laterally. After negative aspiration, injection of contrast under live fluoroscopy is recommended to assure correct needle placement (Fig. 36.3). Barring intravascular spread of contrast, medication can be

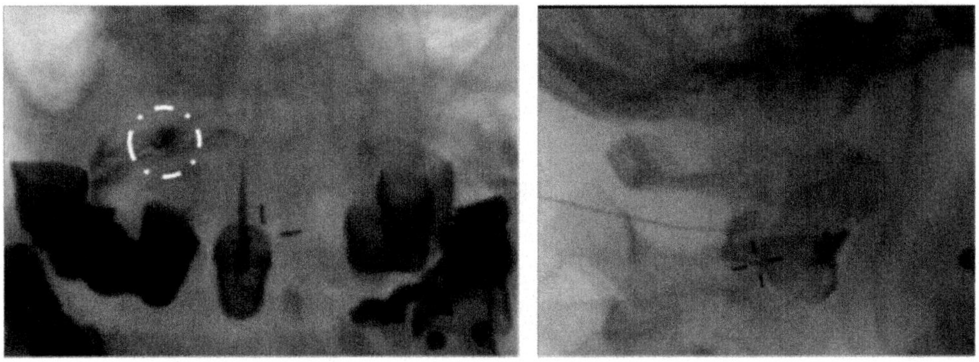

Fig. 36.3 Identifying the vertebral body of C1 and C2. *Left*: Note the vertebral body of C2, with a prominent odontoid process in the midline and coaxial view of the needle hub in the atlantoaxial joint. *White dashed line circle* around the hub. *Right*: Note the contrast dye outlining the *joint lines*. Lateral image demonstrating needle and contrast dye in the atlantoaxial joint

incrementally injected with intermittent aspiration via extension tubing under close scrutiny for neurovascular compromise or change in neurologic status.

Complications

Complications associated with AO/AA injection are related to the close proximity of the target structures to the foramen magnum and the vertebral arteries. Injury to the brain stem and spinal cord may result directly from inadvertent needle placement or indirectly form intravascular injection that leads to compromised blood flow to the brain and spinal cord. Inadvertent intravascular injection of local anesthetic can lead to anesthetic toxicity, presenting as ataxia, dizziness, or seizures. Other signs and symptoms of anesthetic toxicity include a metallic taste in the mouth and ringing in the ears. Injection of particulate steroids may lead to embolic infarction of the central nervous system. Subarachnoid administration of local anesthetic in this region can result in an immediate total spinal anesthetic. These injections are contraindicated in patients with cervical joint hypermobility or joint instability.

Suggested Reading

1. Aprill C, Axinn MJ, Bogduk N. Occipital headaches stemming from the lateral atlanto-axial (C1-2) joint. Cephalalgia. 2002;22(1):15–22.
2. Bogduk N. The anatomical basis for cervicogenic headache. J Manip Physiol Ther. 1992;15:67–70.
3. Busch E, Wilson PR. Atlanto-occipital and atlanto-axial injections in the treatment of headache and neck pain. Reg Anesth. 1989;14(Suppl 2):45.
4. Chua NHL, Halim W, Evers AWM, Vissers KCP. Whiplash patients with cervicogenic headache after lateral atlanto-axial joint pulsed radiofrequency treatment. Anesth Pain Med. 2012; 1(3):162–7.
5. Halim W, Chua NH, Vissers KC. Long-term pain relief in patients with cervicogenic headaches after pulsed radiofrequency application into the lateral atlantoaxial (C1-2) joint using an anterolateral approach. Pain Pract. 2010;10(4):267–71.
6. Narouze SN, Casanova J, Mekhail N. The longitudinal effectiveness of lateral atlanto-axial intra-articular steroid injection in the management of cervicogenic headache. Pain Med. 2007;8:184–8.

Facet Medial Branch Block

37

W. Porter McRoberts

Key Concepts

- The facet joints are well-documented, common sources of spinal pain.
- The medial branch (MB) block of the dorsal primary ramus subserves the facet joints and a chemical or steroidal block of the nerve serves both as a diagnostic predicate to facet joint denervation as well as a potentially therapeutic intervention.
- Facet medial branch block (MBB) can safely be performed in the cervical, thoracic and lumbar spine, but varying level of evidence support MBB possibly because there exists low variability in MB anatomy in the cervical and lumbar spines and more inconsistency the thoracic spine.
- Cervical facet syndromes can contribute to cervicogenic headache particularly with painful joints high in the cervical spine; joints lower may also contribute to shoulder and thoracic pain.
- Thoracic facet joints, while less likely to be diseased secondary to the relative stability yielded by ribs, also respond well to blockade and ablation.
- Lumbar facets are most commonly involved and in addition to the associated low back pain may also generate pain that radiates to the hips and thighs.
- MBB should not be confused with intra-articular injection of the facet. While both address the joint, they serve very different purposes.

Introduction

Interest in the specific course of the posterior or dorsal ramus of the spinal nerve was detailed as early as 1956, and interest in percutaneous rhizolysis of the innervating nerves of the lumbar facets grew in the early 1970s particularly in Australia. Nikolai Bogduk appears to be the first (1979) to perform dissection to specifically elucidate the variability surrounding the neuroanatomy of the facet joints. Since, hundreds of publications have arisen surrounding the joints, their anatomy, and neural supply and how interventions aimed at curbing pain associated with the joints treat patients. The dorsal primary ramus of von Luschka trifurcates into lateral, intermediate, and medial branches. The medial branch serves the multifidus and interspinalis muscle, the facet joint, the interspinous ligaments, as well as other lesser structures. After trifurcation the MB again bifurcates into superior and inferior branches to serve the individual articular surface of the joint. Each joint is largely served by two independent MBs.

Anatomy

True diarthrodial joints, the facets are formed via the articular processes of the inferior and superior laminar projections and are present from C1 inferiorly to the sacrum. Posteriorly, they are capsulated, and when arthritic, joint access angles change considerably. Anteriorly the capsule is formed of ligamentum flavum and is often fenestrated or incompetent, thus allowing the physiologic release of joint fluid. Total joint volume is variable from 1 to 2 cubic centimeters (cc).

W. Porter McRoberts, MD (✉)
Interventional Spine, Pain and Neurosurgery, Holy Cross Hospital, 3111 NE 44th St., Fort Lauderdale, FL 33308, USA
e-mail: portermcroberts@gmail.com

J.E. Pope, T.R. Deer (eds.), *Treatment of Chronic Pain Conditions*, DOI 10.1007/978-1-4939-6976-0_37

MBB Technique and Implications

The actual method of needle delivery is beyond the scope of the chapter; however, understanding the neurophysiology of the block is important (Figs. 37.1 and 37.2). Numbing the skin reduces pain associated with the injection and likely minimally affects the specificity of the block. The needle is then passed down to the corresponding innervating nerve(s) in succession, and an aliquot of local anesthetic is used. The larger the aliquot, the more likely are collateral structures to also be blocked, such as disk and or spinal nerve, and thus specificity suffers. Smaller aliquots increase sensitivity and put onus on the interventionalist's accuracy. Most suggest a half cc of volume per MBB. The duration of blockade is largely dependent on the anesthetic used. The optional addition of corticosteroid dilutes the concentration of the anesthetic and may confound the results not only because of diminished effect of the local, but also because the patient may associate the delayed effects (without immediate effect) with a positive block. The addition of steroid however has been associated with prolonged pain relief, and in some the blocks may also be therapeutic, negating the need for rhizotomy. When removing the needle, some leave a light wake of local anesthetic to diminish the resultant and possibly confounding pain of the procedure itself; however, the contrary opinion argues, painful paraspinal muscles respond to intramuscular local anesthetic well, and this too may confound results. Accurate MBB also chemodenervates nonarticular structures such as the multifidus and interspinalis muscles as well as the interspinal the supraspinal ligaments and other potentially painful structures, and while diminishing the specificity of the block for diagnosing articular pain, it is the most prognostic for successful denervation. Lastly, debate continues regarding the utility of one versus two prognostic blocks and the cutoff percentage of pain relief for "successful." Making denervation contingent upon two blocks or higher percentages while increasing the percentage of successful denervations does diminish the overall treatment success number.

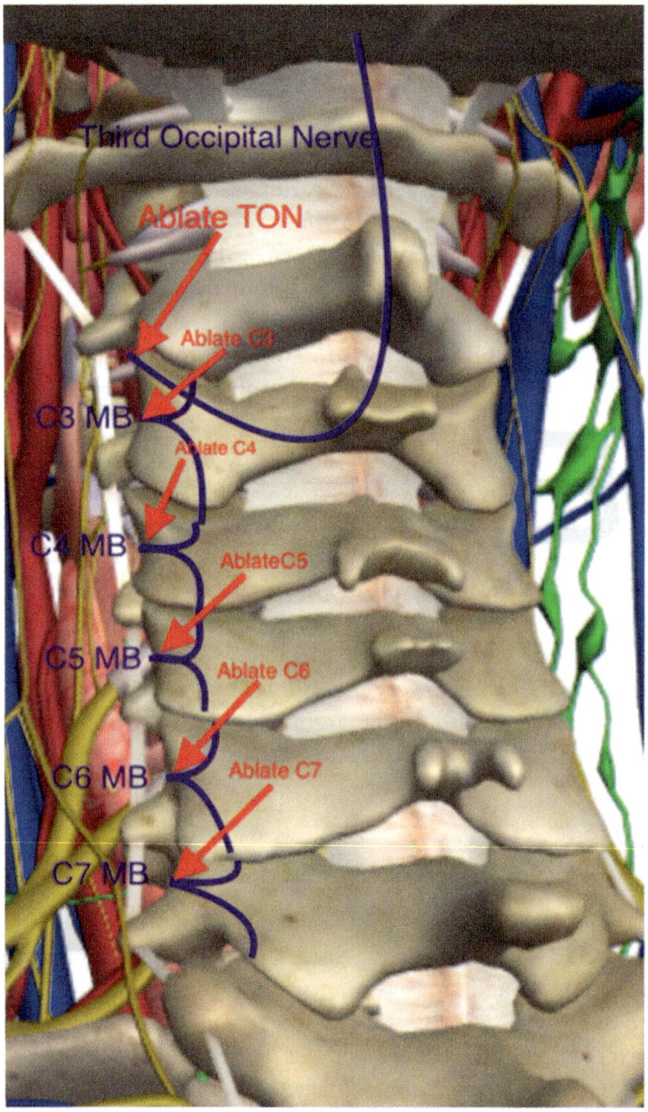

Fig. 37.1 Optimal cervical loci for facet joint denervation

Some argue, however, that the blockade is essentially unnecessary as the rhizotomy is neither detrimental, dangerous, nor expensive, and the blockade serves only to delay treatment, increase medical costs, and cause pain to the patient.

Intra-articular injection is the most specific in diagnosing the intra-articular facet as the source of pain; however, overfill runoff usually runs anteriorly into the epidural posterior lateral recess where the spinal nerve lies. If prediction of successful rhizotomy is the aim, then MBB is best.

Conclusions

Facet joints are a common cause of spinal pain, and MBB remains the best overall prognostic tool for evaluating the potential success of denervation. Accuracy in needle placement increases specificity. Debate ensues regarding the need for prognostic steps, as the denervation is safe and effective.

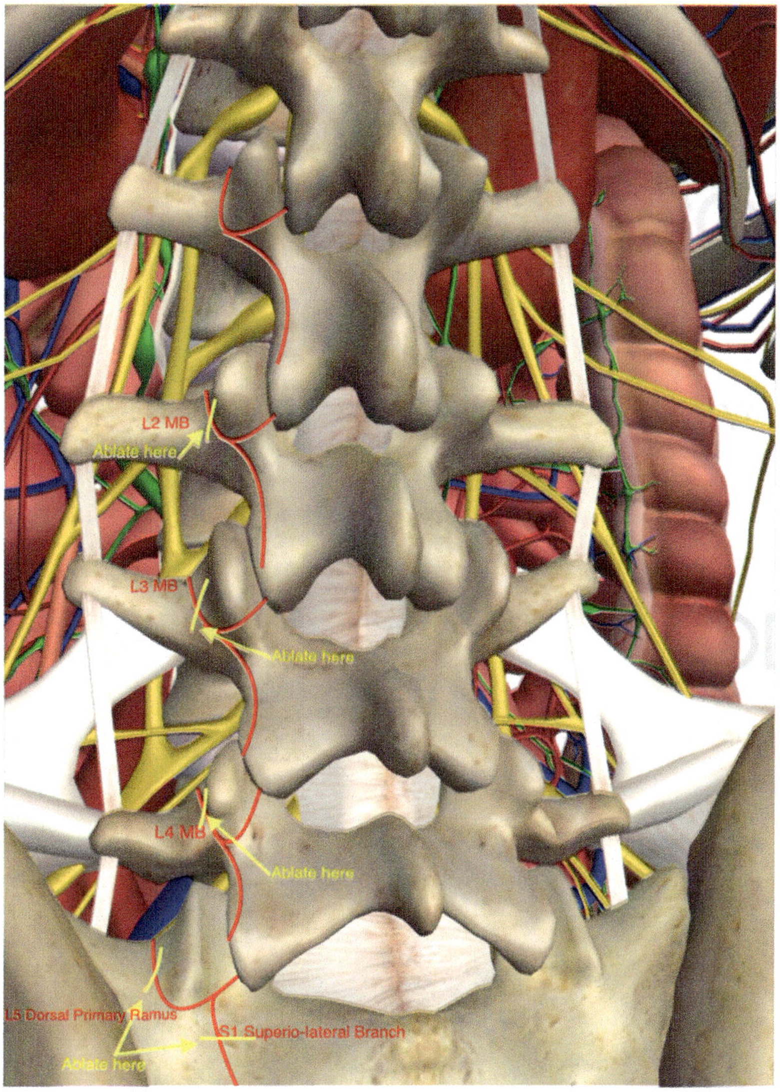

Fig. 37.2 Optimal lumbar loci for denervation

Suggested Reading

1. Bogduk N, Long DM. The anatomy of the so-called "articular nerves" and their relationship to facet denervation in the treatment of low-back pain. J Neurosurg. 1979;51(2):172–7.
2. Civelek E, Cansever T, Kabatas S, Kircelli A, Yilmaz C, Musluman M, Ofluoglu D, Caner H. Comparison of effectiveness of facet joint injection and radiofrequency denervation in chronic low back pain. Turk Neurosurg. 2012;22(2):200–6.
3. Cohen SP, Huang JH, Brummett C. Facet joint pain – advances in patient selection and treatment. Nat Rev Rheumatol. 2013;9(2):101–16.
4. Fenton DS, Czervionke LF, editors. Image-guided spine intervention. Philadelphia: Saunders Elsevier; 2003.
5. Manchikanti L, Pampati V, Fellows B, Bakhit CE. The diagnostic validity and therapeutic value of lumbar facet joint nerve blocks with or without adjuvant agents. Curr Rev Pain. 2000;4(5):337–44.
6. Maslow GS, Rothman R. The facet joints: another look. Bull N Y Acad Med. 1975;51(11):1294–311.
7. Pederson H, Bluncik E, Gardner G. The anatomy of lumbosacral posterior rami and meningeal branches of spinal nerve. J Bone Joint Surg Am. 1956;38A:379.
8. van Kleef M, Barendse GA, Kessels A, Voets HM, Weber WE, de Lange S. Randomized trial of radiofrequency lumbar facet denervation for chronic low back pain. Spine (Phila Pa 1976). 1999;24(18):1937–42.

Facet Medial Branch Ablation

38

W. Porter McRoberts

Key Concepts

- Denervation is typically performed via radiofrequency (RF) ablation but can also be performed with either cryoneurolysis or chemoneurolysis
- Thermal ablation can provide significant relief for the better part of a year for most patients
- Cryoneurolysis yields neuropraxic injury without neurotmesis, temperatures typical of liquid nitrogen yield 3–4 months relief; colder temperatures generate possibly longer periods of pain relief
- Lesion size is directly proportional to nerve injury likelihood, and significant industry energy is aimed at increasing lesion size safely
- Sensory testing may increase accuracy and nerve injury likelihood
- Motor testing may predict safety
- With typical radiofrequency ablation, very little tissue destruction occurs distal to the spindle-shaped lesion, making needle placement and understanding of lesion shape critical to success

Introduction

Early in the 1970s, Rees and later Toakley appear to be among the first to attempt fluoroscopically directed medial branch sectioning via radiofrequency technique. Soon thereafter Norman Shealy reported on electrocoagulation rhizolysis. Toakley's results of 200 sectioned patients revealed a surprisingly excellent outcome of 125 good results and 37 fair results with a follow-up of 6 months to 2 years.

W. Porter McRoberts, MD (✉)
Interventional Spine, Pain and Neurosurgery, Holy Cross Hospital, 3111 NE 44th St, Fort Lauderdale, FL 33308, USA
e-mail: portermcroberts@gmail.com

Techniques

The conventional RF generator provides the following several essential functions:

Function	Purpose
Sensory nerve stimulation (50 Hz)	Proximity to target sensory nerve
Motor nerve stimulation (2 Hz)	Proximity to motor nerve (or spinal nerve)
Temperature monitoring	Ensure appropriate coagula
Impedance monitoring	Confirm physiologic electric circuit

Temperatures	Function
42.5–44 °C	Temporary conduction block
45–50 °C	Early cytotoxic range
70–80 °C	Irreversible lesioning
>90 °C	Carbonization of tissues

Proximity predicts success and, importantly, catastrophe. To serve that end, 0.25 V depolarizes nerve when immediately adjacent, and 2 V depolarizes at 1 cm distant. Lower sensory thresholds indicate increased proximity, and the absence of radicular neural recruitment at high thresholds indicates safe distance. Lesion size can be influenced by injectate, temperature, and gauge of the needle employed. Commonly, a 10 mm active tip is employed for radiofrequency.

Cervical Testing

Motor 2-Hz: 2.0 V without radicular stimulation.

Sensory 50-Hz: 0.25–0.50 V local recruitment suggests good proximity.

Sensory 50-Hz: 1.0 V absence of radicular recruitment indicates safety.

J.E. Pope, T.R. Deer (eds.), *Treatment of Chronic Pain Conditions*, DOI 10.1007/978-1-4939-6976-0_38

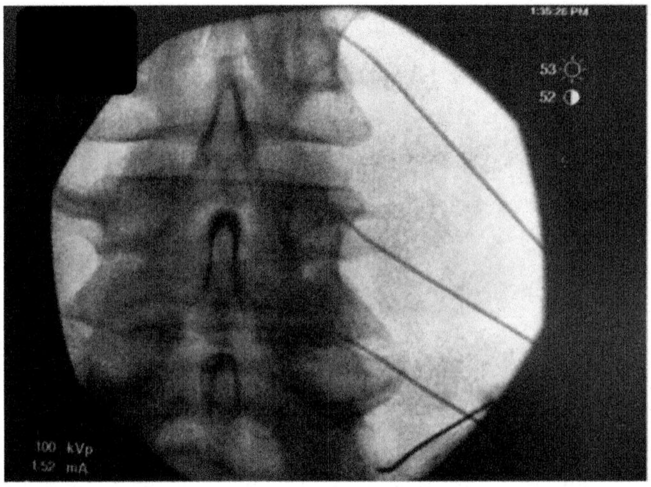

Fig. 38.1 AP lumbar spot film of needle placement for low-threshold sensory testing indicating excellent location

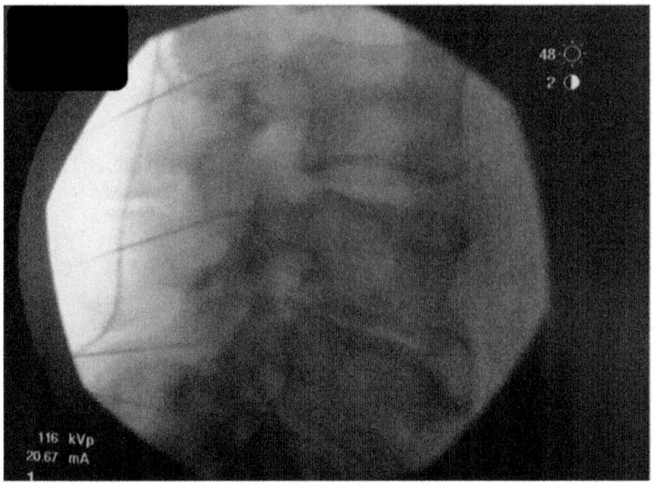

Fig. 38.2 Lateral view lumbar needle placement

Lumbar Testing (Figs 38.1 and 38.2)

Motor 2-Hz: 3.0 V without radicular stimulation.

Sensory 50-Hz: 0.25–0.50 V local recruitment suggests good proximity.

Sensory 50-Hz: 1.0 V absence of radicular recruitment indicates safety.

Conclusions

Facet joints are a common cause of spinal pain, and MBB remains the best overall prognostic tool for evaluating the potential success of denervation. Accuracy in needle placement increases specificity. Debate ensues regarding the need for prognostic steps, as the denervation is safe and effective.

Suggested Reading

1. Brodkey J, Miyazaki I, Ervin F, Mark V. Reversible heat lesions: a method of stereotactic localization. J Neurosurg. 1964;21:49.
2. Kline MT. Radiofrequency techniques in clinical practice. In: Waldman S, Winnie A, editors. Interventional pain management. Philadelphia: W.B. Saunders; 1996. p. 185–217.
3. Moringlane JR, Koch R, Schafer H, Ostertag CHB. Experimental radiofrequency coagulation with computer-based on line monitoring of temperature and power. Acta Neurochir. 1989;96:126–31.
4. Rees W. Multiple bilateral subcutaneous rhizolysis of segmented nerve in the treatment of intervertebral disc syndrome. Ann Gen Pract. 1971;16:126.
5. Toakley J. Subcutaneous lumbar "rhizolysis": an assessment of 200 cases. Med J Aust. 1973;2:490.

39 Epidural Injection in Chronic Pain Management

Ramana K. Naidu

Key Points

- Epidural analgesia has been used for chronic pain management for over a century.
- The anatomy of the spinal epidural space has several misconceptions, and proceduralists should be knowledgeable about the details of this unique space.
- There are several approaches, trajectories, and techniques to enter the epidural space and several needle designs have been employed and modified over time.
- Therapy using local anesthetics, steroids, and normal saline has been widely used for epidural analgesia.
- The risks of epidural analgesia include post-meningeal puncture headache, hematoma, infection, and neurologic complications.
- Outcomes are mixed. Certain conditions that result in radicular pain appear to have short-term benefit.

Introduction

The reported first attempt and successful injection of drug for chronic pain management occurred in 1901 in France by Jean-Athanase Sicard and Fernand Cathelin. The unique features of injection into this relatively small space were the production of *segmental neural blockade* and *influence on neuraxial pathology*. Since then, the epidural space has been used to manage acute, chronic, and cancer pain. This review will focus on its use in chronic pain management.

R.K. Naidu, MD (✉)
University of California at San Francisco, Department of Anesthesia & Perioperative Care, Division of Pain Medicine, 2255 Post St, San Francisco, CA 94115, USA
e-mail: ramana.naidu@ucsf.edu

Anatomy

A discussion regarding epidural analgesia is founded on an understanding of the anatomy, which has gone through several controversies over the past century. It is imperative that practitioners are aware of the details and potential aberrancies of this unique anatomical structure (Fig. 39.1). The spinal epidural space is distinct from the cranial epidural space; the spinal epidural space is often coined a potential space, but the fact that it is filled with fat, arterioles, Batson's venous plexus, and lymphatics with millimeters of thickness which can be viewed with any MRI or CT contradicts the definition of a potential space—it is in fact an actual space (Figs. 39.2, 39.3, and, 39.4). The cranial epidural space is a potential space. The posterior spinal epidural space is between dura and ligamentum flavum and runs from foramen magnum to the sacrococcygeal ligament (Fig. 39.5). On the lateral aspects of the epidural space, rootlets exit the neuroforamina. Injectate flows along rootlets, to the nerve roots and dorsal root ganglia (Fig. 39.6) [1]. The thickest portion of the epidural space is typically at the interlaminar interspace in the posterior midline. The anterior aspect of the epidural space which is between the posterior longitudinal ligament, and the dura is of interest because this is where injectate may have an impact on disc pathology. There is significant heterogeneity of the epidural space with changes in thickness anterior to the spinous process and around pedicles; although often depicted as a contiguous and symmetric sheet based on artists' renderings in textbooks, it is more often not (Fig. 39.7). In rare instances, *plica mediana dorsalis*, a midline septum, can prevent bilateral spread of injectate [2].

Anatomy of Pathology

There are several etiologies for neck and back pain with or without radicular pain. The discs have nerves, including the sinuvertebral and gray rami innervating the annu-

J.E. Pope, T.R. Deer (eds.), *Treatment of Chronic Pain Conditions*, DOI 10.1007/978-1-4939-6976-0_39

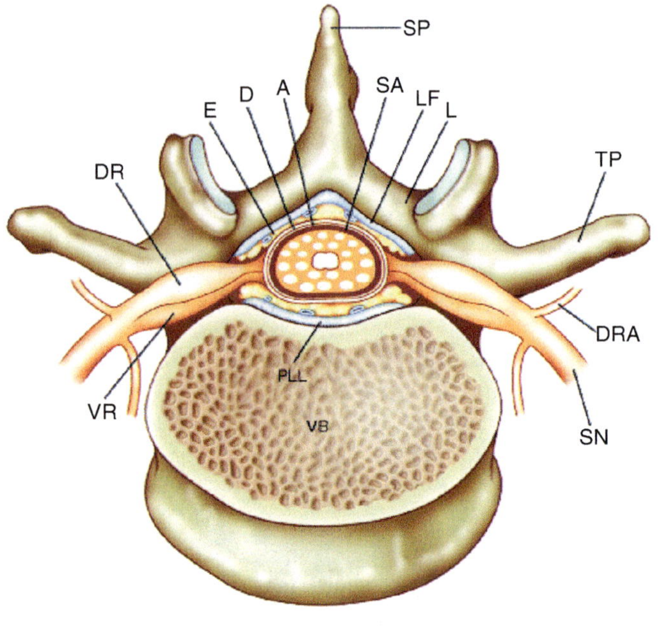

Fig. 39.1 Local anesthetics may abolish sensation in various parts of the body by topical application, injection in the vicinity of peripheral nerve endings and along major nerve trunks, or instillation within the epidural or subarachnoid space. The ensuing sensory block occurs locally and spreads to areas distal along the nerve pathway (With permission from Deer et al. [27]. © American Academy of Pain Medicine 2013)

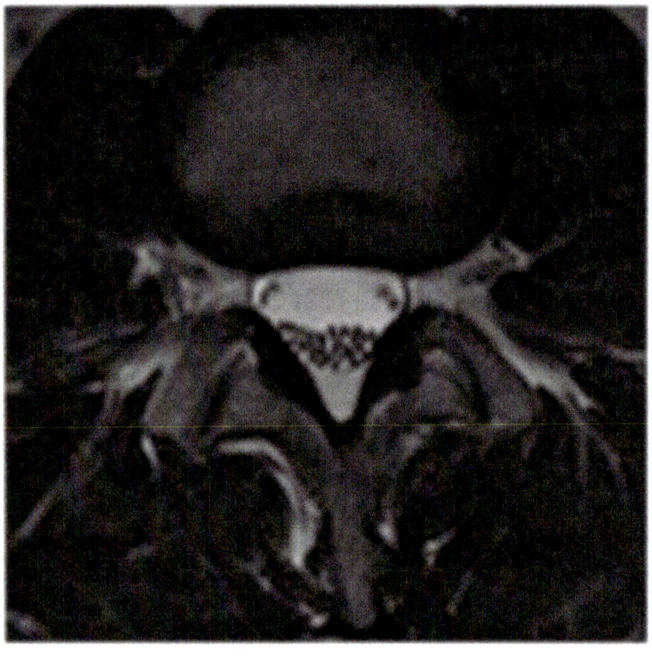

Fig. 39.2 Magnetic resonance imaging of lumbar spine. Axial T2-weighted image demonstrates the dorsal and lateral epidural space (Acknowledgement of Dr. Alex Schabel)

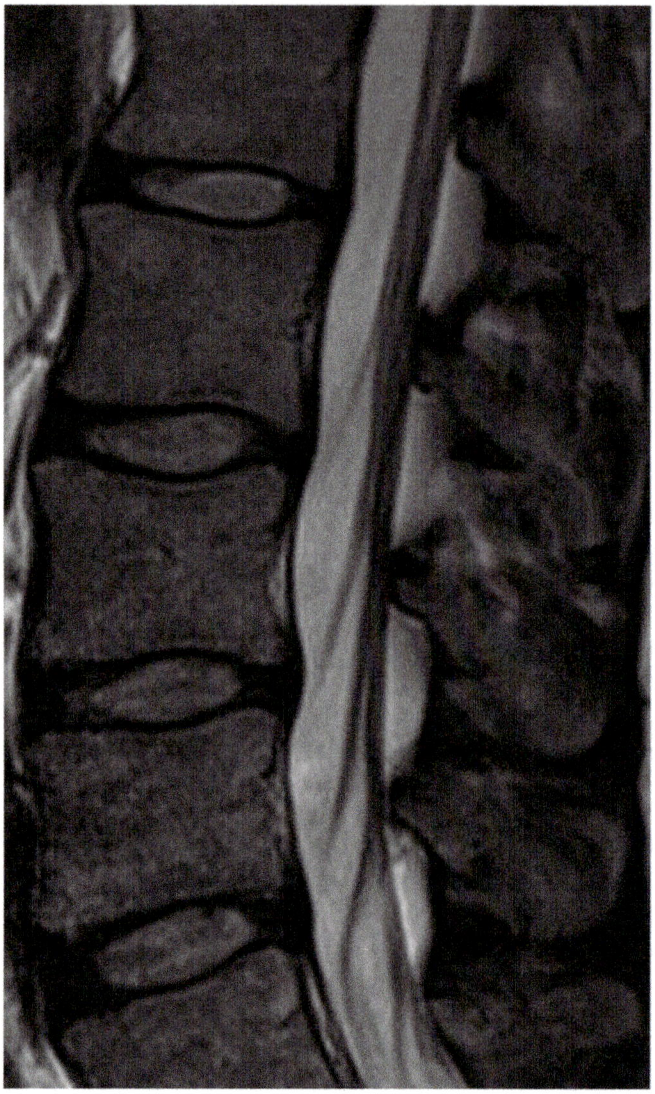

Fig. 39.3 Magnetic resonance imaging of lumbar spine. Sagittal T2-weighted images revealing the typical "sawtooth" pattern of the posterior midline epidural fat (Acknowledgement of Dr. Alex Schabel)

lus fibrosus which can be nociceptive due to inflammation or trauma. When there is a disc herniation, the nucleus pulposus, a vestige of the notochord, may extrude its contents of proteoglycans onto nerves causing significant nociceptive input. The natural history of disc herniation is not as dire as once believed—most patients recover without intervention as discs do protrude, extrude, and absorb over time [3] although predicting where resorption versus continued pathology will occur and in whom is difficult to predict at this time.

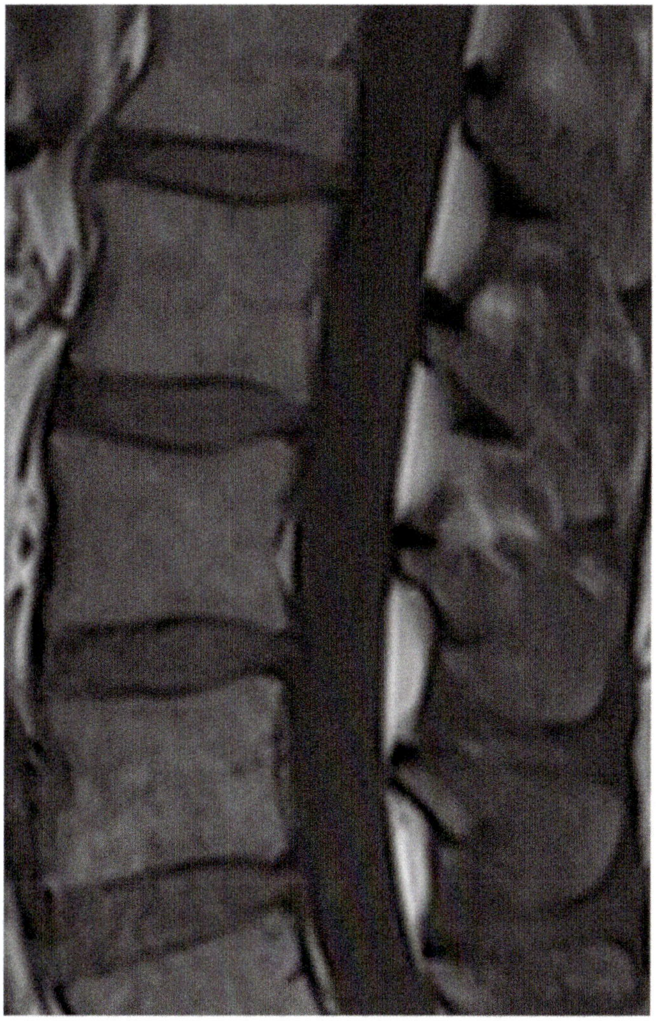

Fig. 39.4 Magnetic resonance imaging of lumbar spine. Sagittal T1-weighted images revealing the typical "sawtooth" pattern of the posterior midline epidural fat (Acknowledgement of Dr. Alex Schabel)

The neuroforamina may be occluded causing lateral stenosis due to disc herniation, facet hypertrophy, synovial cyst, or scarring. Central spinal canal stenosis can be congenital, as in short pedicle syndrome, or due to degeneration which has an estimated prevalence of 19.4% of the US population aged 60–69 years with absolute spinal stenosis based on CT imaging; not all of these patients have symptoms of neurogenic claudication [4]. Stenosis can result from disc herniation, ligamentum flavum hypertrophy, vertebral osteophytosis, posterior longitudinal ligament osteosis, facet hypertrophy, compression fracture, or spondylolisthesis.

In addition to understanding these structural components that may stimulate nociceptive inputs, it is crucial that practitioners understand that pain is an unpleasant sensory and emotional experience [5]. An individuals' genotype, phenotype, and psychological makeup also play a role in what they describe as pain, or suffering.

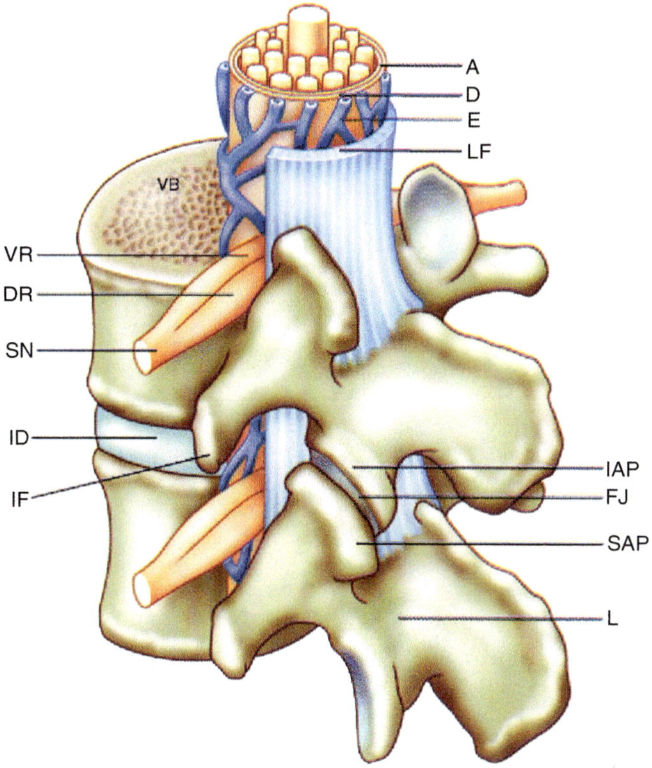

Fig. 39.5 Layers of the neuraxial canal (With permission from Deer et al. [27]. © American Academy of Pain Medicine 2013)

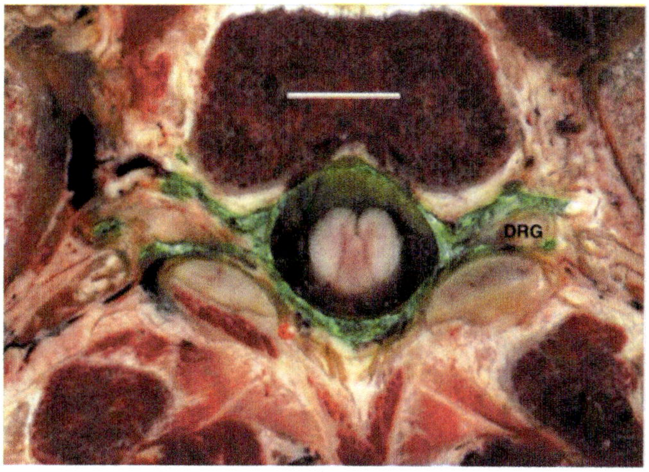

Fig. 39.6 Axial cryomicrotome of the second thoracic vertebrae and spinal nerve. *DRG* dorsal root ganglion (With permission from Hogan [1]. © Wolters Kluwer Health Inc.)

Techniques

The epidural space can be approached via several routes in the sacral, lumbar, thoracic, and cervical spine (Fig. 39.8). The *interlaminar* approach involves a posterior introduction of the needle between the superior and inferior lamina

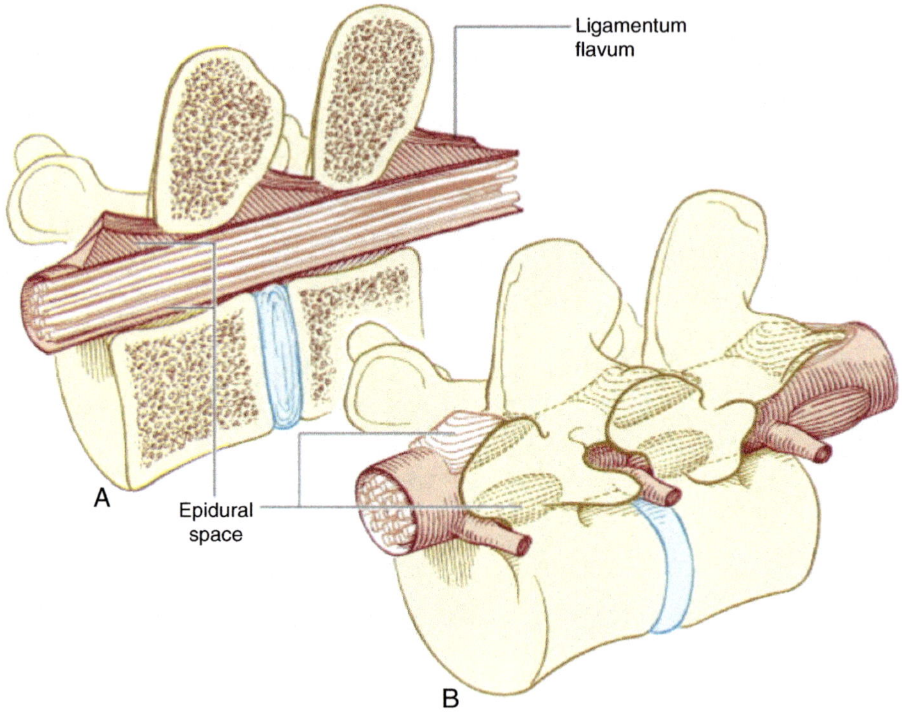

Fig. 39.7 Conceptual model of the epidural space with pockets of incongruity (Image obtained from SlideShare.net)

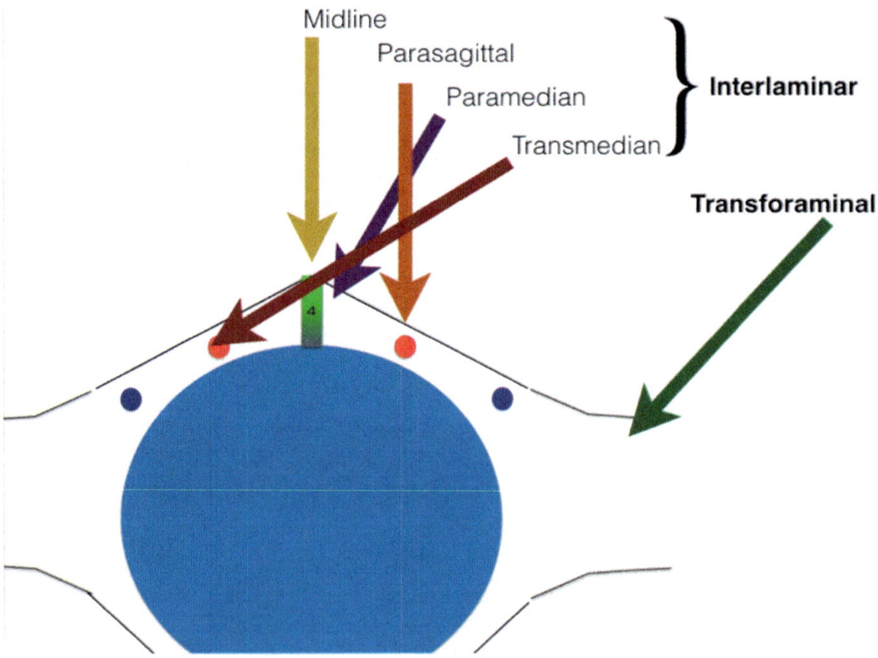

Fig. 39.8 Conceptual approaches to enter the epidural space. The interlaminar approach has four trajectories: midline, paramedian, parasagittal, and transmedian. The transforaminal approach enters laterally in the neuroforamina

of the desired levels of the cervical, thoracic, and lumbar spine. The commonly performed trajectories include the midline and paramedian. Some operators choose to perform a parasagittal or transmedian trajectory to deposit injectate to one side of the epidural space, ideally where the pathology exists. The *caudal* approach enters the epidural space from its most inferior aspect at the sacral hiatus with piercing of the sacrococcygeal ligament. Determination of the approach or interspace to enter and/or target depends on where a patient describes their nociceptive input, which is often corroborated by provocative testing and radiologic imaging. The type of needle used for this approach is generally a more blunt needle so operators can feel the differences in tissue, with particular attention on the pressure gradient on the syringe plunger between the ligamentum flavum and into the epidural space [6]. The Tuohy, Coudé, Weiss, Crawford, or Hustead needles are blunt needles and come in a variety of sizes for entry from 14 gauge for spinal cord stimulator leads to 22 gauge for single-shot injection. Catheters come in various materials and can be steered through needles to the area of pathology. The Tuohy needle was developed by Ralph Huber, DMD, and utilized by Edward Tuohy, MD, for continuous spinal anesthesia in 1945 [7]. This needle has since been used for continuous epidural analgesia, starting with Curbelo on 1949, and has the advantageous property of a scalloped surface on the back of the bevel allowing for laminar sliding.

Entry into the epidural space can be determined via several approaches, most commonly, the loss-of-resistance technique, which was developed by the Italian physician, Achille Mario Dogliotti, in 1933. The loss-of-resistance technique can be accomplished with a low-friction piston/syringe (glass or plastic) using saline or air. Saline is recommended to reduce the potential risk of pneumocephalus if there is intrathecal infiltration, although there may be situations where using air has advantages [8]. Other ways to determine entry into the epidural space include the hanging drop method, catheter insertion, fiber optics, and epiduroscopy.

The *transforaminal* approach starts at a point lateral on a patient's back and enters via the neuroforamen. This technique does not use loss-of-resistance and utilizes a spinal needle (Quincke, Chiba) to end either adjacent to the nerve root or at a point contiguous with the epidural space. All of these techniques are confirmed using contrast media under fluoroscopy to watch spread along nerve roots or with epidural fat delineation and spinous process sparing, to differentiate from intrathecal spread, or a myelogram. The landmark or blind approach has fallen out of favor due to poor reliability in entering the epidural space, although was the pioneering method for entry. Ultrasound can be a useful imaging tool, particularly in pregnant patients where radiation is contraindicated [9].

The epidural space can be used to place catheters for continuous infusion such as in acute or cancer pain, to place leads for dorsal column stimulation, or if adhesions in the epidural space are a source of nociception, adhesiolysis can be performed. The remainder of this chapter will focus on epidural steroid injections.

Therapeutic Injectate

Local anesthetics were the first drugs injected into the epidural space, starting with cocaine in 1901. Even with the longest-acting local anesthetics to date, relief is still on the order of several hours via voltage-gated sodium channel blockade. For this reason, other agents have been added to prolong relief. Steroids were introduced into the epidural space in 1952 by Robecchi and Capra, and despite a voluminous history of epidural steroid injections, steroids are not FDA approved for use in the epidural space today. The North American Spine Society, Agency for Healthcare Research and Quality, and Department of Health and Human Services recognize that epidural steroid injections are part of the management for radicular pain. It is hypothesized that steroids work by decreasing inflammation by inhibiting PLA2 [10], reducing vascular permeability, or by epigenetic mechanisms [11], which may account for the delay (days) in relief. The relief from steroids is variable from patient to patient. Glucocorticoids are preferred for epidural steroid injections because of their greater anti-inflammatory activity (Fig. 39.9). There has been controversy regarding the ability of particulate steroids to aggregate and their potential role in neurologic injury. For this reason, non-particulate steroids are recommended. Greater scrutiny of steroids occurred in 2012 when the New England Compounding Center (NECC) shipped methylprednisolone that was contaminated by fungi leading to 800 individuals developing meningitis—this tragic event led to 64 deaths [12]. Steroid frequency and dose must be monitored; chronic neuraxial steroid use can lead to hypercorticism, adrenal suppression, osteopenia, impaired glucose tolerance, and increased intraocular pressure, among other side effects.

Other adjuvants in chronic pain management have not been as widely explored as compared to acute pain management where adjuvants such as epinephrine, clonidine, neostigmine, cyclooxygenase inhibitors, etc. have been used. One of the unspoken therapeutics in epidural injections is normal saline, a substance that is not benign. Future development of therapeutics in the epidural space to modulate pathology, dorsal root ganglia, or nerves could be impactful in chronic pain management (Table 39.1).

Contraindications and Risks

The contraindications to this procedure include patient refusal, an allergy to any of the substances in contact with the patient, systemic infection or local infection at the needle entry site, bleeding dyscrasia, or on an antithrombotic agent without proper cessation. In a retrospective study of 4265 ESIs, the most common complications were increased pain (1.1%), pain at site of injection (0.33%), persistent numbness (0.14%), and "others" (0.80%) [13].

Meningeal puncture is a risk and can result in postural headache. Bernards expressed that the term post-dural puncture headache (PDPH) is inaccurate because dura mater is actually porous; he advocated the term post-meningeal puncture headache (PMPH) [14]. PMPH appears to be more rare in chronic pain management, with one retrospective analysis

STEROIDS

	Drug	Approximate Equivalent Dose	Relative Anti-Inflammatory Potency	Relative Mineralcorticoid Potency	0-10 micrometers (Benzon)	11-20 micrometers (Benzon)	21-50 micrometers (Benzon)	>50 micrometers (Benzon)	Particle Image (Benzon)
Short	Cortisone	25 mg	0.8	2					
	Hydrocortisone	20 mg	1	2					
Intermediate	Prednisone	5 mg	4	1					
	Prednisolone	5 mg	4	1					
	Triamcinolone	4 mg	5	0	71	8	9	12	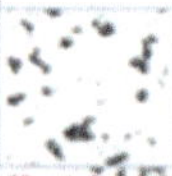
	Methylprednisolone (Depo-Medrol®)	4 mg	5	0	53	11	8	27	
Long	Dexamethasone (Decadron®)	0.75 mg	25-30	0	0	0	0	0	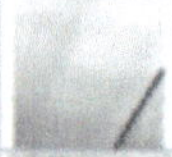
	Betamethasone Sodium Phosphate (Celestone®)	0.6 - 0.75 mg	25	0	61	7	10	22	
	Betamethasone Sodium Phosphate	0.6 - 0.75 mg	25	0	0	0	0	0	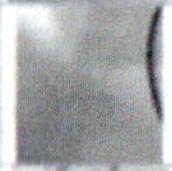
	Betamethasone Sodium Phosphate/ Betamethasone Acetate	0.6 - 0.75 mg	25	0					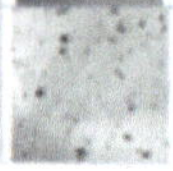

Fig. 39.9 Relative properties of steroids (Adapted from Benzon et al. [26])

Table 39.1 Indications in chronic pain management

Disc herniation
Central spinal canal stenosis
Neuroforaminal stenosis
Facet or nerve root cyst with radicular pain
Compression fracture of the spine with radicular pain
Postherpetic neuralgia

stating an incidence of 0.004% [13], than it is in labor analgesia, approximately 1% [15], due to several factors including imaging and age differences. Management of PMPH is generally time, fluid, caffeine, cyclooxygenase inhibitors, potentially triptans, and epidural blood patch [16].

Risks of epidural injections include bleeding in the epidural space resulting in an epidural hematoma, which could lead to paralysis if not identified and evacuated [17, 18]. In 2015, the American Society of Regional Anesthesia and Pain Medicine (ASRA) developed their guidelines on the use of antithrombotics for interventional pain procedures. [19] It should be noted that even strict adherence to these guidelines does not prevent this complication absolutely. Patients are at rare risk for segmental medullary artery or artery of Adamkiewicz vasospasm or occlusion from transforaminal injections; this can result in anterior spinal artery ischemia and paralysis [20]. Infections can occur locally at the site of injection, cellulitis; into the epidural space, becoming an epidural abscess; or along the meninges, to become meningitis. Needles and catheters have found their way into and around nerve roots, as well as into the spinal cord. Development of cauda equina syndrome has been reported [21]. A review of methods to reduce neurologic complications related to epidural steroid injections was published in *Anesthesiology* and is worth review [22].

Outcomes

The study on the outcomes of epidural steroid injections has historically been poor, and in order to understand the impact of this intervention on individuals and populations, better studies must be conducted and published without bias. Various operators, routes, injectate properties, approaches, pathologies, and individual differences make studying outcomes an extraordinary challenge. After the NECC fungal meningitis outbreak, *The New England Journal of Medicine* published a perspective article that stated "clinicians persist in clinical practices despite weak evidence of efficacy." [23] A review and meta-analysis in *Pain Physician* in 2015 looked at 52 articles that met manuscript criteria (with 72 excluded) and concluded that there is level II evidence for ESI for disc herniation, discogenic pain, postsurgery back syndrome, and spinal canal stenosis [24]. In 2013, Cohen et al. summarized the evidence regarding the use of epidural steroid injections, their impact on patient beneficence, cost-effectiveness, prevention of surgery, return to work, and healthcare utilization [25].

Conclusion

At 115 years since the first epidural for chronic pain management, we are still in our developing stages of understanding the power of the epidural space. Its physiologic purpose is enigmatic, and some interventionists feel its purpose is to provide a conduit to one of the most epidemiologically pressing health problems in humans—low back and neck pain. We have a long way to go to understand which candidates are best for such intervention to improve our currently shaky outcomes. Refining understanding, techniques, and development of drugs will progress the utility of epidural analgesia in chronic pain management.

References

1. Hogan Q. Distribution of solution in the epidural space: examination by cryomicrotome section. Reg Anesth Pain Med. 2002;27:150–6.
2. Gallart L, Blanco D, Samso E, Vidal F. Clinical and radiologic evidence of the epidural plica mediana dorsalis. Anesth Analg. 1990;71:698–701.
3. Benoist M. The natural history of lumbar disc herniation and radiculopathy. Joint Bone Spine. 2002;69:155–60.
4. Kalichman L, et al. Spinal stenosis prevalence and association with symptoms: the Framingham Study. Spine J. 2009;9:545–50.
5. International Association for the Study of Pain (IASP) – Taxonomy. at http://www.iasp-pain.org/Taxonomy.
6. Usubiaga JE, Wikinski JA, Usubiaga LE. A note on the recording of epidural negative pressure. Anesth Analg. 1967;46:119–22.
7. Martini JA, Bacon DR, Vasdev GM. Edward Tuohy: the man, his needle, and its place in obstetric analgesia. Reg Anesth Pain Med. 2002;27:520–3.
8. Verdun AV, Cohen SP, Williams BS, Hurley RW. Pneumocephalus after lumbar epidural steroid injection: a case report and review of the literature. A A Case Rep. 2014;**3**:9–13.
9. Narouze S. Atlas of ultrasound-guided procedures in interventional pain management. New York: Springer; 2011.
10. Saal JS. The role of inflammation in lumbar pain. Spine (Phila Pa 1976). 1995;20:1821–7.
11. Hunter RG, Gagnidze K, McEwen BS, Pfaff DW. Stress and the dynamic genome: steroids, epigenetics, and the transposome. Proc Natl Acad Sci U S A. 2015;112:6828–33.
12. Centers for Disease Control and Prevention. Multistate outbreak of fungal meningitis and other infections - case count. at http://www.cdc.gov/hai/outbreaks/meningitis-map-large.html
13. McGrath JM, Schaefer MP, Malkamaki DM. Incidence and characteristics of complications from epidural steroid injections. Pain Med. 2011;12:726–31.
14. Bernards CM. Sophistry in medicine: lessons from the epidural space. Reg Anesth Pain Med. 2005;30:56–66.
15. Flood P, Li G. A terrible headache in obstetric anesthesia. Anesthesiology. 2012;116:242–3.
16. Turnbull DK. Post-dural puncture headache: pathogenesis, prevention and treatment. Br J Anaesth. 2003;91:718–29.
17. Stoll A, Sanchez M. Epidural hematoma after epidural block: implications for its use in pain management. Surg Neurol. 2002;57:235–40.
18. Williams KN, Jackowski A, Evans PJD. Epidural haematoma requiring surgical decompression following repeated cervical epidural steroid injections for chronic pain. Pain. 1990;42:197–9.
19. Narouze S, et al. Interventional spine and pain procedures in patients on antiplatelet and anticoagulant medications. Reg Anesth Pain Med. 2015;40:182.
20. Wybier M, Gaudart S, Petrover D, Houdart E, Laredo J-D. Paraplegia complicating selective steroid injections of the lumbar spine. Report of five cases and review of the literature. Eur Radiol. 2010;20:181–9.
21. Bilir A, Gulec S. Cauda equina syndrome after epidural steroid injection: a case report. J Manipulative Physiol Ther. 2006;**29**:492.
22. Wallace M, et al. Safeguards to prevent neurologic complications after epidural steroid injections. Anesthesiology. 2015;122:974–84.
23. Outterson K. Regulating compounding pharmacies after NECC. N Engl J Med. 2012;367:1969–72.
24. Kaye AD, et al. Efficacy of epidural injections in managing chronic spinal pain: a best evidence synthesis. Pain Physician. 2015;18:E939.
25. Cohen SP, Bicket MC, Jamison D, Wilkinson I, Rathmell JP. Epidural steroids. Reg Anesth Pain Med. 2013;38:175–200.
26. Benzon H, Chew T, McCarthy R, Benzon H, Walega D. Comparison of the particle sizes of different steroids and the effect of dilution: a review of the relative neurotoxicities of the steroids. Anesthesiology. 2007;106:331–8.
27. Deer TR, et al. Comprehensive treatment of chronic pain by medical, interventional, and integrative approaches. New York: Springer; 2013. p. 258.

Suggested Reading

28. Benzon, H. et al. *Practical management of pain.* (Elsevier Health Sciences, 2013). Philadelphia
29. Cohen, S. P., Bicket, M. C., Jamison, D., Wilkinson, I. & Rathmell, J. P. Epidural steroids. Reg Anesth Pain Med. 38**,** 175–200 (2013).
30. Cousins MJ. Cousins and bridenbaugh's neural blockade in clinical anesthesia and pain medicine. Lippincott Williams & Wilkins; 2012.
31. Hogan, Q. Distribution of solution in the epidural space: examination by cryomicrotome section. Reg Anesth Pain Med 27**,** 150–156 (2002).
32. Kaye, A. D. et al. Efficacy of epidural injections in managing chronic spinal pain: a best evidence synthesis. (2015). Pain Physician 18, E939
33. Narouze, S. et al. Interventional spine and pain procedures in patients on antiplatelet and anticoagulant medications. Reg Anesth Pain Med 2015 40, 182.
34. Wallace, M. et al. Safeguards to prevent neurologic complications after epidural steroid injections. Anesthesiology 122**,** 974–984 (2015).

Stellate Ganglion Blockade

40

Emil H. Annabi, Jimmy Arefieg, and Stephen Shiller

Background

Existing in approximately 80% of cases imaged, the stellate ganglion is formed by the fusion of the inferior cervical and first thoracic ganglia of the sympathetic tract. It is normally located anterior to the transverse process of C7, superior to the neck of the first rib, and inferior to the subclavian artery.

Indications

A blockage of the stellate ganglion is utilized for both diagnostic and therapeutic purposes in pathologies affecting the upper extremities, face and head. As a diagnostic tool, the injection of local anesthetic at this site can potentially reduce pain if it has a sympathetic component.

A stellate ganglion blockade has shown to be an effective treatment for the following conditions:

- Complex regional pain syndrome
- Herpes zoster (shingles)
- Raynaud's phenomenon
- Scleroderma
- Phantom limb pain
- Hyperhidrosis
- Hot flashes
- Intractable hiccups

E.H. Annabi, MD (✉)
Pima Pain Center, Pain Medicine, Tucson, AZ 85712, USA
e-mail: eeannabi@gmail.com

J. Arefieg, MD • S. Shiller, MD
Pima Pain Center, Tucson, AZ 85712, USA

Contraindications

- Allergic reactions to local anesthetics
- Recent myocardial infarction
- Coagulopathies
- Symptomatic bradycardia

Procedure

The stellate ganglion block is performed utilizing either CT, fluoroscopic, or ultrasound guidance. While ultrasound allows for a better visualization of soft tissue anatomy without the radiation exposure, fluoroscopy provides better localization of local anesthetic delivery through the use of a contrast agent.

The most common technique for this procedure is the C6 transverse process approach. After positioning the patient supine, with head slightly turned to the contralateral side and mouth open, the physician locates Chassaignac's tubercle. This easily palpable landmark usually exists between the trachea and the carotid sheath at the level of the cricoid cartilage, medial to the sternocleidomastoid muscle (SCM). The SCM is retracted laterally, and pressure is maintained on the surrounding tissues as the needle is inserted and directed toward the tubercle. One percent lidocaine with sodium bicarbonate is injected creating a skin wheel over the tubercle. Under fluoroscopic guidance, a 22-gauge stellate needle is directed toward the tubercle, and after negative aspiration for heme, air, and CSF, 3 cc of Omnipaque contrast is administered. Once visualization of contrast movement down the paravertebral fascia to the inferiorly located stellate ganglion is achieved, 10 cc of 0.25% Bupivacaine, with/without Kenalog, is injected in 1 ml increments intermittently with negative aspirations under fluoroscopic view.

J.E. Pope, T.R. Deer (eds.), *Treatment of Chronic Pain Conditions*, DOI 10.1007/978-1-4939-6976-0_40

A successful stellate ganglion block is suggested clinically by the onset of Horner's symptoms as well as a relative temperature change in the ipsilateral versus the contralateral hand of ≥ 1.5 °C. As an important side note, if the practitioner achieves a successful block based on the abovementioned symptoms without significant reduction in pain, the possible involvement of Kuntz fibers should be considered. Believed to exist in 10–20% of the population, these T2-nerve fibers contribute to the brachial plexus without traversing the sympathetic trunk. This may necessitate reevaluation for possible neuraxial techniques in an attempt to assess T2–T3 sympathetic involvement.

Complications

The following are possible complications of the stellate ganglion blockade through either of the two approaches discussed:

- Pneumothorax (higher risk with C7 anterior paratracheal approach)
- Dysphagia
- Vocal cord paralysis
- Intra-arterial or intravenous injection
- Epidural placement of local anesthetic

Celiac Plexus Block

41

Emil H. Annabi, Jimmy Arefieg, and Stephen Shiller

Key Points

- Celiac plexus is formed from paired nerves of the greater, lesser, and least splanchnic nerves.
- Techniques described to block the celiac plexus include the retrocrural and anterocrural needle placement.
- Visceral pain involving the intestines, liver, pancreas, gallbladder, and bladder can be treated by the celiac plexus block.
- Celiac plexus denervation strategies have been described for both cancer and non-cancer-related visceral pain.

Introduction

Celiac plexus block (CPB) is an interventional modality used for the purposes of diagnosing and treatment of non-somatic abdominovisceral pain. Although the most common etiology of chronic abdominal pain treated with CBP is pancreatic cancer, chronic abdominal pain secondary to cancer and non-cancerous involvement of many of the visceral structures of the abdominal compartment have been successfully treated with CPB. One may separate non-visceral from visceral etiologies of abdominal pain by positive response to somatic blocks such as intercostal nerve blocks. A Cochran review of CPB in patients with pancreatic cancer had statistically improved pain scores and demonstrated less side effects compared to those patients receiving opioid only. Some mis-analyses have even suggested longer life expectancy with improved pain control following CPB.

E.H. Annabi, MD (✉)
Pima Pain Center, Pain Medicine, Tucson, AZ 85712, USA
e-mail: eeannabi@gmail.com

J. Arefieg, MD • S. Shiller, MD
Pima Pain Center, Tucson, AZ 85712, USA

Background

The celiac plexus is a retroperitoneal structure that is found anterolateral to the aorta, epigastrium, and crus of the diaphragm located typically at L1 vertebral level. However, some variability exists, and plexus may be found anywhere between T12 and L2 vertebral bodies. Splanchnic nerves composed of autonomic afferent and efferent fibers as well as nociceptive fibers of the upper abdominal viscera form the celiac plexus. Parasympathetic contributions via the vagus nerves are also contributory. These nerves travel from the spine in the retrocrural space and pierce the crura of the diaphragm to enter the retroperitoneal cavity (Table 41.1).

Considerations

See Table 41.2.

Techniques

There are many techniques that may be used for CPB. The posterior approach to the splanchnic nerves and celiac plexus using retrocrural and anterocrural techniques, respectively, and transaortic and to endoscopic ultrasound have all been used to successfully block the transmission of pain via the celiac plexus.

The most common technique employed to proceduralists today is the posterior approach with the aid of fluoroscopy, CT, or both. The level of needle insertion is typically L1, identified with fluoroscopy. A 15 cm or longer 20 gauge spinal needle is inserted 6–8 cm lateral of midline, with the left needle placement attempted first. The needle is advanced along the anterolateral aspect of the superior half of the L1 vertebral body with the bevel of the needle pointing superiorly. Care is taken to not make contact with the vertebral body as this can be quit painful. With the c-arm in position

J.E. Pope, T.R. Deer (eds.), *Treatment of Chronic Pain Conditions*, DOI 10.1007/978-1-4939-6976-0_41

Table 41.1 Indications for celiac plexus block

Indications	
Intractable non-somatic abdominal visceral pain that has failed medical management. Cancerous and non-cancerous involvement of the following viscera	
Liver	Gallbladder
Stomach	Spleen
Omentum	Mesentery
Pancreas	
Small intestine	Mid-transverse colon
Kidneys	Adrenal glands
Contraindications	
Contrast allergy	
Abnormal coagulation profile	

Table 41.2 Considerations

Standard ASA monitoring
Intravenous access for medication and fluid administration
Positioning tolerance by the patient (i.e., prone position is poorly tolerated in a patient with large ascites)
Normal coagulation profile

for a lateral view, the needle is advanced until its tip is just ventral to the anterior border of the vertebral body. The right needle is position the same as the left. At this location, the needle is in the retrocrural space where the splanchnic nerves are located just prior to piercing the diaphragmatic crura and forming the celiac plexus. Injection of contrast media at this location will show a cephalic spread along the splanchnic nerves in the retrocrural space. The anterocrural technique is employed by advancing the needle until it pierces through the crura of the diaphragm. If the aorta is contacted during placement of the left needle, a transaortic approach may be utilized using a single needle. With this approach, the needle is advanced through the aorta until blood is no longer aspirated. At this location, the needle is just anterior of the aorta where the celiac plexus is located. Injection of contrast media in the anterocrural space will show spread more caudal and anterior than with retrocrural technique.

Anterior approach utilizes a single needle placement under CT guidance to the periaortic region, possibly traversing the abdominal viscera. This approach may be particularly useful in a patient who cannot tolerate the prone position. This is often performed by interventional radiologists.

Endoscopic ultrasound is an approach in growing popularity today. With this technique, a needle is inserted through the endoscope and through the posterior wall of the stomach to the periaortic region. This is often performed by gastroenterologists.

Regardless of the approach, needle placement is confirmed with the use of contrast media. Extreme care must be taken to ensure there is no vascular uptake, posterior spread in the vicinity of the neuroforamina or epidural space, or contrast uptake within the intima of the aorta.

Medications

Once proper needle placement is confirmed, 5–10 ml of 2% lidocaine is injected through each needle as a test dose. If neurolysis is desired, 10–20 ml of either ethyl alcohol of 60% or greater or phenol of 6% or greater is injected. Both cause neurolysis by similar mechanisms by causing extraction of phospholipids and cholesterol and precipitating lipoprotein and mucoprotein ultimately causing Wallerian degeneration and fibrosis of the nerves. Alcohol is hypobaric, and care must be taken that its injection is not in the epidural or intrathecal space. The limitation of the use of alcohol is the severe burning that the patient feels upon its injection, although dilution with local anesthetic may be used to assuage this effect. The benefit of phenol injection is that it has local anesthetic properties, and therefore additional local anesthetic is not needed. Radiofrequency of the splanchnic nerves has also been described.

Complications

- Diarrhea from increased parasympathetic activity is experienced by approximately 44% of patients. Bowel motility may be beneficial in those who have constipation secondary to chronic opioid use
- Hypotension secondary to splanchnic dilation is experienced by approximately 38% of patients. Administration of IV fluids prior to procedure may ameliorate this
- Respiratory depression may occur if care is not taken to reevaluate patient's opioid requirements. Opioid requirements may be decreased following successful block.
- Vascular injection
- Spinal cord and nerve damage
- Retroperitoneal and visceral hematoma
- Abscess
- Discitis
- Pneumothorax

Lumbar Sympathetic Block

42

Sean K. Graham

Key Concepts

- Lumbar sympathetic block is a diagnostic and therapeutic treatment modality for sympathetically maintained pain to the lower extremities.
- The ideal site for blockade is at the upper third of the L3 vertebral body.

Introduction

Lumbar sympathetic blockade results in interruption of the sympathetic efferent fibers to the lower extremities without affecting the somatic nerve roots. This provides diagnostic information as to the relative sympathetic contribution to the patient's pain syndrome. It also provides analgesia in those patients with a significant sympathetically maintained component to their pain.

Anatomy

The lumbar sympathetic chain consists of sympathetic efferent fibers. The neurons follow somatic nerves or vessels to effect vascular smooth muscle, sudomotor cells, and peripheral nociceptors.

There are five paired lumbar ganglia that lie along the anterolateral border of either side of the five lumbar vertebrae. The majority of sympathetic efferent neurons responsible for vascular tone in the lower extremities pass through the paravertebral ganglia at L2 and L3. These ganglia therefore are the targets for lumbar sympathetic blockade. The lumbar arteries at these levels are known to exit the aorta and travel posteriorly across the middle of the vertebral bodies prior to branching into radicular or segmental medullary arteries. The ideal site then, for blockade of the L2 and L3 ganglia, would be at the upper third of the L3 vertebral, both targeting the ganglia and avoiding the segmental lumbar arteries and their branches.

The lumbar sympathetic chain is well separated from the lumbar somatic nerves by the psoas major muscle and its fascia. This separation is what allows sympathetic blockade to the lower extremities without affecting sensorimotor function. It is important to note however that there is a connection between the sympathetic chain and the somatic nerves via the gray and white rami communicantes. Caution should be taken, especially when performing neurolysis, as the injectate may track posteriorly along these pathways and result in somatic nerve injury.

Candidacy

Indications for lumbar sympathetic blockade include chronic moderate to severe cancer and noncancer pain not controlled by more conservative measures. It is indicated for any painful condition in which there is a significant contribution from the sympathetic nervous system. It can also be used in conditions associated with limited blood flow within the small vessels of the lower extremities.

Indications

See Table 42.1.

Contraindications

The contraindications to lumbar sympathetic blockade include bleeding diathesis and local or systemic infection.

S.K. Graham, MD (✉)
The Spine Diagnostic and Pain Treatment Center, Department of Pain Medicine, Baton Rouge, LA, USA
e-mail: seangrahammd@gmail.com

J.E. Pope, T.R. Deer (eds.), *Treatment of Chronic Pain Conditions*, DOI 10.1007/978-1-4939-6976-0_42

Table 42.1 Indications

Complex regional pain syndrome (I and II)
Acute herpes zoster
Postherpetic neuralgia
Post-amputation stump pain
Phantom limb pain
Radiation neuritis
Peripheral neuropathy
Peripheral ischemia due to: Atherosclerosis Frostbite Erythromelalgia Raynaud's disease Buerger's disease

Technique

The patient is placed in the prone position, and the skin is marked at a site approximately 7–9 cm lateral to the spinous process of L3. A skin wheal is raised, and local anesthetic is infiltrated in an oblique path directed toward the L3 vertebral body. A 22-gauge 6-inch needle is then inserted and advanced under fluoroscopic guidance toward the target just below the inferior border of the transverse process of L3 and just lateral to the L3 vertebral body. Once passing underneath the transverse process, the needle is angled in such a way to move along the lateral surface of the vertebral body and advanced until the tip lies at the anterolateral edge and the upper third of L3. Lateral fluoroscopic imaging is then used to advance the needle until the tip sits exactly at the most anterior border of the vertebral body.

With appropriate needle position confirmed, 2–3 mL of contrast is injected and should be visualized tracking in a cephalocaudal direction along the anterolateral surface of L3, without vascular uptake and without tracking posteriorly toward the somatic nerve root. Once contrast spread is deemed appropriate, a test dose of 5 mL 2% lidocaine is injected to facilitate a rapid onset of the sympathetic block and production of subsequent changes in skin temperature. When skin temperature has started to increase in the affected lower extremity, a volume of 15–20 mL of 0.375% bupivacaine is injected.

Suggested Reading

1. Boas RA. Sympathetic blocks in clinical practice. In: Stanton-Hicks M. International anesthesia clinics. Regional anesthesia: advances in selected topics, vol 16, no 4. Boston: Little, Brown; 1978.
2. Brown EM, Kunjappan V. Single-needle lateral approach for lumbar sympathetic block. Anesth Analg. 1975;4:725.
3. Hatangdi VS, Boas RA. Lumbar sympathectomy: a single needle technique. Br J Anaesth. 1985;57:285.
4. Rocco AG, Palombi D, Raeke D. Anatomy of the lumbar sympathetic chain. Reg Anesth. 1995;20(1):3–19.
5. Tran KM, Frank SM, Raja SN. Lumbar sympathetic block for sympathetically maintained pain: changes in cutaneous temperatures and pain perception. Anesth Analg. 2000;90:1396–401.
6. Umeda S, Toshiyuki A, Hatano Y. Cadaver anatomic analysis of the best site for chemical lumbar sympathectomy. Anesth Analg. 1987;66:643–6.

Superior Hypogastric Plexus Block

43

Emil H. Annabi, Jimmy Arefieg, and Stephen Shiller

Key Points

- Superior hypogastric plexus is a target for lower abdominal pain of visceral origin.
- Posterior approach is the most common technique and requires fluoroscopy.
- Neuroablative techniques have been described.

Background

The superior hypogastric plexus is a culmination of nerves formed by the aortic plexus and the splanchnic nerves. It is located in the retroperitoneum anterior to the vertebral bodies of the lower one-third of L5 to the upper one-third of S1 bilaterally. It consists of both outgoing (efferent) sympathetic fibers and incoming (afferent) pain fibers.

Indications

A superior hypogastric plexus blockade has been shown to be efficacious in reducing pelvic pain associated with metastatic cancers and nonmalignant pathologies that do not respond to medication management related to the following anatomic sites:

- Bladder
- Descending colon
- Penis
- Prostate
- Rectum
- Testes
- Urethra
- Uterus
- Vagina
- Vulva

Contraindications

- Recent myocardial infarction
- Coagulopathies

Procedure

A superior hypogastric plexus blockade can be done under CT guidance but is more commonly done under fluoroscopy due to decreased radiation exposure to the patient and availability of equipment. Both an anterior and posterior approach have been documented, with the posterior approach commonly utilized unless spinal pathology renders this approach impossible.

When performing the posterior approach, the patient is placed in the prone position with a cushion under the pelvis to decrease physiologic lumbar lordosis. One percent lidocaine is used to create a skin wheel at the site in intended injection, approximately 1–2 mm superior to the sacral alae, bilaterally. Under fluoroscopic guidance, the needle is advanced in an oblique direction to allow passage inferiorly to the transverse process of L5. The final location for the needle tip is immediately anterior to the L5-S1 intervertebral disk. At this site, 3 cc of Omnipaque contrast is administered to assure localization followed by 10 cc of 0.25% bupivacaine with/without Kenalog injected in 1 ml increments intermittently with negative aspirations.

E.H. Annabi, MD (✉)
Pima Pain Center, Pain Medicine,
6226 E Pima St #3, Tucson, AZ 85712, USA
e-mail: eeannabi@gmail.com

J. Arefieg, MD • S. Shiller, MD
Pima Pain Center, Tucson, AZ 85712, USA

J.E. Pope, T.R. Deer (eds.), *Treatment of Chronic Pain Conditions*, DOI 10.1007/978-1-4939-6976-0_43

Complications

Complications for the posterior approach of the superior hypogastric plexus blockade are incredibly rare but do include:

- Bleeding
- Local infection
- Injury to iliac vessels
- Injury to organs of the region

Ganglion Impar Block

44

Emil H. Annabi, Jimmy Arefieg, and Stephen Shiller

Key Points

- Perineal pain can be managed with injection of the ganglion impar.
- The ganglion impar is the most caudal visceral plexus.
- A trans-sacrococcygeal ligament approach is the most common described.

Introduction

The ganglion impar supplies nociceptive and sympathetic innervation of the perineum, distal rectum, perianal region, distal urethra, vulva/scrotum, and distal third of the vagina. Blockade of the ganglion impar has classically been utilized for treatment of malignant pelvic and perineal pain when it was first described in 1990. However, there are many benign etiologies of visceral and sympathetically maintained pain of the pelvis and perineum that have been successfully treated with ganglion impar block without the need for neurolysis.

Indications

See Table 44.1.

Contraindications

Contrast allergy

Abnormal coagulation profile

E.H. Annabi, MD (✉)
Pima Pain Center, Pain Medicine, Tucson, AZ 85712, USA
e-mail: eeannabi@gmail.com

J. Arefieg, MD • S. Shiller, MD
Pima Pain Center, Tucson, AZ 85712, USA

Technique

Blockade of the ganglion impar was first described in 1990 and is practiced among many proceduralists today. It is performed with the patient in the lithotomy position, lateral decubitus position with the knees flexed, or the prone position with a pillow under the abdomen or flexion of the operating table to allow flexion of the lumbosacral spine. The technique includes bending, usually at two different locations, or curving the needle with the insertion site being midline through the anococcygeal ligament under fluoroscopic guidance. Needle advancement is directed anterior to the coccyx and into the retroperitoneal space to the level of the sacrococcygeal joint. At this location, contrast media is injected, and spread is observed to be both cephalad and caudad along the anterior board of the sacrum and coccyx forming the classic "comma sign." Since the needle is directed within the retroperitoneal space, there is risk of rectal injury. If this is of considerable concern, the proceduralist may place his index finger of his non-dominant hand within the patient's rectum and directing it anteriorly to increase the space between the anus and tip of the coccyx. Once correct needle placement has been confirmed, local anesthetic is injected and the patient is asked about relief of pain. If the etiology is malignant, neurolysis may be employed. For benign etiologies, neurolysis may not be necessary. Since this technique involves inducing multiple bends or pronounced curvature to the needle, the proceduralist may find it difficult to withdraw the stylet of the needle, and this should be practiced at the beginning of the procedure prior to needle insertion.

Since the original description of the above technique, there have been alternative approaches that have been offered in the literature with reported success. These include trans-sacrococcygeal and intercoccygeal approaches where needle through needle technique is employed through the sacrococcygeal ligament and intercoccygeal ligaments, respectively, under fluoroscopic guidance. For example, a

J.E. Pope, T.R. Deer (eds.), *Treatment of Chronic Pain Conditions*, DOI 10.1007/978-1-4939-6976-0_44

Table 44.1 Indications

Malignant	
	Pelvic organ cancer pain (cervix, colon, bladder, rectum, endometrium)
	Perineal metastatic cancer pain
	Perianal malignant pain
Benign (potential indications)	
	Idiopathic perineal pain
	Coccydynia
	Sacroiliitis
	Sacrococcygeal pain
	Post-traumatic perianal pain
	Vulvovaginitis
	Post-episiotomy pain
	Chronic anal pain
	Pain of the glans penis
	Tenesmoid pain
	Chronic prostatitis
	Chronic proctitis
	Sacral postherpetic neuralgia
	Spinal cord malformations
	Failed back surgery
	Postsurgical thrombosis of perineal veins
	Vaginal protrusion
	Testicular ablation
	Perineal pain of unknown origin

22-gauge 38-mm needle is used as an introducer, while a 25-gauge 50-mm needle is advanced to the location of the ganglion impar. The main benefits reported include not needing to induce bends or curves to the needle to allow use of stylet, and therefore less blockage occurs. It is also reported that there is less discitis or fistula formation and is better tolerated by patients since there is no need for the proceduralist to place his finger in the rectum. Potential difficulty is that the sacrococcygeal ligament is calcified and fused in over 50% of patients. Intercoccygeal fusion is only seen in approximately 12% of patients.

Medications

- Local anesthetics
- Steroids
- Clonidine
- Neurolytics (minimal volume since ventral ramus of the sacral nerve runs close the to the ganglion)
- Botox

Complications

- Rectal perforation
- Needle breakage with multiple bends
- Periosteal injection
- Needlestick injury to proceduralist
- Fistula formation

Suggested Reading

1. Lee JE, Kwak KH, Hong SW, Jung H, Chung SY, Park JM. Treatment of radiation-induced cystitis and vulvodynia via a ganglion impar block using a lateral approach under computed tomography guidance: a case report. Korean J Anesthesiol. 2017;70(1):81–5. doi:10.4097/kjae.2017.70.1.81. Epub 2017 Jan 26.
2. Patijn J, Janssen M, Hayek S, Mekhail N, Van Zundert J. van Kleef M.14. Coccygodynia. Pain Pract. 2010;10(6):554–9. doi:10.1111/j.1533-2500.2010.00404.x. Epub 2010 Sep 6 Review.
3. Lin CS, Cheng JK, Hsu YW, Chen CC, Lao HC, Huang CJ, Cheng PH, Narouze S. Ultrasound-guided ganglion impar block: a technical report. Pain Med. 2010;11(3):390–4. doi:10.1111/j.1526-4637.2010.00797.x.

Vertebral Augmentation

45

Jonathan D. Carlson

Key Points

- Vertebral body augmentation is typically performed in the presence of an acute or non-healing vertebral compression fracture.
- MRI with STIR or CT scan with contrast may be helpful in evaluating the location and age of the fracture.
- Retropulsed fragment architecture is a contraindication for vertebral body augmentation.
- Employing a fitted brace is a conservative care approach.
- Care and vigilance should be exercised when performing the procedure.

Introduction

Vertebral augmentation is a percutaneous fluoroscopic-guided procedure of which orthopedic cement or polymethyl methacrylate (PMMA) is injected into a vertebral compression fracture (VCF) to minimize pain and decrease morbidity. Pain can be severe, and associated morbidity may include decreased lung functional residual capacity, spine deformity, and decreased movement/ambulation.

Vertebral augmentation was first reported in 1987 by a French radiologist and neurosurgeon, Deramond and Galibert, who injected orthopedic cement into a painful C2 hemangioma. The patient received significant relief.

Vertebral augmentation (VA) can be done either as a vertebroplasty or kyphoplasty. Vertebroplasty is when the PMMA is injected via carefully placed trocars within the vertebral body (Fig. 45.1). The thought is the trabeculation of the cement stabilizes the fracture.

Kyphoplasty is when trocars are placed in the same fashion as vertebroplasty, but balloons are first inflated to reduce the fracture and possibly decrease the associated kyphosis. Subsequent PMMA is injected after the balloons are removed (Fig. 45.2).

Diagnosis

Adequate history and physical are imperative. Physical exam usually notes marked pain with percussion at the concordant level of the suspected fracture. The ideal imaging is typically MRI: T1 fat suppressed and T2 STIR (Fig. 45.3). MRI is useful, especially STIR images, because they can help to determine the age of the fracture. Acute/subacute VCF typically showed radiographic changes. Repair of fractures with bone edema noted on MRI or increased uptake on a bone scan is more likely to produce pain relief than chronic VCF repair.

Indications

The primary indication in the United States is for painful osteoporotic compression fractures. Malignancy is the other main indication. Repair of VCF in younger patients is typically avoided due to lack of insurance coverage and the need for surgical intervention.

Conservative treatment would include pain medications/adjuvants and spine bracing such as a Jewett brace. Most would agree that physical therapy should be avoided as this may worsen the fracture. Some providers would further suggest facet joint procedures at, above, and below the level of the VCF.

Local coverage determination (LCD) as of 2013 is fairly ubiquitous and states that conservative measures should be exhausted, the fracture should not be older than 4 months, and there must not be any retropulsion into the spinal canal visualized on imaging. Failure to adhere to these guidelines may result in lack of payment of the procedure.

J.D. Carlson, MD (✉)
Arizona Pain/Pain Doctor, Glendale, AZ, USA
e-mail: jcarlsonmd@gmail.com

J.E. Pope, T.R. Deer (eds.), *Treatment of Chronic Pain Conditions*, DOI 10.1007/978-1-4939-6976-0_45

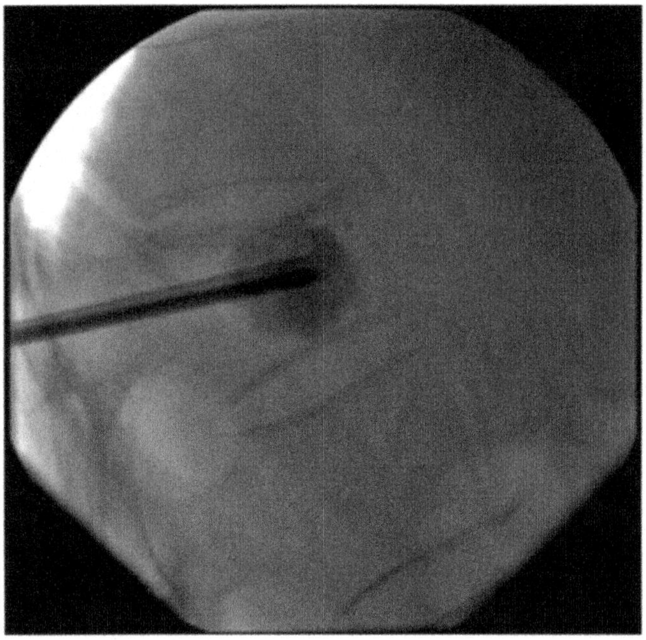

Fig. 45.1 Vertebral augmentation via vertebroplasty

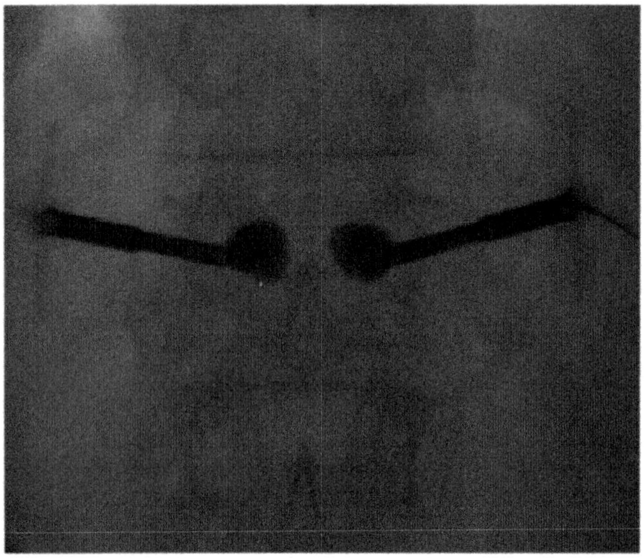

Fig. 45.2 Vertebral augmentation via kyphoplasty

Technique

1. Proper patient selection: a painful fracture refractory to conservative treatment.
2. Expert hands-on training and supervision are essential.
3. Seek out spine surgical consult in patients with new-onset myelopathy or in younger patients with traumatic VCF.
4. Avoid repair of severe VCF or "bow-tie" fractures.
5. Limit VA to mid-thoracic (T6 or lower) and lumbar regions.

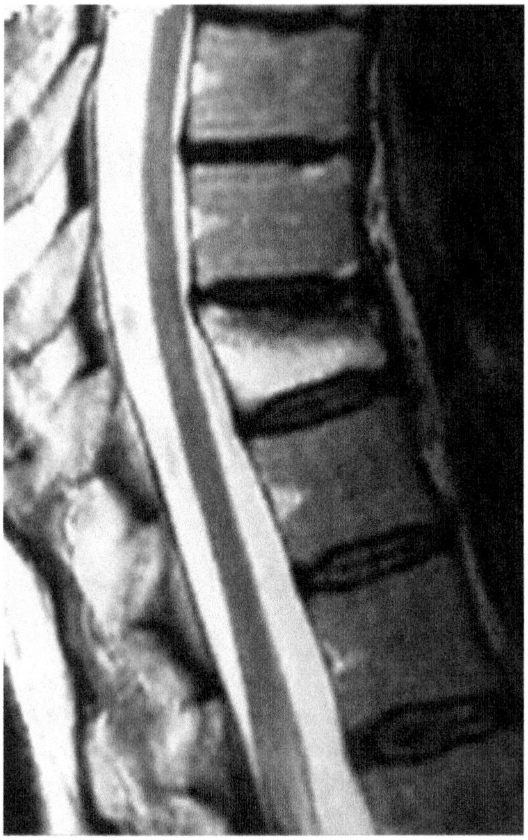

Fig. 45.3 T1 fat suppressed with gadolinium enhances VCF; T2 STIR is most sensitive for water content and will elucidate bone edema

6. Confirm that there are adequate radiographic landmarks in all views before starting the procedure.
7. The transpedicular approach seems to be the safest entry route.
8. Unilateral midline trocar placement or bilateral trocar placement are considered by many experts the best manner in which to stabilize the VCF.
9. In AP fluoroscopic view, do not violate medial border of the pedicle until the trocar has entered the cortex of the vertebral body in a lateral view. This will assure, with a high degree of confidence, that you are not in the spinal canal.
10. Allow for adequate setup time for PMMA; it should have the consistency of toothpaste.
11. Inject PMMA slowly, always under live fluoroscopy.
12. Use no more than 2–4 ml of PMMA per vertebral level.
13. In lateral fluoroscopic view, once the trocar is in the anterior one-third of the vertebral body, do not allow PMMA to enter the posterior one-third of the vertebral body, or there may be risk of spinal canal compromise.
14. No more than two to three levels should be repaired in one sitting. General rule of thumb: for every 1 ml of

cement injected, 1 ml of bone marrow fat is potentially displaced. The higher the volume of PMMA injected, the higher the risk for pulmonary fat emboli.

Contraindications

- Adequate response to conservative treatment
- New-onset myelopathy
- Burst fractures
- Standard neuraxial spine procedures contraindications
- Retropulsed fracture architecture

Complications

Subsequent adjacent VCF can occur 12.4–21% of the time after VA. Other complications include extravasation of cement, improper trocar placement, and the usual complications of bleeding, infection, and nerve damage.

Vertebroplasty Versus Kyphoplasty

A meta-analysis with over 21 studies and over 1000 patients showed that both techniques reduced vertebral compression pain in the immediate postoperative period greater than 50%. A smaller prospective study showed that, again, both methods were similar in reducing pain but that kyphoplasty showed a significant increase in the angle of kyphosis and decreased cement leakage.

Controversy

In 2009, two randomized controlled studies published in the *New England Journal of Medicine* stated that there was minimal difference with VA versus placebo. These studies were highly publicized lending to the controversy of whether or not VA should be done at all. Advocates of these studies underscored the conclusion that VA was not efficacious and the procedure imposed unnecessary risk to the patient. Opponents argued that the studies were highly flawed and were potentially putting patients at risk for increased pain and morbidity. They further argued that VA was not compared to a true sham but rather another pain procedure (facet procedures), thus nullifying the term "placebo." Furthermore, the power analysis was not met and nearly all of the initial sham patients crossed over for VA treatment. Regardless, the salient message was that both views acknowledged that overutilization of VA was more than likely occurring and should be curtailed.

Conclusion

In properly selected patients, vertebral augmentation, when done by a proficient interventionalist, may be of valuable benefit in reducing pain and decreasing morbidity as well as being more efficacious and cost-effective than conservative treatment alone.

Suggested Reading

1. Chandra RV, et al. Vertebral augmentation: update on safety, efficacy, cost-effectiveness, and increased survival. Pain Physician. 2013;16:309–20.
2. Gill JB, et al. Comparing pain reduction following kyphoplasty and vertebroplasty for osteoporotic vertebral compression fractures. Pain Physician. 2007;10(4):583–90.
3. Glazen CA, et al. Vertebroplasty versus conservative treatment in acute osteoporotic vertebral compression fractures (Vertos II): an open-label randomised trial. Lancet. 2010;376(9746):1085–92.
4. Schofer MD, et al. Comparison of kyphoplasty and vertebroplasty in the treatment of fresh vertebral compression fractures. Arch Orthop Trauma Surg. 2009;129(10):1391–9.
5. Syed MI, Shaikh A. Vertebroplasty: a systematic approach. Pain Physician. 2007;10:367–80.

Discography

46

Sherif Zaky

Key Concepts

- Provocative discography is a modality that correlates symptoms with pathological findings identified with other imaging tools.
- Discography is usually indicated for patients with persistent back pain with high suspicion of discogenic origin, in whom surgery is a viable option.
- During discography, physician must assess at least one normal disc to compare with the suspected disc.
- Measuring the amount and type of pain provoked, pressure measures, volume of the contrast injected, and the radiographic findings evaluate each disc.
- Discitis is the most feared serious complications following discography.
- Other potential complications include nerve root injury, epidural hematoma, trauma to retroperitoneal structures, and pneumothorax.

Introduction

Discography was first introduced in 1948 as a diagnostic modality for herniated nucleus pulposus in patients with axial low back pain. Although different diagnostic modalities such as magnetic resonance imaging (MRI) and computed tomography (CT) can diagnose pathological or morphological changes of the intervertebral disc, yet they fail to correlate these changes to pain. Provocative discography on the other hand is not only an imaging modality but also a tool that correlates symptoms with pathology.

S. Zaky, MD, MSC, PhD (✉)
Pain Management Service, Firelands Regional Medical Center, Case Western Reserve University, Sandusky, OH, USA
e-mail: zakys1@gmail.com

Indications

Discography is usually indicated in:

1. Patients with persistent back pain for at least 3 months, in whom conservative treatment measures failed to provide relief.
2. Patients in whom surgical intervention is a viable option where there is a high index of suspicion for discogenic pain.
3. Patients with failed back surgery syndrome to distinguish between painful pseudoarthrosis and a symptomatic disc.
4. Patients who have previous lumbar fusion to identify whether the levels above and below the fusion are the source of pain.

Contraindications

Contraindications to discography include (1) bleeding disorder or anticoagulation therapy, (2) systemic infection or skin infection at the puncture site, (3) pregnancy, (4) allergy to contrast dye, and (5) severe psychiatric conditions where the patient cooperation and pain reporting are impaired.

Lumbar Discography Technique

Different techniques have been described for lumbar discography. Posterolateral approach is commonly used today and is described below.

The patient is positioned in the prone with a pillow under the abdomen. Surgical prep and full-body drapes should be utilized. Antibiotic prophylaxis is recommended before the beginning of the procedure. For L5–S1 disc, a cranial tilt of the C-arm at about 45° is usually required. The C-arm is then moved oblique until the superior articular process is seen at the midpoint of the disc. The presence of the iliac crest in the

J.E. Pope, T.R. Deer (eds.), *Treatment of Chronic Pain Conditions*, DOI 10.1007/978-1-4939-6976-0_46

needle trajectory sometimes causes difficulty approaching this disc. L4–L5 disc usually requires less cranial tilt. A straight anteroposterior view is usually sufficient for L3–L4 and L2–L3 discs, and even some caudal tilt might be required. At any disc, the superior articular process (SAP) should be at the midpoint of the disc space.

After skin infiltration, an 18-gauge angiocath is inserted under fluoroscopy lateral to the SAP at the midpoint between the endplates. A 22-gauge 7-inch spinal needle is then inserted via the 18-gauge angiocath. Resistance is typically encountered when passing through the annulus. Leg pain usually suggests contact with the nerve root and requires needle redirection. Final needle position should be confirmed in the anteroposterior and lateral views, which should show the tip of the needle in the middle of the disc in both views (Figs. 46.1 and 46.2). The same steps should be repeated for each level tested. When all needles are in place, water-soluble contrast is injected at each level in increments of 0.2–0.6 ml.

Physician must assess at least one normal (control) disc to compare with the suspected disc. Each disc is evaluated by five measures: amount of pain provoked, type of pain (concordant or discordant), pressure measures (opening pressure, pressure at the onset of pain, and maximum pressure), volume of the contrast injected, and the radiographic findings.

Pressure Interpretation

Disc pressure should be measured by connecting each needle to a manometer as the disc is pressurized. Opening pressure is the pressure at which the dye starts to appear in the disc. Each disc is pressurized until pain is elicited or until reaching 90–100 psi (pound per square inch). Pain that starts at pressure between 0 and 15 psi is typically related to chemical sensitivity. This means that the pain is triggered from contact of the contrast dye with the nerve endings. Pain with pressure between 15 and 50 psi correlates with the disc being mechanically sensitive. Pain with a pressure between 51 and 90 psi is inconclusive, and other sources of pain should be investigated. Pain with pressure above 90 psi is considered negative.

Radiographic Interpretation

Computed tomography (CT) scan should be performed immediately after discography. This is important to evaluate the spread of the contrast in the nucleus as well as the degree of the annular disruption. The grade of annular degeneration is evaluated by the extent of the spread of contrast into the annulus using the modified Dallas discogram scale:

- Grade I: the contrast reaches the inner third of the annulus.
- Grade II: the contrast reaches the middle third of the annulus.
- Grade III: the contrast reaches the outer third of the annulus.
- Grade IV: when the fissure spreads circumferentially.
- Grade V: when the fissure has completely ruptured the outer layers of the disc and is leaking contract material out of the disc. This type can cause a chemical radiculopathy.

Complications

The most common serious side effect following discography is discitis. The incidence of discitis is variable and reported between 5:2000 and 1:30. Other rare but serious complications following discography include epidural hematomas or abscesses. Discography can also lead to nerve root trauma or even trauma to the spinal cord or cauda equina. Other complications related to the site of discography include retropharyngeal hematoma or abscess with cervical epidural, pneumothorax with thoracic discography, and trauma to retroperitoneal structures with lumbar discography (Figs. 46.1 and 46.2).

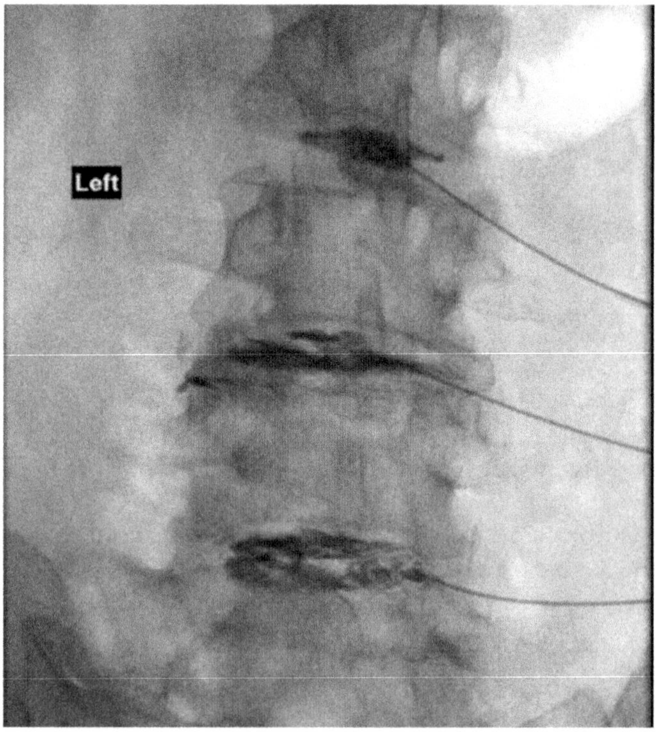

Fig. 46.1 Discogram of L3–L4, L4–L5, and L5–S1 showing needle position with contrast dye spread in anteroposterior view

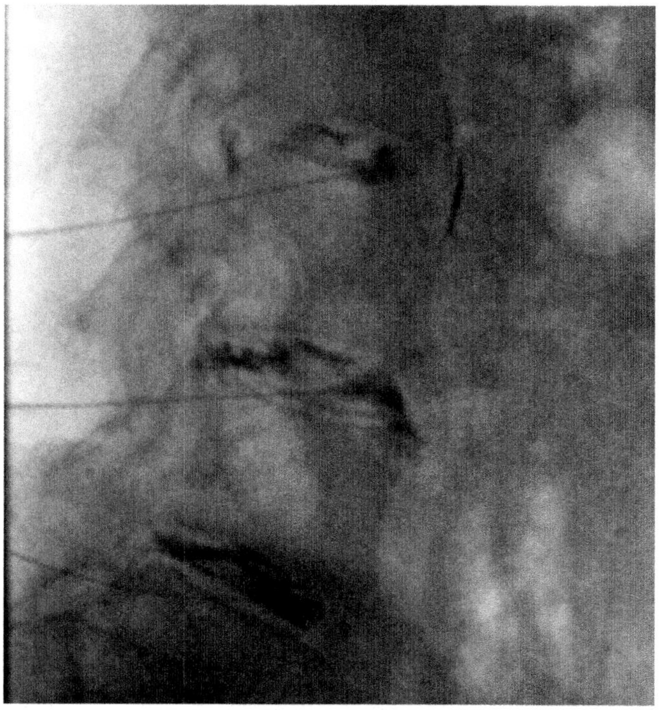

Fig. 46.2 Discogram of L3–L4, L4–L5, and L5–S1 showing needle position with contrast dye spread in lateral view

Suggested Reading

1. Bogduk N, Aprill C, Derby R. Lumbar discogenic pain: state of the art review. Pain Med. 2013;14:813–36.
2. Cohen SP, Larkin TM. Lumbar discography. In: Raj's practical management of pain. 4th ed. Philadelphia: Elsevier Press; 2008.
3. Joseph Walker III, El Abd O, Isaac Z, Muzin S. Discography in practice: a clinical and historical review. Curr Rev Musculoskelet Med. 2008;1:69–83.
4. O'Neill C, Kurgansky M. Subgroups of positive discs on discography. Spine. 2004;29:2134–9.
5. Waldman SD. Lumbar discography. In: Atlas of interventional pain management. 3rd ed. Philadelphia: Elsevier press; 2009.

Management of Iatrogenic Emergencies in Interventional Pain Management

47

Michael Grille, George C. Chang Chien, and Jiang Wu

Key Concepts

- Complications in interventional pain management are overall quite rare; the interventional pain physician should be adept at minimizing complications and identifying the early warning signs of complication and keen at understanding the acute and post-acute management of these complications.

Introduction

Iatrogenic emergencies in interventional pain management are overall quite rare. According to one multicenter review analysis of 26,151 procedures, less than 0.1% of the procedures resulted in a transfer to an emergency department (ED) or an aborted procedure. Importantly, each procedure has a unique risk and safety profile. According to the ASA Closed Claims Project, epidural steroid injections accounted for 40% of all claims involving pain management cases that occurred between 1970 and 1999. Early identification of iatrogenic complications is imperative to preventing significant morbidity and mortality.

In this review, we discuss the more common iatrogenic emergencies into broad categories: cardiovascular, neurologic, and other (Table 47.1).

M. Grille, MD
Cleveland Clinic, Anesthesiology Institute, Cleveland, OH, USA

G.C. Chang Chien, DO (✉)
Cleveland Clinic, Anesthesia Institute Pain Management, 9500 Euclid Ave, Dept C-25, Cleveland, OH 44195, USA
e-mail: gchangchien@gmail.com

J. Wu, MD
University of Washington Medical Center, Department of Anesthesiology & Pain Medicine, Seattle, WA, USA

Anaphylaxis

Anaphylaxis is an acute, life-threatening allergic reaction. In anaphylactic reactions, exposure to an allergen (food, medication, insect, or chemical compound) causes a severe immune reaction. During an anaphylactic episode, activated mast cells and basophils release potent inflammatory mediators including: histamine, TNF, and IL-4. The excessive release of these acute inflammatory mediators results in rapidly progressive vasodilatation, increased vascular permeability, and bronchoconstriction.

Signs and Symptoms

Providers should have high suspicion for anaphylaxis when patients present with rapidly progressive and severe symptoms involving the skin, respiratory, and cardiovascular systems after exposure to known or possible allergens. Integumentary involvement is seen in about 90% of cases and is characterized by urticaria and itching. These symptoms may be absent due to the use of antihistamines or not apparent due to draping of procedural patients. Respiratory symptoms are apparent in a majority of cases. Progressive airway swelling can lead to airway obstruction and acute respiratory failure. Tachycardia and hypotension are typically observed, but, in severe cases, cardiovascular collapse can occur.

Immediate in Office Management

Symptoms in patients with anaphylactic reactions progress rapidly over minutes. Initial management should focus on activation of emergency resources, airway protection, and early administration of epinephrine. Upon recognizing an anaphylactic reaction, the provider should immediately stop patient exposure to the suspected allergen, call for help, and activate emergency response systems. Continuous monitoring

J.E. Pope, T.R. Deer (eds.), *Treatment of Chronic Pain Conditions*, DOI 10.1007/978-1-4939-6976-0_47

Table 47.1 Complications in interventional pain management

Cardiovascular	Neurologic	Other
Anaphylaxis	*Local anesthetic toxicity and iatrogenic seizure*	Post-dural puncture headache
Vasovagal syncope	Subarachnoid anesthetics injection (high/total spinal block)	
Pneumothorax	Epidural hematoma	

of vital signs, cardiac telemetry, and pulse oximetry should be instituted, and supplementary 100% oxygen should be provided. Large bore IV access should be obtained, and IV fluid bolus should be started for patients with hypotension. Elevation of the patient's legs facilitates venous return, and a partial head-up position may improve respiratory mechanics.

Respiratory compromise can progress rapidly. Patients who are experiencing stridor, who have neck swelling or angioedema, or rapidly progressing symptoms, may be in danger of imminent respiratory obstruction. Intubation for airway protection by an experienced provider should be strongly considered in these cases.

The primary goal, in addition to supportive care, is early treatment with epinephrine to halt progression of the reaction and to minimize respiratory and circulatory involvement. Intramuscular epinephrine (1:1000) in a dose of 0.2–0.5 mg should be given on the mid-anterior-lateral thigh. This dose can be repeated every 5–15 min depending on the response. All other agents (antihistamines, B2 agonists, steroids) should be considered second-line therapies and may have minimal effects on severe respiratory and cardiovascular symptoms. Many patients respond to a single dose of epinephrine. Despite initial improvement, some patients may show recurrent symptoms hours later, so all patients should be transferred to a monitored setting.

Neurocardiogenic (Vasovagal) Syncope

Mechanism

Neurocardiogenic or vasovagal syncope is a common cause of syncope. It is a transient and self-limited episode of syncope which is mediated by neural reflexes. These episodes are induced by exposure to a trigger (pain, sight of blood or needle, rapid changes in position, or stress). These triggers can cause a paradoxical increased parasympathetic and decreased sympathetic tone which can result in bradycardia and/or a drop in blood pressure. This subsequent drop in blood pressure can cause loss of consciousness due to decreased brain perfusion.

Signs and Symptoms

Sudden vasovagal syncope is often preceded by prodromal symptoms lasting seconds to minutes. Early signs include diaphoresis, nausea and vomiting, flushing, tinnitus, and palpitations. Later signs include visual disturbances (blurry vision, dark spots, tunnel vision), anxiety, skin pallor, paresthesia, and confusion. Loss of consciousness may follow and the patient may fall. The subsequent change to horizontal position results in restoration of perfusion and usually return of consciousness.

Immediate in Office Management

Objectives in treating neurocardiogenic syncope involve restoration of normal perfusion, supportive care, and evaluation of etiology. Normal perfusion can most rapidly be restored by placing the patient in a supine or Trendelenburg position. Evaluation of the circulation, airway, breathing (CABs), vital signs, and mental status should be conducted, as well as evaluation for injuries if a fall occurred. Supportive care including supplemental oxygen, IV access, blood glucose monitoring, and discontinuation of inciting medications should be instituted. In more severe cases, IV fluid administration, pharmacological heart rate, and blood pressure support may be indicated. Most patients will recover spontaneously with minimal intervention after perfusion is restored. In these instances, avoid reexposure to the inciting trigger, and slowly return patients to the upright position. If rapid recovery is not observed or if the patient is at high risk, consider transfer to a higher level of care.

Workup

Workup for neurocardiogenic syncope includes 12-lead EKG (obtained at the time of the event if possible) and may include Holter monitoring and tilt table testing. Referral for outpatient workup may also include cardiology and neurology consultations for evaluation of the underlying cause of the syncope.

Treatment

Long-term treatment options include maintenance of intravascular volume, avoidance of triggers, desensitization therapy, vasoconstricting medications, or pacemakers.

Local Anesthetic Toxicity and Iatrogenic Seizure

Mechanism

Local anesthetics are commonly used in pain management practices for both therapeutic and diagnostic applications. Local anesthetics interrupt neuronal transmission by blocking voltage-gated sodium channels. High dosages and unrecognized intravascular injection can lead to elevated plasma concentrations with undesirable effects. Local anesthetic systemic toxicity (LAST) is related to non-specific blockage of sodium channels in the central nervous system and myocardium.

Providers giving local anesthetics should give particular attention to avoiding systemic toxicity with local anesthetics. Careful attention to toxic dosing is advisable. If large quantities of local anesthetics are required, they should be given in divided doses with observation for signs of toxicity. Unintentional intravenous injection of local anesthetic should be avoided. Negative aspiration after needle or catheter placement and between doses does not always exclude intravascular placement. If applicable, test doses with a pharmacological marker (i.e., epinephrine) or radiological contrast can be helpful. Despite these safeguards, systemic local anesthetic toxicity can occur.

Signs and Symptoms

Early signs and symptoms of local anesthetic toxicity are caused by the effects on the central nervous system (CNS). First signs of LAST may be reported as altered sensation by the patient such as perioral numbness, vision changes, metallic taste, and tinnitus. Patients may report light-headedness or dizziness as well. Objective signs usually begin with an initial excitation phase. Altered mental status, including agitation and confusion, is usually present; however, these symptoms may be attenuated by periprocedural sedation. Muscle twitching may be observed. Progression of CNS symptoms may finally result in generalized seizure. Following the excitation phase and possible seizure, CNS depression may develop with drowsiness progressing to nonresponsiveness and even coma. Respiratory depression and apnea further augment the central toxic effects.

Following neurological symptoms, the cardiovascular effects of LAST may develop. A hyperdynamic state with hypertension and tachycardia can be seen first. Progression of cardiovascular toxicity results in hypotension and slowed cardiac conduction leading to brady-arrhythmias. Ventricular arrhythmia and hemodynamic collapse are the final stages of LAST and can be resistant to resuscitative efforts.

Immediate in Office Management

Upon recognizing the development of LAST, the provider should focus on activation of emergency resources, avoidance of further symptom progression, and preparation for severe neurological and cardiovascular manifestations. Activation of emergency medical resources and obtaining assistance are critical. Local anesthetic infusions should be immediately stopped. Supplementary 100% oxygen should be provided, IV access obtained, and vital sign and cardiac monitoring initiated. If CNS symptoms are progressing or severe, seizure prophylaxis should be instituted by giving a benzodiazepine such as midazolam. Ventilation support with positive pressure should be provided if breathing becomes inadequate.

Although most patients do not develop to severe symptoms and cardiovascular effects, delayed progression can be seen, so transfer to a monitored setting is indicated. While awaiting a higher level of care, preparation for advanced cardiovascular life support (ACLS) is wise, and cardiac medications including epinephrine and atropine should be made immediately available.

Workup

Avoidance of systemic toxicity is obviously the best approach to reducing LAST. After an episode of systemic toxicity, providers should consider performing a root cause analysis to evaluate the factors which may have contributed including excessive dosing, unrecognized intravascular injection, selection of local anesthetic, solution concentrations, and patient factors (comorbidities, age). Assessment of preparedness for recognizing and treating LAST should be conducted. Providers should examine their practices and use of medications and contrast to identify intravascular injection.

Treatment

Advanced treatment of LAST is best provided in a highly monitored and well-equipped environment. Seizures are managed with repeated dosages of benzodiazepines. The cardiovascular effects, particularly in the case of bupivacaine, can be resistant to treatment. ACLS protocols primarily guide management. According to the American Society of Regional Anesthesia and Pain Medicine (ASRA), epinephrine doses should be limited to less than 1 mcg/kg when treating hypotension and vasopressin, calcium channel blockers, and beta-blockers, and additional local anesthetics should be avoided. ASRA guidelines recommend Intralipid, a 20% lipid emulsion, for treatment of severe LAST. An initial bolus of 1.5 ml/kg given over 1 min (which can be repeated if refractory), followed by an infusion of 0.25 ml/kg/min for at least 10 min, is recommended. Longer infusions and increased rates to 0.5 ml/kg/min can be used for persistent hypotension up to 10 ml/kg of lipid emulsion.

Pneumothorax

Pneumothorax is an abnormal collection of air or gas in the pleural space that causes an uncoupling of the lung from the chest wall which may interfere with normal breathing. This interference with normal respiratory function has potential for severe morbidity and mortality depending on the size of the lesion and the physiologic reserve of the patient. According to the American Society of Anesthesiology closed claims database on liability related to chronic pain management, of the 284 chronic pain management claims between 1970 and 1999, the most common complication of blocks was iatrogenic pneumothorax, accounting for 51% of all block claims. On reexamination of the ASA closed claims database from 2005 through 2008, the percentage of iatrogenic pneumothorax was drastically down to less than 0.1% due to significantly increased cervical procedure-related complications. Among all pain interventions, trigger point injections and facet injections are associated with majority of pneumothorax incidents. Iatrogenic pneumothorax can occur when patients are treated with trigger point injections in the neck region, trapezius muscle, rhomboid major, or minor muscles. The highest risk for iatrogenic pneumothorax is associated with the rhomboid major muscle due to the variability in thickness of the skin, subcutaneous fat layer, and other soft tissues in this area between individuals. One study investigated an appropriate depth of needle insertion during trigger point injection into the rhomboid major muscle using ultrasonography and suggested the safe margin was 1.4–1.7 cm in the underweight or normal group (BMI <23) and 2.1–2.1 cm in the obese group (BMI > 25) to deliver a safer and more efficient procedure.

Mechanism of Iatrogenic Pneumothorax

The visceral pleura covers the surface of the lung, and the parietal pleura lines the inside of the chest wall. Between the two layers, there is only a small amount of lubricating serous fluid. If the integrity of the two layers is violated, air is allowed to enter and accumulate between the visceral and parietal pleura, and a one-way valve is formed; pneumothorax develops.

Signs and Symptoms

Symptoms of iatrogenic pneumothorax include sharp and sudden-onset chest pain at the same side of intervention during the procedure. The pain is made worse by a deep breath or a cough, leading to feelings of tightness in the chest. Shortness of breath, rapid heart rate, rapid breathing, cough, and fatigue are other symptoms of pneumothorax. Examination of the chest with a stethoscope may reveal decreased or absent breath sounds over the affected lung if the size is large enough. The diagnosis is usually confirmed by chest X-ray. In office examination by a trained provider with ultrasound is also an efficient method to evaluate the integrity of the pleura. If a pneumothorax is suspected, M-mode ultrasound can detect small air collections with high sensitivity.

Immediate in Office Management

Immediate in office management depends on a number of factors, e.g., the size, the mechanism of trauma, the clinic stability of patient, and the physician managing the patient. The treatment of pneumothorax may vary from discharge with early follow-up, to immediate needle decompression and transfer to a higher level of care for chest tube placement.

Most of iatrogenic pneumothoraces by needle injury are very small (defined 1 cm or less air rim) or small (defined as <15% of the volume of the hemithorax). These pneumothoraces are unlikely to progress to respiratory failure or tension pneumothorax. They resolve by resorption at a rate of 1.25% per day, although the rate may be increased by the administration of supplement oxygen. Patients who have no associated breathlessness, increased O2 requirement (O2 Sat > 94% on room air) or underlying lung disease, do not always require treatment, and their pneumothorax will likely resolve spontaneously. A case-by-case evaluation is needed and careful follow-up of these patients is critical. If patients are asymptomatic and hemodynamically stable, a short-stay observation is an option for these patients, and they should be given clear instructions to return to hospital if there are worsening symptoms. Outpatient follow-up includes repeated X-rays to confirm improvement.

In the case of a large pneumothorax (>15%) or a symptomatic patient with breathlessness, increased oxygen requirement, and decreased oxygen saturation (<94% without O2 therapy), immediate reduction of the pneumothorax by urgent aspiration or insertion of a chest tube should be considered in the office under fluoroscopic guidance.

Advanced Treatment

It has been observed that when compared to tube drainage, first-line aspiration in iatrogenic pneumothorax significantly reduces the number of patients requiring hospital admission, without increasing the risk of complications. The remainder of the treatment can be conservative. However, ongoing observation in hospital is required even after a successful procedure. A chest tube (or intercostal drain) is the most definitive initial treatment of a pneumothorax. If the patient has respiratory or hemodynamic compromise, tension pneumothorax should be suspected. This is characterized by shifting of the mediastinum and potentially life-threatening compression of the contralateral lung and great vessels. In cases of tension pneumothorax, the needle or cannula is left in place to provide continuous decompression, maintain ventilation, and restore cardiac output. Rarely, in extreme cases, video-assisted thoracoscopic surgery (VATS) or pleurodesis may be necessary in some refractory pneumothorax.

Aftercare

If iatrogenic pneumothorax occurs in a smoker, it may be advisable for the patient to remain off work for up to a week after this incident. Air travel is discouraged for up to 7 days after complete resolution of a pneumothorax if recurrence does not occur. Underwater diving is considered unsafe after an episode of pneumothorax unless a preventative procedure has been performed.

Subarachnoid Local Anesthetics Injection (High or Total Spinal Block)

Background

According to the ASA closed claims database review from 2005 through 2008, among 294 chronic pain management claims, about 1% of the cases were directly related to cervical dural puncture during ESI. The incidence of accidental dural puncture during a labor epidural needle placement is 1–1.5%, but the incidence of accidental dural puncture during epidural steroids injection under fluoroscopy guidance is unknown and probably much lower.

Depending on the dose and level of LA delivered, iatrogenic subarachnoid local anesthetic injection leads to spinal anesthesia, which can be classified into three categories:

1. Surgical spinal anesthesia: anesthetic block reaches to desired anatomic level for planned surgery.
2. High spinal: clinical block well above the level required for surgical anesthesia but without significant sequelae (such as respiratory compromise or bradycardia).
3. Complete spinal block: anesthetic block involving the cervical spine and above (such as brain stem and cranial nerves).

It may be a rare event, particularly under fluoroscopy guidance, but unexpected extensive spinal anesthetic from ESI could be a life-threatening and devastating event requiring emergent cardiopulmonary resuscitation.

Pathophysiology of Total Spinal Anesthesia

Intrathecal local anesthetics block the transmission of afferent nerve signals from peripheral nociceptors and efferent nerve signals from the central nervous system. The degree of neuronal blockade is determined by the amount and concentration of local anesthetic used and the properties of the axon. Heavily myelinated, small preganglionic sympathetic fibers are blocked first. Thin unmyelinated C-fibers associated with pain are blocked later, while thick, heavily myelinated A-alpha motor neurons are blocked last.

Total spinal anesthesia occurs when excessive doses of anesthetic intended for epidural administration are delivered into the subarachnoid space and interfere with normal neuronal function in the cervical spinal cord and brain stem.

Signs and Symptoms

Symptoms and signs usually occur within minutes of ESI; however, delay up to 30 min has been reported. Clinical progression usually occurs over the subsequent several minutes. Nausea and high sensory level block (>T1) may be early signs. The impairment of ventilatory function and hemodynamic instability are the indicators for emergent resuscitation. The clinical manifestations of complete spinal block include some or all of those listed in Table 47.2.

Table 47.2 Clinical manifestations of complete spinal block

Cardiorespiratory	Neurological
Hypotension[a]	Nausea and anxiety[a]
Bradycardia[a]	Arm/hand dysaesthesia or paralysis[a]
Respiratory compromise[a]	High sensory level block
Apnea[a]	Cranial nerve involvement
Reduced oxygen saturation	Loss of consciousness[a]
Difficulty speaking/coughing	
Cardiac arrest (asystole)	

Adapted from www.totw.anaesthesiologists.org
[a]Commonly reported or "classical"

Prevention of Intrathecal Injection

Prevention of injury is the most reliable means to assure the safety during image-guided pain interventions. The precise placement of the epidural needle with the assistance of fluoroscopic guidance is mandatory. Practitioners must learn to recognize the characteristic patterns of epidural and intrathecal contrast spread. It is also important to recognize unusual contrast patterns that signal subdural placement. During epidural steroid injection, it is wise to abort the procedure before placing steroid when either subdural or intrathecal needle position is suspected. The clinician should limit a single epidural bolus of anesthetic to the maximum reasonable dose to administer as a single intrathecal injection, particular at the cervical level. A resuscitation cart with adequate equipment and medication stored should be readily available; associated training and rehearsal should be regularly scheduled in preparation for this kind of emergent scenario.

Immediate in Office Management

Once injection of intrathecal local anesthetic and particulate steroid has occurred, immediate, on-site supportive care should be given dependent on degree and height of block. The management may include induction of general anesthesia and intubation. Early recognition is vital as block progression may be mitigated (reverse Trendelenburg/head raised) and serious cardiorespiratory compromise avoided. Severe respiratory dysfunction or apnea may occur without loss of consciousness. Appropriate psychological reassurance must be provided and an induction agent administered before intubation to minimize distress and the chance of awareness. Sedation and mechanical ventilation need to be continued until there is clear evidence of adequate spontaneous respiratory function. Hemodynamic changes should progressively improve as the block resolves.

Aftercare

With the appropriate cardiopulmonary resuscitation, usually the patient can be recovered completely without any untoward sequelae. Postoperative discussion with the patient is prudent. This provides the opportunity to assess the potential for psychological distress, provide an explanation of the event, and answer any questions. Unless there is clinical suspicion of an anatomical abnormality, there is no evidence further investigation is beneficial. While the topic of ongoing debate, intrathecal injection of particulate steroid preparations may lead to neurotoxicity.

Post-Dural Puncture Headache (PDPH)

Background

Post-dural puncture headache (PDPH) is a puncture of the dura mater and a complication during spine procedures. Leakage of cerebrospinal fluid through the dura mater puncture causes reduced fluid levels and pressures in the brain and spinal cord and may lead to the development of PDPH hours or days later. The headache is severe and described as "searing and spreading like hot metal," involving the back and front of the head and spreading to the neck and shoulders, sometimes involving neck stiffness. It is exacerbated by movement and sitting or standing and relieved to some degree by lying down.

The incidence of accidental dural puncture during a labor epidural needle placement is 1–1.5%, but the incidence of accidental dural puncture during epidural steroids injection under fluoroscopy guidance is unknown and probably much lower. Generally speaking, the smaller needle diameters correlated with a lower incidence of PDPH, lower incidence of PDPH with a large-diameter blunt-tip needle when compared with a smaller-diameter cutting needle, and the incidence rate reduction of PDPH using the parallel orientation technique to the long axis of the spinal cord comparing to the perpendicular insertion technique. The independent risk factors of PDPH include a higher incidence in women versus men, pregnancy, a higher incidence in the age group 20–50 years, and a higher incidence in patients with lower body mass index.

Pathophysiology of PDPH

The pathophysiology of the PDPH is not completely understood. Through a known dural puncture, cerebral spinal fluid (CSF) escapes at a rate that exceeds CSF production. The Monro-Kellie rule speculates that in an intact skull, the sum of the volumes of brain, CSF, and intracranial blood is constant; therefore, the headache results from CSF volume loss, compensatory vasodilatation, and venous hypervolemia. In contrast, due to the reduction in CSF total volume, especially in the spinal region, the brain shifts caudally. The direct traction hypothesis states that the headache is from placing traction on the pain-sensitive intracranial structures and causing cerebral vasodilatation as a result of the brain shifting.

Signs and Symptoms

An orthostatic bilateral headache following recent history of meningeal puncture is the pathognomonic symptom for PDPH. The headache is characteristically occipital and/or frontal and always bilateral, worse within 15 min after standing or sitting, and improves within 15 min after lying down flat (The International Headache Society). The absence of an orthostatic component should lead to a search for other causes. 75% of PDPH occurs within 48 h following a dural puncture and 72% of PDPH spontaneously resolved within 7 days and 87% by 6 months. Symptoms associated with PDPH can include neck stiffness, nausea, vomiting, photophobia, diplopia, scalp paresthesia, upper and lower limb pain, auditory changes including tinnitus, and hypoacousia and can include mental status changes. PDPH is a clinic diagnosis largely based on a thorough history and physical examination.

Immediate in Office Management

In the event of unintended dural puncture during epidural steroid injection and based upon the fact that 85% of PDPHs last less than 5 days, the initial treatment for PDPH is conservative and supportive therapy. In addition to bed rest and oral or intravenous hydration and analgesics, pharmacological treatment with caffeine is beneficial in the treatment of PDPH. Caffeine, a potent central nervous system stimulant, causes cerebral vasoconstriction and the reduction of cerebral blood volume and is the most widely used pharmacologic therapy. Caffeine is administered as an oral dose of 300 mg or intravenously as 500 mg in 500–1000 ml normal saline over 2 h; the intravenous dose can be repeated over the next 2–4 h. The effect of caffeine is transient, and the dose must be repeated because it does not address the underlying pathology.

Proposed preventive procedures of PDPH include prophylactic EBPs and epidural saline injections and infusions or intrathecal injection of 10 ml normal saline. A Cochrane review did not recommend prophylactic EBP and determined that therapeutic EBP to be beneficial.

Advanced Treatment

Once pharmacologic and other noninvasive options have been exhausted without improvement and the patient is unable to wait for the natural resolution of the headache, more invasive treatment can be explored. The gold-standard epidural treatment for PDPH is an epidural autologous blood patch (EBP). The optimal time to place an epidural blood patch is >24 h after the development of the PDPH, as there is a 71% failure rate if the epidural blood patch is done within 24 h of dural puncture as compared to a 4% failure if done after 24 h. The initial relief can be as high as 100%. Bed rest for 2 h in the supine position after EBP provided 100% relief in contrast 60% relief in patients who remained supine for only 30 min. The overall long-term relief of PDPH from an initial EBP is between 61 and 75%. In these recurrent cases, repeated EBP might be required. The contraindications to an EBP are similar to those for any spinal or epidural procedure.

As the pathophysiology of PDPH is not completely understood, the mechanism of EBP is also controversial. The early mass effect provides rapid relief following an EBP. In agreement with the mechanical traction hypothesis, the initial early epidural mass effect leads to the reduction in the spinal intradural volume, which subsequently shifts the CSF cephalad, thus resuspending the brain and reducing mechanical traction. In agreement with the Monro-Kellie rule, this intracranial shift in CSF also reduces the intracranial blood volume and cerebral vasodilatation. A second, more lasting effect is due to sealing of the dural/arachnoid tear with a gelatinous plug. This sealing of the dural/arachnoid hole prevents further loss of CSF and allows for regeneration and restoration of the CSF volume. The plug acts as a bridge until permanent repair of the dural/arachnoid hole occurs. The occurrence of this second effect is more variable and accounts for the failure of the EBP despite initial relief.

Aftercare

Complications after an EBP are rare. The most common complication is mild low back and radicular pain following the procedure that resolves spontaneously in a few days and can be treated with nonsteroidal anti-inflammatory drugs (NSAIDs). Other possible complications include epidural hematoma, infection, iatrogenic intracranial hypertension, and arachnoiditis due to unintentional subdural/subarachnoid injection of the blood.

Spinal Epidural Hematoma

Spinal epidural hematoma (SEH) is an accumulation of blood in the potential space between the dura and the bone surrounding the spinal cord. It is typically the result of trauma such as lumbar puncture or epidural analgesia but may also occur spontaneously. Spontaneous spinal epidural hematoma may be associated with anticoagulation, thrombolysis, blood dyscrasias, coagulopathies, thrombocytopenia, neoplasms, or vascular malformations. Early identification of SEH is important as delayed intervention may result in irreversible morbidity such as permanent neurological deficits.

The incidence of spinal epidural hematoma (SEH) has been estimated to be 1:220,000 after a spinal block, 1:150,000 after an epidural block, 1:190,000 after epidural anesthesia, and 1:250,000 in the obstetrical population. However, the incidence of SEH specifically as a complication of ESI has not been defined. Large case series of serial cervical ESIs ranging from 141 to 790 patients have reported no associated serious neurologic complications, including SEH.

Pathophysiology

Various mechanisms have been suggested to account for SEH including unrestrained epidural venous and arterial bleeding, as well as bleeding from arteriovenous malformations. Other theories include bleeding from the posterior internal vertebral venous plexus, although some have argued that venous pressure is less than intrathecal pressure, and thus venous bleeding should not be capable of causing acute spinal cord compression. In support of an arterial origin of SEH, three cases have been reported of SEH with bleeding arising from arteries in the posterior longitudinal ligament following anterior discectomy.

Spinal epidural hematoma has a bimodal distribution with peaks during childhood and during the fifth and sixth decades of life. Increasing age has been noted as a risk factor for postoperative spinal epidural hematoma. Risk factors for SEH due specifically to ESIs have not been clearly described, but are likely similar to those reported for epidural anesthesia. Cervical ESI may be associated with a higher relative incidence of SEH compared to thoracic or lumbosacral ESI. From an anatomic standpoint, the spinal cord is most vulnerable to compression in the cervical region given the relatively smaller diameter of the spinal canal including a smaller-diameter peridural space in this area compared to thoracic and lumbar levels. A study of ten cadaver specimens suggested that cervical ESIs may also pose a relatively higher risk of hemorrhagic complication due to an observed high frequency of anatomical variation of arteries within the spinal canal in this area compared with the thoracic and lumbar regions.

Signs and Symptoms

Spinal epidural hematoma typically causes severe localized back pain with delayed radicular radiation that may mimic disk herniation. Associated symptoms may include weakness, numbness, urinary incontinence, or fecal incontinence. Spinal epidural hematoma may have variable findings on physical examination, determined by the level of the lesion. A thorough examination for neurologic changes is paramount in cases of suspected SEH. New-onset motor weakness or sensory disturbances may be unilateral or bilateral. Acute changes in myotatic reflexes and asymmetry should be noted, as well as any alterations of bladder or anal sphincter tone. Any reports of ascending paralysis should not be dismissed and unequivocally attributed to anesthetic motor block from neuraxial procedure.

Immediate in Office Management

SEH is a rare complication following interventional neuraxial procedures. However, unrecognized SEH can lead to permanent neurologic sequelae. The interventionalist should be wary of evolving signs and symptoms such as excessive pain or progressive extremity weakness and should refer these patients for emergent imaging. Early decompression, within 8 h of onset of symptoms, increases the likelihood of favorable outcomes. In office management includes monitoring of vital signs, monitoring for progressive neurologic change, and inclusion of total spinal anesthesia within the differential.

Advanced Treatment

Emergent evaluation for SEH includes complete blood count (CBC) with platelets to assess for infection, hematocrit, and platelets to identify potential causes for hemorrhage, as well as prothrombin time (PT), activated partial thromboplastin time (aPTT), and international normalized ratio (INR) to evaluate for derangements in the clotting cascade. Blood chemistries, including electrolytes, blood urea nitrogen (BUN), creatinine, and glucose are helpful to characterize metabolic derangements that may complicate clinical course. Emergent imaging with MRI or computer tomography (CT) is necessary to identify the epidural hematoma. A neurosurgical consultation is necessary for possible emergent evacuation of a spinal epidural hematoma. Early decompression will decrease the likelihood of any neurological sequelae.

Aftercare

If the patient has any resultant neurological deficits from the spinal epidural hematoma such as paraplegia or tetraplegia, intense rehabilitation with physical and occupational therapy will reduce the long-term disability for the patient.

Conclusion

Iatrogenic complications in interventional pain management office are rare but have potential to cause significant morbidity and mortality. Proper planning including emergency protocols and early recognition of potential complications are necessary to promote safety in the interventional pain practice.

Suggested Reading

1. Morjaria JB, Lakshminarayana UB, Liu-Shiu-Cheong P, Kastelik JA. Pneumothorax: a tale of pain or spontaneity. Ther Adv Chronic Dis. 2014;5(6):269–73.
2. Scavone BM. Timing of epidural blood patch: clearing up the confusion. Anaesthesia. 2015;70(2):119–21.
3. Sheldon RS, Grubb 2nd BP, Olshansky B, Shen WK, Calkins H, Brignole M, Raj SR, Krahn AD, Morillo CA, Stewart JM, Sutton R, Sandroni P, Friday KJ, Hachul DT, Cohen MI, Lau DH, Mayuga KA, Moak JP, Sandhu RK, Kanjwal K. 2015 heart rhythm society expert consensus statement on the diagnosis and treatment of postural tachycardia syndrome, inappropriate sinus tachycardia, and vasovagal syncope. Heart Rhythm. 2015;12(6):e41–63.

Regenerative Medicine

48

Richard M. Rosenthal, Enrique Galang, and George C. Chang Chien

Key Concepts

- Regenerative medicine is a branch of medicine that attempts to change the course of chronic disease by healing damaged tissues and organs that are beyond repair by current technology.
- Regenerative medicine modalities include platelet-rich plasma and various types of mesenchymal stem cells including adipose-derived stem cells, bone marrow aspirate concentrate, and amnion-derived stem cells.
- Regenerative medicine modalities are an enticing alternative to injectable forms of local anesthetics and corticosteroids which have both demonstrated chondrotoxic potential.
- Level 1 evidence supports PRP for the treatment of lateral epicondyle tendinopathy.
- Regenerative medicine for the treatment of numerous musculoskeletal conditions including degenerative disc disease are on the horizon.

Introduction

Current medical treatments are increasingly unable to keep pace with patients' needs, and there are few effective ways to treat the root causes of many diseases, injuries, and congenital conditions. Regenerative medicine is defined as the "process of creating living, functional tissues to repair or replace tissue or organ function lost due to age, disease, damage, or congenital defects." Regenerative sciences have made major advances in understanding how tissues repair after injury; and the signaling mechanisms involved are being progressively understood. Recent developments in the emerging fields of stem cell science and regenerative medicine may allow the use of stem cells to repair tissue damage. Because of these advances, regenerative medicine therapies have seen a dramatic increase in breadth and frequency of use for orthopedic conditions. Currently, regenerative medicine therapies are showing promise in the treatment of osteoarthritis, acute and chronic soft tissue injuries, ligament and tendon injuries, and enhancement of healing after reconstructive ligament surgeries. Promising clinical and surgical applications in the future include improved outcomes of spinal fusion and improved treatment of degenerative joint and disc disease. The current clinical evidence on many regenerative therapies is mixed regarding efficacy. This in part is due to the variability in study protocols and treatment parameters. However, this realm of biomedical research is growing rapidly, and there are numerous ongoing studies.

To understand a therapeutic treatment focused on accelerating healing, the clinician must be knowledgeable in the physiological processes of wound healing and tissue repair. Regenerative medicine encompasses a wide array of therapeutic modalities and may be overwhelming to the clinician who is beginning to incorporate regenerative medicine in their medical practice. Regenerative treatment includes the use of but not limited to autologous platelet-rich plasma (PRP) and mesenchymal stem cells (MSCs) such as amniotic stem cells and those found in the bone marrow and adipose (Table 48.1).

Platelet-Rich Plasma (PRP)

Platelet-rich plasma therapy is currently the most common form of regenerative medicine practiced in the United States. PRP is a volume of plasma containing a concentrated platelet count that is four to eight times above that in whole blood.

R.M. Rosenthal, MD
Regenerative Medicine Applications in Pain, Provo, UT, USA

E. Galang, MD
Orthopaedic and Rheumatologic Institute, Cleveland Clinic, 9500 Euclid Ave, Cleveland, OH 44195, USA

G.C. Chang Chien, DO (✉)
Cleveland Clinic, Anesthesia Institute Pain Management, 9500 Euclid Ave, Dept C-25, Cleveland, OH 44195, USA
e-mail: gchangchien@gmail.com

J.E. Pope, T.R. Deer (eds.), *Treatment of Chronic Pain Conditions*, DOI 10.1007/978-1-4939-6976-0_48

Table 48.1 Summary of common regenerative medicine modalities

Modality	Source
Platelet-rich plasma (PRP)	Whole blood is separated into cellular components either by centrifuge or density gradient cell separator. The buffy coat/plasma (leukocytes and platelets) can then be extracted for use as PRP
Mesenchymal stem cells (MSCs)	*Adipose-derived MSCs (ADMSCs):* A small amount of fat is removed from the waist via a minimally invasive procedure. The fat is subsequently centrifuged and stems cell separated *Bone marrow aspirate concentrate (BMAC):* commonly removed from the iliac crest via a minimally invasive procedure. BMAC is subsequently centrifuged and stem cells separated *Amniotic mesenchymal stem cells (AMSC):* commercially prepared stem cells sourced from a tissue bank. The cells are derived from the placenta of live healthy donors prescreened for disease during the pregnancy. As opposed to ADMSC and BMAC (which are autologous), amniotic stem cells are allogenic

PRP is an autologous blood product that is derived by drawing a sample of venous blood (usually 60 cc) and spinning it in a centrifuge in order to separate and harvest the platelet fraction. It is delivered via image-guided injection to damaged joints, ligaments, and tendons to promote healing. PRP produces an anabolic state in tissues as a result of the platelets releasing growth factor proteins including transforming growth factor-β1, insulin growth factors 1 and 2, vascular endothelial growth factor (VEGF), basic fibroblast growth factor, and hepatocyte growth factor (HGF). These growth factors stimulate cell division and promote angiogenesis, tissue granulation formation, and growth of the extracellular matrix.

Currently, PRP is primarily used for soft tissue injuries (tendons, ligaments, bursa) and osteoarthritis of the three major joints (shoulder, hip, knee). There is also an unpublished study on its use for treatment of annular disruption of the lumbar disc. There are many controversies surrounding the use of PRP that remain to be solved. These include but are not limited to preparation method, ideal platelet and leukocyte concentration, timing of injection to injury, and patient-specific factors such as general health, age, and sex. As an example, it has been found that a leukocyte-rich PRP preparation creates a greater pro-inflammatory response as compared to leukocyte-poor PRP. The consequences of this effect are currently unclear, with studies currently underway to differentiate the impact on outcomes of this variable.

Mesenchymal Stem Cells (MSC)

A stem cell is an undifferentiated cell that is capable of self-renewal through mitotic cell division while remaining in an undifferentiated state and can differentiate into a variety of specialized cells when needed. There are three basic types of stem cells – adult, embryonic, and induced pluripotent stem (iPS) cells. Adult stem cells are found in all organs and tissues of the body and serve to replace dying cells and regenerate damaged tissues. Because they are derived from adult tissue, their use is not considered controversial. Adult stem cells can be further subdivided based on differentiation potential into mesenchymal stem cells, hematopoietic stem cells, neural stem cells, etc. The largest number of publications listed in the US National Library of Medicine for MSK disorders is on mesenchymal stem cells.

Mesenchymal stem cells are a specific type of adult stem cell. They are multipotent cells that differentiate into a variety of connective tissue types (adipose, bone, tendon, cartilage, muscle). As such, they are ideally suited for musculoskeletal procedures. They can be derived from autologous sources such as the bone marrow and adipose tissue or allogenic sources such as commercially prepared stem cells. When injected into a targeted tissue, they induce an anabolic response through paracrine effects on the surrounding cells. MSCs actively secrete cytokines and growth factors that turn on cellular processes resulting in healing. While PRP is most commonly used to treat damaged ligaments and tendons, MSCs are more often used to treat cartilage damage associated with osteoarthritis or degenerative disc disease. As such, there are multiple studies examining the chondrogenic potential of various subtypes of cells, e.g., bone marrow vs adipose-derived MSCs. The preponderance of the evidence supports bone marrow-derived MSCs as the best choice for treating cartilaginous disorders.

Regenerative Treatments for Tendon and Ligament Disorders

Chronic tendinopathy is characterized by failure of the normal tendon repair mechanism and is a common malady that leads to chronic pain. Multiple studies have demonstrated the efficacy of PRP in the treatment of chronic tendinopathy and ligamentous injuries. Currently, the most compelling data to date have been in elbow lateral epicondyle tendinopathy, for which numerous randomized controlled trials have demonstrated therapeutic benefit and superiority over both local anesthetic and corticosteroid for pain and function. According to one randomized controlled study, a single autologous PRP injection produced better and longer-lasting relief than a single corticosteroid injection for the treatment of tennis elbow. In another study looking at the use of PRP in the treatment of grade 2 hamstring muscle injuries, PRP in combination with a rehabilitation program was significantly more effective than rehabilitation program alone.

As with any emerging treatment, continued diligence in the medical community to further evaluate the efficacy and safety of regenerative therapies is paramount. One RCT showed "no clinical and ultrasonographic superiority of platelet-rich plasma injection over a placebo injection in chronic Achilles tendinopathy at 1 year combined with an eccentric training program." One limitation of this study included differences in the natural healing response between load-bearing tendons and non-load-bearing tendons. Thus, current regenerative medicine technology does not work universally across chronic degenerative injuries.

Regenerative Treatments for Osteoarthritis

PRP has been demonstrated to be an effective treatment for mild to moderate osteoarthritis of the knee. In one prospective study in patients with degenerative knee cartilage lesions and osteoarthritis, intra-articular injections of PRP demonstrated superiority over hyaluronic acid viscosupplementation at 6-month follow-up. In this study, as well as other regenerative medicine studies, younger patients with milder forms of disease tended to fair better.

Regenerative Therapy for Discogenic Pain

Low back pain is a major cause of disability and of particular interest to the pain physician. Degenerative disc disease (DDD) is one of the most common causes of low back pain. Regenerative therapy trials for degenerative disc disease are currently underway. Results from a prospective, double-blind, randomized controlled trial studying the efficacy of lumbar intradiscal PRP demonstrated statistically significant and clinically relevant improvements in pain and function. Potential sources for cell therapy for discogenic pain are described in Table 48.2.

Conclusion

The future for regenerative treatments in pain medicine is promising. Future research is necessary to identify appropriate protocols for specific purposes.

Table 48.2 Potential sources for cell therapy

Cell types	Source	Advantages	Disadvantages
Embryonic stem (ES) cells	Early embryo	Pluripotent stem cells with high capacities of self-renewal, proliferation, and differentiation	Ethical barriers
Induced pluripotent stem (iPS) cells	Artificially derived from somatic cells by reprogramming with transcription factors	Pluripotent stem cells with high capacities of self-renewal, proliferation, and differentiation	Safety issues, especially caused by potential tumor genesis
Mesenchymal stem cells (MSCs)	Bone marrow	The technology for isolation and expansion is mature, and basic research has documented its role in discogenesis	More invasive procedure required to obtain cells from donors
	Adipose	Abundance Ease to harvest Low immunogenicity Well-documented research on its role in disc regeneration	Questions remain regarding the capacity of differentiation in chondrocytes No head-to-head efficacy comparisons with BM-MSCs efficacy
	Nucleus pulposus	Can be stimulated to proliferate and differentiate, in situ	Low yield in number, decreased viability, and expression of proteoglycan and type II collagen in the setting of DDD
	Umbilical cord	Pluripotent No ethical barriers	Further studies to establish the immunologic safety of allogeneic human umbilical cord MSC transplantation are needed
	Amniotic	Pluripotent No ethical barriers	Further studies needed to establish efficacy in the treatment of cartilaginous tissues

Suggested Reading

1. A Hamid MS, Mohamed Ali MR, Yusof A, George J, Lee LP. Platelet-rich plasma injections for the treatment of hamstring injuries: a randomized controlled trial. Am J Sports Med. 2014;42(10):2410–8.
2. Centeno CJ. Clinical challenges and opportunities of mesenchymal stem cells in musculoskeletal medicine. Phy Med and Rehab. 2014;6:70–7.
3. Gou S, Oxentenko SC, Eldrige JS, Xiao L, Pingree MJ, Wang Z, Perez-Tercic C, Qu W. Stem cell therapy for intervertebral disk regeneration. Am J Phys Med Rehabil. 2014;93(Suppl):S122–31.
4. National Institutes of Health Facts Sheet: Regenerative Medicine. http://report.nih.gov/nihfactsheets/viewfactsheet.aspx?csid=62.
5. Sharma P, Maffulli N. Tendon injury and tendinopathy: healing and repair. J Bone Joint Surg Am. 2005;87(1):187–202.

Sacroiliac Joint Dysfunction

49

George C. Chang Chien, Radhika P. Grandhe,
and Joseph D. Fortin

Key Concepts

- The sacroiliac joint (SIJ) joins the sacrum to the pelvis transmitting the forces from the axial skeleton above to the lower extremities. SIJ dysfunction is a common cause of low back pain.
- History will reveal pain with maneuvers that stress the pelvic ring.
- Look for contributing factors such as a history of pelvic girdle trauma, repetitive asymmetric axial loading, pregnancy, or spondyloarthropathy (ankylosing spondylitis).
- No single physical exam maneuver is indicative of sacroiliac joint dysfunction, but a composite of exam maneuvers has been positively correlated to confirmatory diagnostic joint injection.
- The diagnostic gold standard remains image-guided intra-articular joint injection.
- There are myriad treatment options including corticosteroid injection and radiofrequency ablation.

Introduction

Sacroiliac joint (SIJ) arthropathy is a common cause of acute and chronic low back pain. It is estimated to be the cause of up to 30% of low back pain. In a recent multicentric study, Cher and colleagues found that the overall health burden endured by chronic SIJ pain sufferers was greater than cohorts with COPD, coronary artery disease, and asthma.

The SIJ is a mechanical relay station – transmitting loads to and from the trunk and lower extremities while simultaneously providing logic functions as position sense and loading behavior. As such, it provides a unique role in human locomotion and serves as the driving impulse of truncal counterrotation.

SIJ pathology is commonly associated with other conditions including: trauma to the pelvis, ankylosing spondylitis, psoriatic arthritis, Reiter's syndrome, inflammatory bowel disease, and pregnancy.

Anatomy

The sacroiliac joints are a pair of diarthrodial L-shaped joints that join the sacrum to the ilium bones. The articular surface of the ilium is made up of fibrocartilage, while the sacral surface is made up of much thicker hyaline cartilage. There are interosseous sacroiliac ligaments that maintain tight adherence between the sacrum and ilium. In addition to the primary SI ligaments, the sacrotuberous and sacrospinous ligaments further stabilize the sacrum to the pelvic girdle. These ligaments have also been implicated as potential pain generators. The orientation of the SIJs within the pelvis renders them particularly vulnerable to axial loading to failure. In fact, Miller found the SIJ to be twenty times more susceptible to axial overloading than the lumbar motion segments. Commensurate with Miller's report, Fortin and Roberts observed a high incidence of SIJ pain in competitive figure skaters – who repetitively land their jumps on the same lower extremity.

Normal motion within the paired joints include a small amount of movement (2–18°) in the transverse plane called nutation (forward rotation of the sacrum between the ilia) and counternutation (backward rotation of the sacrum between the ilia). In addition to the amount of nutation/

G.C. Chang Chien, DO (✉)
Cleveland Clinic, Anesthesia Institute Pain Management,
9500 Euclid Ave, Dept C-25, Cleveland, OH 44195, USA
e-mail: gchangchien@gmail.com

R.P. Grandhe, MD, MBBS
Cleveland Clinic, Department of Pain Management,
Cleveland, OH, USA

J.D. Fortin, DO
Spine Technology and Rehabilitation, Indiana School of Medicine,
Fort Wayne, IN, USA

J.E. Pope, T.R. Deer (eds.), *Treatment of Chronic Pain Conditions*, DOI 10.1007/978-1-4939-6976-0_49

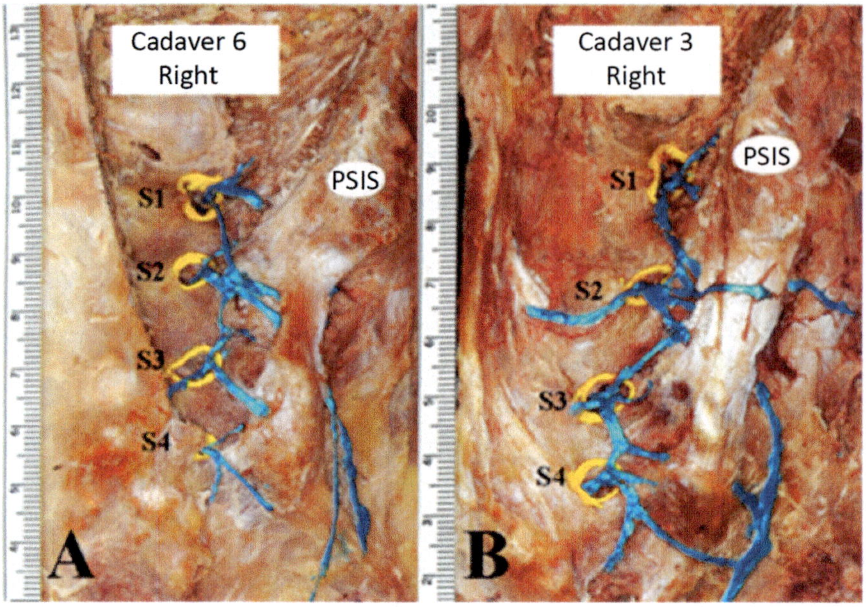

Fig. 49.1 (a, b) Cadaveric specimens demonstrating dense SIJ innervation inferior and medial to the PSIS. Lateral branches of the dorsal rami emanate from the S_1 to S_4 dorsal foramina (Reproduced with permission from Cox and Fortin [2]. © American Society of Interventional Pain Physicians)

counternutation, the existence of an oblique axis (implicated in normal reciprocal gait mechanics) has been the subject of debate.

Innervation

The common pathways of innervation revealed by recent investigations include: the lateral branches of the sacral dorsal rami, the medial branch of the L5 dorsal rami, and variable innervation from the superior gluteal nerve (Fig. 49.1). Several investigators have also reported on the branches from the lumbosacral plexus and obturator nerve. Innervation of ventral rami origin has been questioned by the absence of ventral receptors in fetal SIJ capsules. This complex innervation pattern has implications for the treatment of SIJ arthropathy.

Physical Examination

Patients with symptomatic sacroiliac joints often present to their physicians pointing at the SIJ (immediately medial and inferior to the PSIS) as the source of their pain (i.e., a positive Fortin finger test or FFT). Upon experimental stimulation of the SIJ capsules of asymptomatic volunteers, Fortin and co-workers observed that all volunteers referred evoked symptoms below their PSIS with some extending toward the ipsilateral greater trochanter. These observations are congruent with the aforementioned cadaveric reports demonstrating dense innervation in the same area below the PSIS. While primary buttock pain is the most common presentation, it is not unusual for patients with symptomatic SIJ's to report symptoms radiating as far distal as the foot. Accordingly, Fortin and colleagues employed arthrography, post-arthrography CT, and capsular immunohistochemical techniques to link the SIJ to sciatica.

There are a number of physical examination provocative maneuvers for identifying symptomatic sacroiliac joints including: Gillet's test, Patrick's maneuver (FABER), Gaenslen's test, anterior-posterior compression, thigh thrust, and sacral compression (Table 49.1). While no single exam maneuver is diagnostic for SIJ pathology, Laslett and others have demonstrated that combining multiple stress tests greatly enhances the diagnostic yield. As the pelvic girdle is a ring (consider Pascal's principle), examine patients with putative SIJ pain for tenderness of the surrounding ligaments, as well as the pubic symphysis.

Diagnostic Modalities

Plain films (X-rays) are a common screening method for suspected sacroiliac joint pathology, but are often nondiagnostic for early stages of degenerative or inflammatory pathology. They do play an important role in the setting of trauma; when evaluating a patient for gross fracture, dislocation, or dynamic instability. CT can show evidence of degenerative, erosive, or destructive joint changes earlier than radiographs. While MRI is more sensitive than CT or scintigraphy for evaluating the evolution of marrow space pathology (associated with stress fracture or inflammatory sacroiliitis), CT outperforms MRI when assessing osseous contour abnormalities. Structural findings on imaging studies are not prima facie evidence of pain. In fact, degenerative changes in asymptomatic SIJs are common, after the age of 30.

Table 49.1 Provocative physical exam maneuvers

Exam maneuver	Description	Patient position	Action	Findings
Distraction or anterior-posterior compression	This test applies anterior-posterior shear stress on the bilateral sacroiliac joints	Supine, legs in neutral position	Apply gradual, sustained downward pressure on the bilateral anterior-superior iliac spine.	Reproduction of pain localized to the sacral sulcus or sacroiliac joint
Thigh thrust	This test applies anterior-posterior shear stress on unilateral the sacroiliac joint	Supine, hip flexed to 90° with the knee relaxed	Apply gradual, sustained, vertically directed force through the femur	Reproduction of pain localized to the sacral sulcus or sacroiliac joint
Sacral thrust	This test applies forces to the bilateral sacroiliac joint	Prone, legs in neutral position.	Apply gradual, sustained downward pressure on the superior sacrum	Reproduction of pain localized to the sacral sulcus or sacroiliac joint
Patrick's maneuver (FABER)	This test applies tensile forces to the anterior sacroiliac joint ligaments	Supine, the hip flexed, abducted, and externally rotated and the foot resting on the opposite knee	The examiner then applies gradual, sustained downward pressure on the flexed knee	Reproduction of pain localized to the sacral sulcus or sacroiliac joint, NOT the anterior groin which would suggest femoral-acetabular dysfunction
Fortin finger test	The patient is asked to point to the area of maximum pain	Standing	The patient points with one finger	Patient points immediately posteromedial to PSIS

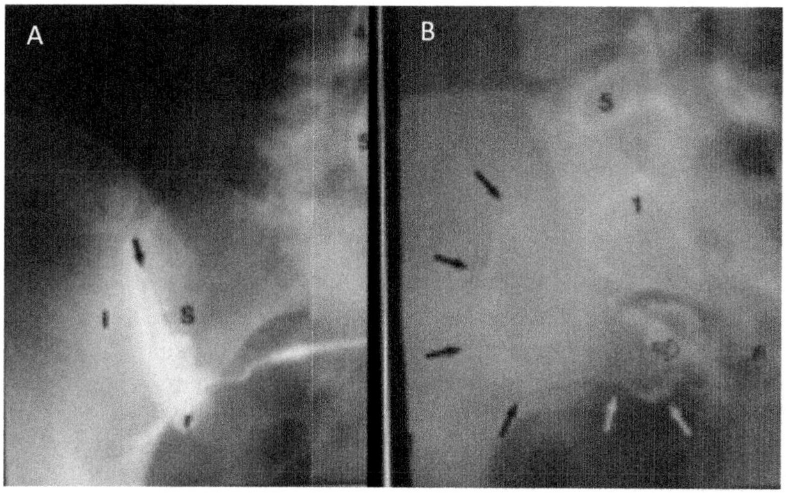

Fig. 49.2 SIJ injection and arthrography injection. (**a**) AP arthrography S (sacrum) I (ilium) r (inferior recess of capsule) *arrow* – bead of contrast in joint margin. (**b**) Enface oblique arthrography. *Arrows* indicate the capsule – delineating the auricular shape of the synovial joint (Reproduced with permission from Fortin and Sehgal [16])

While image-guided anesthetic blockade of a putatively painful joint is the standard for diagnosis (as no single physical exam maneuver is indicative of sacroiliac joint dysfunction), the intervention should be considered an extension of a careful history and physical.

Treatment Options

Conservative treatment should include cold application, anti-inflammatory medication or anti-inflammatory nutritional supplements, and relative rest (in the acute stage). Once pain has subsided, further efforts should be employed to restore normal mechanics, including manual medicine techniques, pelvic stabilization exercises to allow dynamic postural control, and muscle balancing of the trunk and lower extremities. SIJ belts or pelvic stabilization orthoses will provide confidence and proprioceptive awareness for sacroiliac joint dysfunction sufferers. A properly positioned cinch-type pelvic stabilization orthotic (worn directly superior to the greater trochanters) can significantly limit sacroiliac motion and thereby decrease pain.

If conservative treatment fails, SIJ intra-articular injections should be considered, not only as a therapeutic intervention but also to confirm the diagnosis (Fig. 49.2). Mitigation of symptoms by analgesic block is the most reliable and reproducible means by which a painful SIJ can be identified.

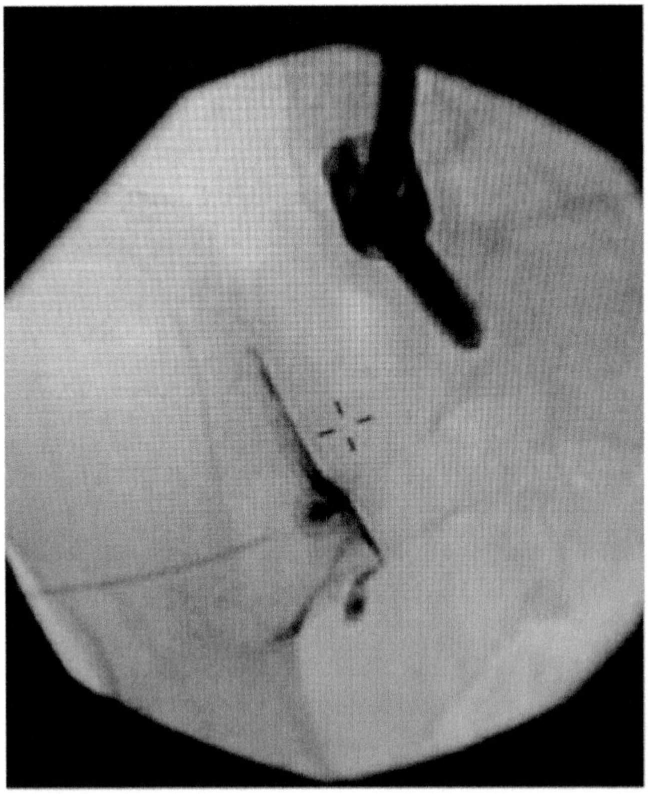

Fig. 49.3 AP plain film projection. Radiofrequency probes (with 10 mm tips) are oriented across the S1 to S4 dorsal foramina (medial to lateral)

Once the diagnosis is confirmed by profound relief of symptoms (lasting at least as long as the duration of the local anesthesia) following a diagnostic block, long-standing relief can often be obtained by radiofrequency ablation treatment of the sacral lateral branches and dorsal ramus of the L5 nerve (Fig. 49.3).

Dorman and co-workers observed in vitro that injecting chemical irritants into ligamentous tissue incites collagen proliferation. Theoretically, scarring and tightening of the ligaments results in stabilization of the joint. Hence, proliferant therapies may have a role in addressing an unstable SIJ.

Autologous mesenchymal stem cells (which morph in to bone, cartilage, and connective tissue) combined with platelet-derived growth factors have also been the subject of considerable research focus for joint conditions, including the SIJ. These biologic media are generally administered by image-controlled injections. While more research and development of this technology is warranted, regenerative approaches to SIJ pathology hold great promise.

Arthrodesis of the sacroiliac joint for chronic, non-traumatic, painful dysfunction is controversial but may be considered if all nonsurgical treatments have failed. Moore found a 75% success rate employing an open, modified Smith-Petersen fusion technique with AO hardware. Since Moore's study there have been at least ten reports in the peer review literature suggesting that minimally invasive ("closed") fusion with instrumentation approaches are also effective for a subset of patients. Clinical judgment should be used if lumbar spine pathology coexists with sacroiliac joint dysfunction, as this information should factor in the treatment algorithm.

Summary

On balance, look for a history of trauma to the pelvic ring or repetitive asymmetric axial loading. Many patients with SIJ dysfunction present with primary buttock pain, as well as some who point directly at the joint as the source of their symptoms (i.e., positive FFT). Some patients will report symptoms suggestive of instability – the so-called "slipping clutch" syndrome. Palpatory examination reveals sacral sulcus, joint line, and surrounding ligamentous tenderness. Pubic symphysis tenderness further implicates pelvic girdle versus primary lumbar pathology. Several PE stress maneuvers also substantiate the diagnosis of SIJ dysfunction.

The history and physical findings should be confirmed by an image-guided direct intra-articular diagnostic block. Treatment options range from anti-inflammatory medications and physical therapy to radiofrequency ablation, stem cell therapy, and surgical fusion.

Suggested Reading

1. Cher D, Polly D, Berven S. Sacroiliac joint pain: burden of disease. Med Devices (Auckl). 2014;7:73–81.
2. Cox RC, Fortin JD. The anatomy of the lateral branches of the sacral dorsal rami: implications for radiofrequency ablation. Pain Physician. 2014;17:459–64.
3. Dorman T. Pelvic mechanics and prolotherapy. In: Vleeming A, Mooney V, Dorman T, Snijders C, Stoeckart R, editors. Movement, stability, and low back pain: the essential role of the pelvis. New York: Churchill Livingstone; 1997. p. 501–22.
4. Elgafy H, Semaan HB, Ebraheim NA, Coombs RJ. Computed tomography findings in patients with sacroiliac pain. Clin Orthop Relat Res. 2001;382:112–8.
5. Fortin JD. An algorithm for understanding spine imaging. Pain Physician. 2002;5(1):102–9.
6. Fortin JD, Dwyer A, West S, Pier J. Sacroiliac joint pain referral patterns upon application of a new injection/arthrography technique – Part I, asymptomatic volunteers. Spine. 1994;19(13): 1475–82.
7. Fortin JD, Falco FJE. The fortin finger test: an indicator of sacroiliac joint pain. Am J Orthop. 1997;26(7):477–80.
8. Fortin J, Falco F, Washington W. Three pathways between the sacroiliac joint and neural structures exist. Am J Neuroradiol. 1999; 20(8):1429–34.
9. Fortin JD, Roberts D. Competitive figure skating injuries. Pain Physician. 2003;6(3):313–8.
10. Fortin JD, Vilensky JA, Merkel GJ. Can the sacroiliac joint cause sciatica? Pain Physician. 2003;6(3):269–71.

11. Fortin JD, Wahezi SE, Mintz D, Chang A. Diagnostic imaging of painful sacroiliac Jioints. In: DePalma MJ, editor. iSpine evidence-based interventional spine care. New York: Demos Medical; 2013.
12. Laslett M, Young SB, Aprill CN, McDonald B. Diagnosing painful sacroiliac joints: a validity study of a McKenzie evaluation and sacroiliac provocation tests. Aust JPhysiother. 2003;49:89–97.
13. Miller JAA, Schultz AM, Anderson GBJ. Load-displacement behavior or sacroiliac joints. J Orthrop Res. 1987;5:92–101.
14. Moore MR. Surgical treatment of chronic painful sacroiliac joint dysfunction. In: Vleeming A, Mooney V, Dorman T, Snijders C, Stoeckart R, editors. Movement, stability, and low back pain: the essential role of the pelvis. New York: Churchill Livingstone; 1997. p. 563–72.
15. Nakagawa T. A study on the distribution of nerve filaments of the iliosacral joint and its adjacent region in the Japanese. J Jap Orthop Assoc. 1966;40:419–30.
16. Fortin JD, Sehgal N. Sacroiliac joint injection and arthrography with imaging correlation. In: Lennard TA, editor. Pain procedures in clinical practice. 2nd ed. Philadelphia: Hanley & Belfus; 2000.

Platelet-Rich Plasma

50

Hector Miranda-Grajales

Key Concepts

- Platelet-rich plasma (PRP) injection therapy has evidence-based medicine supporting its use for certain tendinopathies: lateral epicondylitis, Achilles tendinopathy, and plantar fasciitis.
- PRP rarely has any complications.
- There are multiple PRP isolation techniques described in the literature.

Introduction

Platelet-rich plasma is a therapeutic technique used to treat tendinopathies. It is mostly used to treat chronic pain secondary to the following conditions: lateral epicondylitis, Achilles tendinopathy, and plantar fasciitis. PRP is used to treat other conditions as well: patellar tendinopathy, medial epicondylitis, and rotator cuff tendinopathy, although evidence base for the benefit of PRP to treat these conditions is lacking. The use of PRP rarely has any complications. One side effect of using this technique is worsening of the patient's pain at the site of injection. This usually lasts no more than 48 h. If this side effect happens, it should not be treated with nonsteroidal anti-inflammatory drugs as this would counteract the effects of the platelet-rich plasma pro-inflammatory mechanism of action. It should not be treated with local anesthetic injection as this has been shown to decrease efficacy of the healing properties of PRP. It can be treated with a short course of short-acting narcotics or with ice therapy.

Platelet-rich plasma can be isolated with a centrifuge in multiple different ways: single-spin process at 1500 revolutions per minute (RPM) for 5 min, single-spin process at 3200 RPM for 15 min, and double-spin process. The double-spin process involves centrifugation of whole blood for 5 min at 1500 RPM, and then the plasma containing the platelets is centrifuged a second time for 20 min at 6300 RPM. The single-spin process at 1500 RPM yields a lower platelet-rich plasma concentration (PRPLP), single-spin process at 3200 RPM yields high platelet and white blood cell plasma concentrations (PRPHP), double-spin process yields a higher platelet plasma and lower white blood cell concentration (PRPDS). PRPLP increases cell proliferation osteocytes, myocytes, and tenocytes. PRPDS increases cell proliferation of osteoblasts and tenocytes, but not of myocytes. PRPHP increases cell proliferation of tenocytes but not of myocytes. The studies done thus far to test the efficacy of PRP injections have not determined superiority among any of the mentioned PRP isolation techniques.

A total of 25–30 mL of whole blood is required to isolate at least 3 mL of PRP. After this is done, 2–3 mL of PRP is injected into the affected area.

Background

The proposed mechanism of action of PRP is that it assists in the healing process of an injured tendon. Tendon connective tissue has poor blood supply and, hence, decreased healing properties. Platelets contain endogenous growth factors within alpha granules. These growth factors are transforming growth factor-β1 (TGF-β1), insulin-like growth factors (IGF) 1 and 2, vascular endothelial growth factor (VEGF), basic fibroblast growth factor (BFGF), and hepatocyte growth factor (HGF). These factors are released upon degranulation of the alpha granules; degranulation is precipitated by calcium, thrombin, or collagen. It is worth mentioning that the first phase of wound repair involves the arrival of the platelet/fibrin complex to initiate the healing cascade.

Once injured, tendons and ligaments don't completely regain the biomechanical properties they had prior to the injury. This makes tendons/ligaments susceptible to reinjury.

H. Miranda-Grajales, MD (✉)
Medical Injury Rehabilitation Specialists, Gainesville, FL 32653, USA
e-mail: hmirandamd@medinjury.net

J.E. Pope, T.R. Deer (eds.), *Treatment of Chronic Pain Conditions*, DOI 10.1007/978-1-4939-6976-0_50

Chronic ligament injuries generally represent chronic instability from failure of acute ligament healing and may have an inflammatory component. Inserting PRP into the injured tendon accelerates the healing process by increasing the platelet concentration by 5–8 times the normal concentration.

Indications

1. Lateral epicondylitis
2. Medial epicondylitis
3. Achilles tendinopathy
4. Plantar fasciitis
5. Patellar tendinopathy
6. Rotator cuff tendinopathy

Suggested Reading

1. Hayter CI, Guffre BM. Overuse and traumatic injuries of the elbow. Magn Reson Imaging Clin N Am. 2009;17:617–38.
2. Khan KM, Cook JL, Bonar F, et al. Histopathology of common tendinopathies. Update and implications for clinical management. Sports Med. 1999;27:393–408.
3. Kon E, Filardo G, Delcogliano M, et al. Platelet-rich plasma: new clinical application. A pilot study for treatment of jumper's knee. Injury. 2009;40:598–603.
4. Mazzocca, et al. The positive effects of different platelet-rich plasma methods on human muscle, bone, and tendon cells. Am J Sports Med. 2012;40:1742.
5. de Mos M, van der Windt AE, Jahr H, van Schie HT, Weinans H, Verhaar JA, et al. Can platelet-rich plasma enhance tendon repair? A cell culture study. Am J Sports Med. 2008;36:1171–8.
6. Peerbooms JC, Sluimer J, Bruijn DJ, et al. Positive effect of an autologous platelet concentrate in lateral epicondylitis in a double-blind randomized controlled trial: platelet-rich plasma versus corticosteroid injection with a 1-year follow-up. Am J Sports Med. 2010;38:255–62.
7. Pietro R, Paolo A, Ragone V, Aliprandi A, Cabitza P. Platelet rich plasma in arthroscopic rotator cuff repair: a prospective RCT study, 2-year follow-up. J Shoulder Elb Surg. 2011;20: 518–28.
8. Sanchez M, Anitua E, Azofra J, et al. Comparison of surgically repaired Achilles tendon tears using platelet-rich fibrin matrices. Am J Sport Med. 2007;35:245–51.
9. Ventura A, Terzaghi C, Borgo E, et al. Use of growth factors in ACL surgery: preliminary study. J Orthop Traumatol. 2005;6: 76–9.
10. de Vos RJ, Weir A, van Schie HTM, et al. Platelet-rich plasma injection for chronic Achilles tendinopathy: a randomised controlled trial. JAMA. 2010;303:144–9.

Part VIII

Advanced Pain Care Therapies: VIII. Intrathecal Drug Delivery

Intrathecal Drug Delivery Indications

51

Jason E. Pope

Key Concepts

- Intrathecal therapy is moving away from its position as a pain care salvage therapy to one earlier in the pain care algorithm.
- Morbidity and mortality surrounding intrathecal therapy is largely iatrogenic.
- Intrathecal therapy requires vigilance and ancillary support.

Introduction

The historic contention that bulk flow plays a large role in CSF mixing and solute dispersion has proven to be inaccurate, as recent work into cerebrospinal fluid (CSF) flow dynamics of the intrathecal space has offered an insight into pharmacokinetic modeling. The locomotives behind the nonhomogenous, discrete regions of mixing, with bidirectional cranio-caudal oscillatory movement, are cardiac and pulmonary in origin. Animal models suggest that dispersion from the catheter tip within the CSF by slow infusion is rather limited, dependent on the physiochemical properties of the drug, rate, and volume delivered, suggesting that site-specific catheter placement congruent with area of pain within the IT space is important for optimal efficacy.

Candidacy

Indications for intrathecal therapy include chronic moderate to severe cancer and noncancer pain uncontrolled by more conservative measures. The geriatric population, where opioid analgesics provide pain reduction but complicated by side effect (including constipation or altered mentation), are excellent candidates.

Indications

See Table 51.1.

Patients should be medically compliant and undergo a psychological screen to determine psychological tolerability of implanted therapies. The patient should be medically stable and have no systemic infection, untoward bleeding risks, or local skin infections at the site of the proposed implant. The patient should have the intellectual capacity to manage the therapy (Fig. 51.1).

Suggested Reading

1. Bernards CM. Cerebrospinal fluid and spinal cord distribution of baclofen and bupivacaine during slow intrathecal infusion in pigs. Anesthesiology. 2006;105:169–78.
2. Coffey RJ, Owens ML, Broste SK, et al. Mortality associated with implantation and management of intrathecal opioid drug infusion systems to treat noncancer pain. Anesthesiology. 2009;111:881–91.
3. Deer TR, Prager J, Levy R, Rathmell J, Buchser E, Burton A, Caraway D, Cousins M, De Andres J, Diwan S, Erdek M, Grigsby E, Huntoon M, Jacons MS, Kim P, Kumar K, Leong M, Liem L, McDowell GC, Panchal S, Rauck R, Stanton-Hicks M, Stears L, Wallace M, Willis KD, Witt W, Yaksh T, Mekhail N. Polyanalgesic consensus conference 2012: recommendations for the management of pain by intrathecal (intraspinal) drug delivery: report of an interdisciplinary expert panel. Neuromodulation. 2012;15(5):420–35.
4. Smith TJ, Staats PS, Deer T, et al. Randomized clinical trial of an implantable drug delivery system compared with comprehensive medical management for refractory cancer pain: impact on pain, drug-related toxicity, and survival. J Clin Oncol. 2002;20(19):4040–9.

J.E. Pope, MD (✉)
Summit Pain Alliance, 392 Tesconi Ct, Santa Rosa, CA 95401, USA
e-mail: popeje@me.com

J.E. Pope, T.R. Deer (eds.), *Treatment of Chronic Pain Conditions*, DOI 10.1007/978-1-4939-6976-0_51

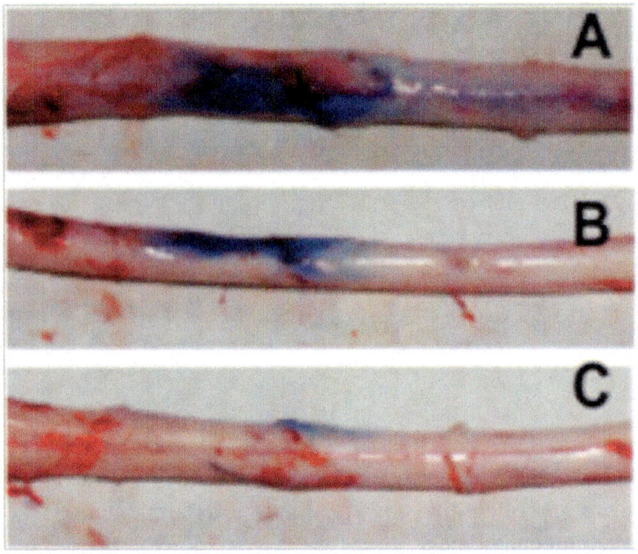

Fig. 51.1 Methylene blue dye spread after chronic infusion in an animal model demonstrating A: posterior, B lateral, and C anterior spread. Taken with permission from [1]

Table 51.1 Indications

Axial back pain Multiple compression fractures Arthritis pain Spinal stenosis Multilevel degenerative disc disease
Complex regional pain syndrome
Abdominal pain
Failed back surgery syndrome
Connective tissue disorders
Trunk pain Postherpetic neuralgia
Cancer pain Primary tumor invasion Bone metastasis Nerve plexus invasion Chemotherapy-induced neuropathy Radiation-induced neuritis
Analgesic efficacy with systemic opioid Delivery with intolerable side effects

Intrathecal Drug Delivery Trialing Strategies

52

Jason E. Pope

Key Concepts

- Trialing for chronic intrathecal infusion has been described employing many different routes of delivery, and while there is little evidence to suggest a superior one, it is recommended to dose within the epidural space.
- Outpatient dosing has been recommended by the PACC, with the importance of vigilance and conservative dosing.
- Cardiopulmonary depression can occur with intrathecal opioid dosing.
- Ziconotide is a non-opioid-based therapy that does not cause cardiopulmonary compromise.

Introduction

The trial procedure is typically performed in one of two ways. Both trialing methods require a 23-h inpatient observation to determine efficacy and monitor for untoward events, namely, respiratory depression. An example of typical 23-h orders is in the appendix. Importantly, an appreciation for predictable side effects helps mitigate complications. In my practice, during the 23-h observed stay, we discontinue all of non-analgesic sedating medications (benzodiazepines, sleep aids, etc.) to avoid complicating the presentation of intrathecal overdose. All of the patient's outpatient analgesic medications are continued, but listed as "prn" status. All patients must urinate prior to discharge. Side effects are dose related, but not linearly. Success is gauged by at least 50% pain reduction with no intolerable side effects.

Intrathecal Medication Side Effects

See Table 52.1.

Itching can be mitigated by Atarax 25 mg BID.

Urinary retention can be mitigated by bethanechol 25 mg BID.

Single-Shot Trial Procedure

Patients are positioned prone in an operating room or injection suite, and strict sterile precautions and drape are followed. Using fluoroscopy, after appropriate topicalization, a 3.5 inch 22 or 25G needle is advanced using AP and lateral guidance to enter into the intrathecal space at the L-2 interspace. After free flow CSF is obtained, 1–2 cc of Isovue is injected to demonstrate myelogram and to survey the intrathecal space. Then, the medication is injected with barbotage. The needle is removed, a Band-Aid is placed over the puncture site, and they are monitored for 23 h.

> Dose calculation opioids: (Oral route converted to morphine equivalents)/300/2.

- The denominator of the equation (2) will increase with escalating doses of medications.

Typical intrathecal morphine dose trials range from 0.1 to 0.5 mg. See Table 52.2 for conversion from morphine to other opioids. Conversions are not exact and require clinical judgment. Prialt dosing typically is initiated as a 2mcg bolus and increased intervally to a maximum dose of 8 mcg with each subsequent trial.

J.E. Pope, MD (✉)
Summit Pain Alliance, 392 Tesconi Ct, Santa Rosa, CA 95401, USA
e-mail: popeje@me.com

J.E. Pope, T.R. Deer (eds.), *Treatment of Chronic Pain Conditions*, DOI 10.1007/978-1-4939-6976-0_52

Table 52.1 Intrathecal medication side effects

Opioid-related side effects	Pruritus, urinary retention, pedal edema, sedation, respiratory depression
Ziconotide	Nausea, headache, urinary retention, confusion, dizziness, sedation, psychosis (rare), hallucinations (rare)

Table 52.2 Conversion from morphine to other opioids

Morphine (mg)	Dilaudid (mg)	Fentanyl (mcg)
0.1 mg	0.02	10mcg

Catheter Trial Procedure

The patient preparation positioning is the same. Under fluoroscopic guidance, a 17G Tuohy needle is then advanced into the epidural space with the standard "loss of resistance" technique, localizing the epidural space. Under lateral fluoroscopic guidance, the needle is placed with careful attention to paresthesias. Once cerebrospinal fluid is obtained, the flexible catheter is threaded, avoiding paresthesias, and then the needle is removed. The catheter is then secured, and slow infusion of medication is then initiated and titrated to clinical effect up to a maximal ceiling dose.

Site of Service

Historically, IT therapy was proposed to be performed in an inpatient or 23-h observational setting. This allowed an opportunity to monitor for delayed respiratory depression. However, in practice, many clinicians performed outpatient low-dose opioid trials with no untoward events. Recently, the Polyanalgesic Consensus Conference (PACC) of 2017 described strategies for intrathecal trialing in the outpatient setting. Patient selection criteria include previous opioid exposure, medical comorbidities, age of the patient, and medication intrathecal dose.

Suggested Reading

1. Deer TR, Hayek SM, Pope JE, et al. The Polyanalgesic Consensus Conference (PACC): Recommendations for Trialing of Intrathecal Drug Delivery Infusion Therapy. Neuromodulation. 2017;20(2): 133–54. doi:10.1111/ner.12543. Epub 2017 Jan 2. Review.
2. Deer TR, Pope JE, Hayek SM, et al. The Polyanalgesic Consensus Conference (PACC): Recommendations for Intrathecal Drug Delivery: Guidance for Improving Safety and Mitigating Risks. Neuromodulation. 2017;20(2):155–76. doi:10.1111/ner.12579. Epub 2017 Jan 2. Review.
3. Deer TR, Pope JE, Hayek SM, et al. The Polyanalgesic Consensus Conference (PACC): Recommendations on Intrathecal Drug Infusion Systems Best Practices and Guidelines. Neuromodulation. 2017;20(2):96–132. doi:10.1111/ner.12538. Epub 2017 Jan 2. Review.

Intrathecal Drug Delivery: Available Technologies

53

Jason E. Pope

Key Concepts

- Innovation surrounding intrathecal therapy includes new implantable programmable infusion systems.
- The Medtronic SynchroMed II programmable pump employs a peristaltic roller delivery strategy.
- The Flowonix SynchroMed II programmable pump employs a piston valve delivery strategy.
- Both pumps carry MRI compatible conditional labeling at 1.5 Tesla. The Medtronic system restarts after a predictable motor stall while exposed to the MRI, while the Flowonix Prometra II exposure to an MRI trips the flow activated valve (FAV), which requires the device to be reset by removing the medication in its entirety and programming a bolus to reopen the FAV pump, with subsequent replacement of the medication.
- The Flowonix Prometra I programmable pump requires all the medication to be removed from the pump in its entirety prior to MRI exposure, as there is no flow activated valve and the contents of the reservoir are emptied through the catheter into the patient.

Introduction

Intrathecal therapy is a powerful tool in the armamentarium of the pain provider. It serves as a treatment strategy for both nociceptive and neuropathic pain, with sustainable outcomes and cost-effectiveness that is superior to spinal cord stimulation. New platforms have entered into the market, and we will review some of the differences in turn.

Available Devices

Implantable programmable infusion systems have been an advanced pain care option for nearly 30 years. The current offering available, at the time do this writing, are the Medtronic SynchroMed II (Fig. 53.1) and the Flowonix Prometra II (Fig. 53.2). Each offers different attractive features and advancements. A clear understanding of the differences will improve device troubleshooting, management, and patent safety and efficacy.

The Medtronic SynchroMed II pump is the most commonly used implantable, programmable pump in use today. It uses a roller, geared, rotor system that delivers reservoir agents by a seemingly peristaltic sequence along an internal catheter that ultimately leads to the external catheter. It allows for the use of a patient therapy manager, or PTM, which serves as a patient-controlled bolus device. It is an MRI conditional system for 1.5 and 3.0 Tesla, but not for open, sitting, or standing. A predictable motor stall occurs, with imitation and recovery commonly within 20 min. Motor stall scan infrequently take up to 90 min to recover.

Combination therapy caused corrosion of the internal tubing resulting in mechanical failure of the pump, as reported within a series of warning letters, with others surrounding bolus delivery and over-infusion. The pump life is suggested to be 5–7 years.

The Prometra II system represents a new delivery strategy and is an implantable, programmable intrathecal delivery device. It employs a valve-gated regulation system that allows for a very accurate delivery, even at small volumes, delivering small bolus. This has been hypothesized to reduce granuloma formation. The pump has a delivery strategy that does not corrode with placement of combination therapy within the device. The pump is MRI conditional for 1.5 Tesla. Once exposed to a magnetic field, the flow activated valve (FAV) is closed, preventing the contents of the reservoir to be emptied in the patient, which could have occurred in the Prometra I.

J.E. Pope, MD (✉)
Summit Pain Alliance, 392 Tesconi Ct, Santa Rosa, CA 95401, USA
e-mail: popeje@me.com

J.E. Pope, T.R. Deer (eds.), *Treatment of Chronic Pain Conditions*, DOI 10.1007/978-1-4939-6976-0_53

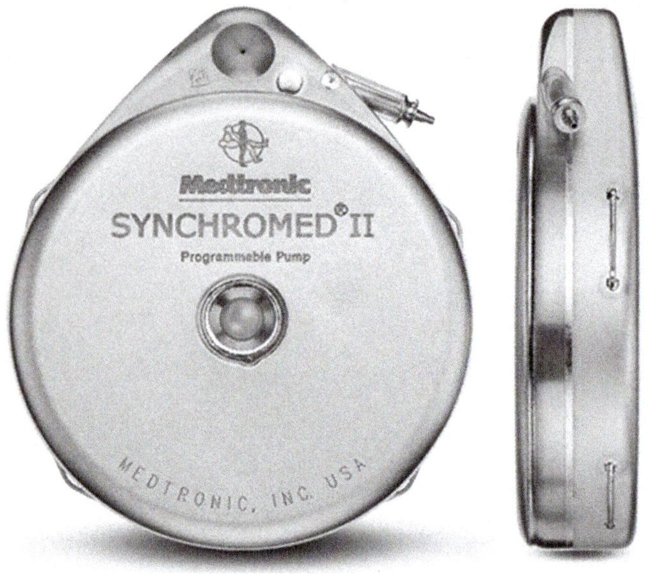

Fig. 53.1 Medtronic SynchroMed II (From http://professional.medtronic.com/pt/neuro/itb/prod/synchromed-ii/index.htm#.V2t5GFZ_dUs)

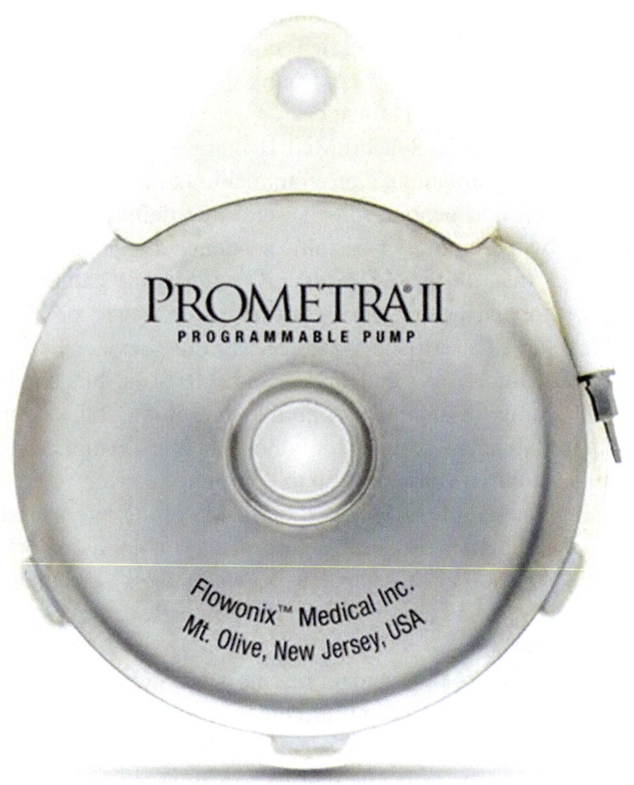

Fig. 53.2 Flowonix Prometra II (From http://www.flowonix.com/sites/default/files/Prometra-Practice-Brochure.pdf)

Once the FAV trips, the contents of the reservoir have to be removed and then replaced, within the reservoir in order for the valve to be reset. Further, there is no reading to inform the clinician or the patient if the valve trips. The pump also has a positive pressure refill reservoir, where once the refill needle is placed correctly within the septum, once deployed, if the refill syringe is left in place, it will refill with reservoir contents, adding a layer of safety to the refill procedure. The side port needle cannot be exchanged for the reservoir refill needle, which makes accurate placement of either needle for the intended procedure more likely. The pump also supports a PTC (Patient Therapy Controller) which allows for patient-controlled boluses. Pump longevity has been estimated to be as high as 10 years.

Table 53.1 Comparison of the latest technologies

	Prometra® II	SynchroMed II
Motor/rotor	None	Yes
Flow rate	0.0–28.8 ml/day	0.048–24 ml/day
Pump mechanism	Valve gated	Peristaltic
Material	Titanium	Titanium/plastic
Refill septum	Raised 3 mm	Inverted septum
Refill septum	25 psi	3–5 psi
MRI conditional[a]	1.5 Tesla; removal of medicine after MRI is required	1.5 and 3.0 Tesla, no removal of medicine needed
Patient-controlled bolusing strategy	Yes	Yes

[a]The Prometra I and Prometra II requires all reservoir contents to be removed BEFORE MRI

Table 53.1 defines the comparison of the latest technologies. Although the Codman 3000 and the Codman Medstream are commercially available historically, they are mentioned for completeness, although not included in this writing.

Conclusion

Intrathecal therapy is a needed component in the pain offerings to patient suffering. With innovation and multiple platforms available, it is essential to understanding the subtle differences surrounding their delivery.

Suggested Reading

1. Coffey RJ, Owens ML, Broste SK, et al. Mortality associated with implantation and management of intrathecal opioid drug infusion systems to treat noncancer pain. Anesthesiology. 2009;111:881–91.
2. Deer TR, Prager J, Levy R, Rathmell J, Buchser E, Burton A, Caraway D, Cousins M, De Andres J, Diwan S, Erdek M, Grigsby E, Huntoon M, Jacons MS, Kim P, Kumar K, Leong M, Liem L, McDowell GC, Panchal S, Rauck R, Stanton-Hicks M, Stears L, Wallace M, Willis KD, Witt W, Yaksh T, Mekhail N. Polyanalgesic consensus conference 2012: recommendations for the Management

of Pain by intrathecal (Intraspinal) drug delivery: report of an interdisciplinary expert panel. Neuromodulation. 2012;15(5): 436–64.
3. Pope JE, Deer TR. Intrathecal drug delivery for pain: a clinical guide and future directions. Pain Manag. 2015;5(3):175–83. doi:10.2217/pmt.15.12.
4. Pope JE, Poree L, McRoberts WP, et al. Consent decree: physician and institution ramifications. Neuromodulation. 2015; 18(8):653–6.
5. Pope JE, Deer TR, Bruel B, et al. Clinical uses of intrathecal therapy and its placement in the pain care algorithm. [Epub ahead of print]. Pain Pract. 2016; 9 Feb 2016.

Intrathecal Drug Delivery Implantation

54

Jason E. Pope

Key Concepts

- Intrathecal therapy is an important tool for malignant and nonmalignant pain treatment.
- The implantation procedure is typically performed in the right lateral decubitus position.
- When placing the needle, it should be performed below the spinal cord in most scenarios.
- Catheter introduction into the intrathecal space should be performed carefully, and patient should be able to report any new radicular or axial complaints.

Implant Procedure

After a successful trial, the patient is positioned in the lateral decubitus position, with the back flush to the end of the table. The patient should receive antibiotic within 30 min of incision. The patient is marked and draped in the manner depicted in the following figure, marking the lower most palpable rib and the iliac crest. The reservoir site is marked on the abdomen, away from the belt line, on a flat horizontal plane. The site for the paraspinal incision is marked adjacent to the spinous process ipsilateral to the abdominal reservoir site (Fig. 54.1). Sidedness of intrathecal pump reservoir placement is under the discretion of the implanter and deserves mention (Table 54.1).

After appropriate topicalization, a 3.5 inch incision overlying the paraspinal site is created and carried down to the lumbodorsal fascia using blunt dissection and electrocautery. It is identified by the glossy fascia appearance. A weitlaner is commonly used to aid in visualization. Once this is accomplished, a small pocket is formed by horizontal dissection along the fascia to accommodate the anchor and stress relief loop.

Using AP and lateral fluoroscopic guidance, an introducer needle is placed contacting the lamina of the vertebral body ipsilateral to the reservoir site. It is then walked off cephalad and medial into the IT space with serial checks in the lateral projection to determine depth while the patient is conversant. Once free flow CSF has been obtained, the catheter is then advanced into the CSF, again, while the patient is conversant. If paresthesias are felt, the catheter is withdrawn and repassed. Further, if resistance is met while threading the catheter, the catheter is withdrawn. Once the catheter is in place, the needle and stylets are removed, leaving the catheter within the CSF. It is then secured to the lumbodorsal fascia using an anchor and a nonabsorbable suture. The catheter distal end is then clipped to the drape, and a sterile wet lap is placed within the incision.

Attention is then directed to the reservoir site. A 5–6 cm incision is then created to accommodate the diameter of the intrathecal pump. Small rake retractors are used on the caudal side of the incision and pulled outward to create a dissection plane to Scarpa's fascia and then replaced by army-navy retractors on either side of the formed pocket. Once the pocket is created to accommodate the pump, hemostasis is confirmed, and a saturated lap is placed inside the incision.

Attention is then directed to the pump for preparation. Commonly, the pump is shipped with sterile water within the reservoir. This should be removed in its entirety and then discarded. The pump is then refilled with the designed therapeutic medication. Common medication starting doses, maximum concentrations, and maximum daily doses are highlighted in Tables 54.2, 54.3 and 54.4.

Ziconotide requires a rinse of the pump as the medication binds to the internal tubing. The reader is directed to the manufacturer's information for further information.

Attention is then directed to the operative sites. Both laps are removed, and the tunneler is utilized from the paraspinal incision to the abdominal incision with care to remain superficial to the transversus abdominus plane. The catheter is then placed through the tunneler and then the tunneller is

J.E. Pope, MD (✉)
Summit Pain Alliance,
392 Tesconi Ct, Santa Rosa, CA 95401, USA
e-mail: popeje@me.com

J.E. Pope, T.R. Deer (eds.), *Treatment of Chronic Pain Conditions*, DOI 10.1007/978-1-4939-6976-0_54

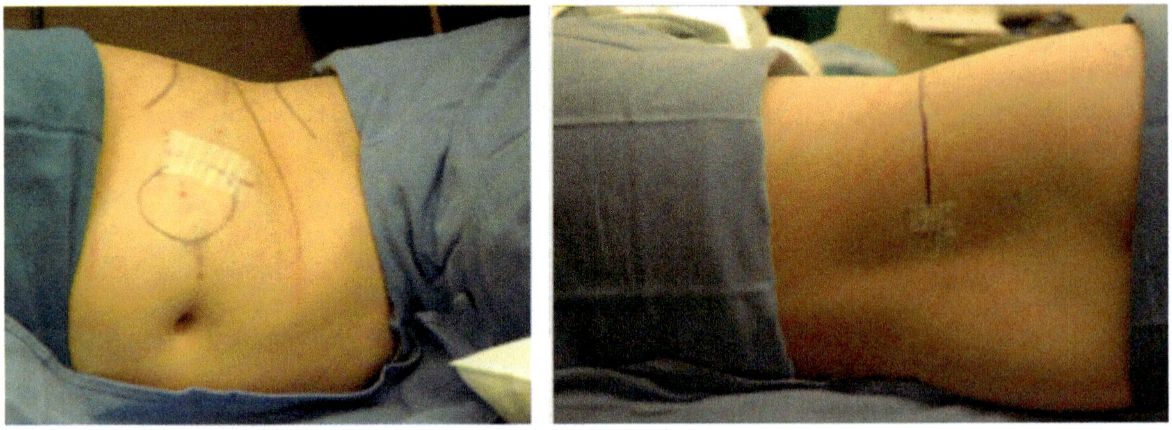

Fig. 54.1 Placement of intrathecal therapy in a patient

Table 54.1 Considerations for sidedness of IT pump placement

	RIGHT side	LEFT side
Intrathecal needle placement	Normal, right-handed driving anatomic placement	Opposite, left-handed, or backhand driving needle placement
Masking of pt comorbid presentations	Appendicitis	Diverticulitis, constipation, diverticulosis

Table 54.2 Recommended starting dose ranges

Drug	Recommendation of starting dose
Morphine	0.1–0.5 mg/day
Hydromorphone	0.01–0.15 mg/day
Ziconotide	0.5–1.2 mcg/day
Fentanyl	25–75 mcg/day
Bupivacaine	0.01–4 mg/day
Clonidine	20–100 mcg/day
Sufentanil	10–20 mcg/day

Table 54.3 Recommended bolus starting doses

Drug	Recommended dose
Morphine	0.1–0.5 mg
Hydromorphone	0.025–0.1 mg
Ziconotide	1–5 mcg
Fentanyl	15–75 mcg
Bupivacaine	0.5–2.5 mg
Clonidine	5–20 mcg
Sufentanil	5–20 mcg

Table 54.4 Recommended maximal daily doses and medication concentrations

Drug	Maximum concentration	Maximum dose per day
Morphine	20 mg/mL	15 mg
Hydromorphone	15 mg/mL	10 mg
Fentanyl	10 mg/mL	2000 mcg
Sufentanil	5 mg/mL	500 mcg
Bupivacaine	30 mg/mL	10 mg
Clonidine	1000 mcg/mL	600 mcg
Ziconotide	100 mcg/mL	19.2 mcg

removed. The catheter is then cut to the proper limit, which allows for slack to be created within both incisions. Importantly, it is handed off the device representative for measurement. The catheter is then secured onto the pump. Both incisions are then irrigated and the pump is internalized with the aspiration side port at approximately the 10:00 position. The incisions are closed with 3-O vicryl and 4-O monocryl in a running fashion. A sterile dressing is then applied and an abdominal binder is placed.

Typically, the dressings are maintained for at least 48 h, along with the abdominal binder with close vigilance. In the outpatient setting, it is advocated to watch the patient for at least 8 h prior to discharge with a responsible adult. In the inpatient setting, they are observed in the 23-h setting.

Conclusions

The implant procedure needs to be approached with appropriate preoperative planning and intraoperative execution of the surgical plan with excellent tissue management. In a closed claims analysis recently published in 2016, most claims for intrathecal therapy were surrounding the implant procedure and the maintenance of the therapy. Iatrogenic error, including programming, can result in overdose and death. Vigilance is imperative to deliver this necessary pain care therapy safely.

Suggested Reading

1. Coffey RJ, Owens ML, Broste SK, Dubois MY, Ferrante FM, Schultz DM, Stearns LJ, Turner MS. Mortality associated with implantation and management of intrathecal opioid drug infusion systems to treat noncancer pain. Anesthesiology. 2009;111:881–91.
2. Deer TR, Pope JE. Factors to consider in the choice of intrathecal drug in the treatment of neuropathic pain. Expert Rev Clin Pharmacol. 2015;8(5):507–10.
3. Pope JE, Deer TR. Intrathecal drug delivery for pain: a clinical guide and future directions. Pain Mange. 2015;5(3):175–83.
4. Prager J, Deer T, Levy R, et al. Best practices for intrathecal drug delivery for pain. Neuromodulation. 2014;17(4):354–72. discussion 372

55 Intrathecal Drug Delivery: Maintenance

John Hau

Key Concepts

- Routine maintenance of intrathecal drug delivery systems is critical to the safety and effectiveness of the therapy.
- Medication management, pump refill, and pump programming are vital aspects of intrathecal drug delivery maintenance.
- Vigilance for adverse events related to intrathecal drug delivery is paramount to patient safety.
- Medication administration adverse events are a significant source of intrathecal drug delivery complications.
- Delayed identification of granuloma formation at the tip of the catheter can lead to significant morbidity.

Introduction

Intrathecal drug delivery for the treatment of chronic refractory pain has grown since its introduction in the 1980s. After appropriate patient selection, trialing, and implantation, routine maintenance of the intrathecal drug delivery system is critical to the efficacy of the therapy as well as to patient safety.

Medications

The available medications for intrathecal drug delivery are extensive. Currently in the United States, the Food and Drug Administration (FDA) has only approved morphine, ziconotide, and baclofen for intrathecal use. However, many other agents have been utilized by pain management practitioners. Current therapy can be broadly divided into opioid and non-opioid-based therapy. The Polyanalgesic Consensus Conference has published recommended care algorithms with separate arms for neuropathic, nociceptive, and mixed pain states. The recommended care algorithms can assist providers in choosing the appropriate medication therapy for patients.

Refills

Routine maintenance of intrathecal drug delivery systems includes the interval refilling of the reservoir. Typical refill intervals range from 1 to 6 months. The US Food and Drug Administration requires intrathecal pumps to be refilled at least every 6 months regardless of remaining reservoir volume. Each device manufacturer will have unique refill kits. Intrathecal pump refills are performed under sterile technique. Refills can typically be performed with palpation and proper alignment of the template provided in the refill kits. The use of image guidance with ultrasound or fluoroscopy can help to reduce the incidence of refill errors.

Programming

Improving technology with intrathecal drug delivery systems has helped to advance the safety and versatility of the therapy. Previously, constant flow pumps delivered a continuous infusion at a set rate. However, with the programmability of the newer devices, providers can adjust flow rates and administer boluses. A personal therapy manager (PTM) can also be used by patients to deliver boluses in a patient-controlled manner. Instead of continuous infusion rates, intermittent bolus dosing has gained popularity as an alternative means of delivering the medications. There are currently no prospective studies to define the best rate and type of drug delivery. Continuous intrathecal delivery has long been the standard mechanism, but intermittent bolus dosing may be associated with reduced incidence of granuloma formation.

J. Hau, MD (✉)
Summit Pain Alliance, 392 Tesconi Ct, Santa Rosa, CA 95401, USA
e-mail: summitpainalliance@gmail.com

J.E. Pope, T.R. Deer (eds.), *Treatment of Chronic Pain Conditions*, DOI 10.1007/978-1-4939-6976-0_55

Adverse Events

Intrathecal drug delivery systems provide practitioners a powerful tool to help manage chronic refractory pain. Due to the nature of the therapy, adverse events can cause significant morbidity and mortality. Therefore, vigilance for possible adverse events is a critical component of therapy maintenance.

Medication administration adverse events are a significant source of intrathecal drug delivery complications. Incorrect medication, programming error, pocket fill, and accessory port fill are potential complications that can arise during maintenance of the intrathecal pump. Respiratory depression from the delivered medications is a serious adverse event that is usually due to inadequate patient monitoring. Having another provider verify medication, dosing, and programming may reduce these errors. Utilizing image guidance during pump refills may also help minimize adverse events.

Mechanical issues with the intrathecal pump itself may arise during the course of the therapy. The internal components of the pump may malfunction. Catheter-related issues such as displacement, kinking, or disconnect may also occur. If there are any concerns for catheter-related issues, a dye study under fluoroscopy can be performed. This is usually performed by injecting radiographic contrast through the side port under fluoroscopic guidance.

Granuloma formation is a significant complication of intrathecal therapy. Granuloma formation at the catheter tip can lead to neurological compromise. Delay in identifying granuloma formation can lead to significant morbidity, including paralysis. Patients will typically present with increased back pain or increasing lower extremity weakness. Patients may also present with decreased therapeutic response. The time to granuloma formation is variable, and in most cases of granuloma formation, opioids are implicated. Morphine and hydromorphone are the most commonly implicated agents in granuloma formation. No reports of fentanyl-related granuloma formation exist, although there are reports of baclofen-related granulomas. The administration of high concentrations of opioids has been associated with granuloma formation. Some providers advocate low concentration and low-dose therapy, but this should be balanced with refill frequency as lower concentrations will require more frequent refills. The diagnosis of granuloma is usually made with MRI with and without gadolinium with closely spaced images through the catheter tip.

Suggested Reading

1. Deer TR, Prager J, Levy R, et al. Polyanalgesic consensus conference 2012: recommendations for the management of pain by intrathecal (intraspinal) drug delivery: report of an interdisciplinary expert panel. Neuromodulation. 2012;15:436–66.
2. Deer TR, Prager J, Levy R, et al. Polyanalgesic consensus conference 2012: consensus on diagnosis, detection, and treatment of catheter-tip granulomas (inflammatory masses). Neuromodulation. 2012;15:483–95.
3. Deer TR, Prager J, Levy R, et al. Polyanalgesic consensus conference 2012: recommendations to reduce morbidity and mortality in intrathecal drug delivery in the treatment of chronic pain. Neuromodulation. 2012;15:467–82.
4. Fitzgibbon DR, Stephens LS, Posner KL, et al. Injury and liability associated with implantable devices for chronic pain. Anesthesiology. 2016;124:1384–93.
5. Hayek SM, Deer TR, Pope JE, et al. Intrathecal therapy for cancer and non-cancer pain. Pain Physician. 2011;14(3):219–48.
6. Prager J, Deer T, et al. Best practices for intrathecal drug delivery for pain. Neuromodulation. 2014;17(4):354–72.

56 PACC Guideline Statements

Andrea C. Wong

Key Concepts

- The PACC guidelines of 2012 created algorithms for treatment approaches to neuropathic and nociceptive pain. The algorithms were established based on the best available evidence from published reports and from interdisciplinary expert panel discussions.

Introduction

Table 56.1 outlines an algorithm for treatment of neuropathic pain with intrathecal therapy. Of note, morphine and ziconotide are the only FDA-approved medications for intrathecal therapy directed at neuropathic and nociceptive pain. Table 56.2 outlines an algorithm for treatment of nociceptive pain with intrathecal therapy. Patients often present with a combination of neuropathic and nociceptive pain. There is no specific algorithm outlined by the PACC 2012 guidelines for this mixed picture. It is suggested that the clinician base decision making on the clinical scenario to determine appropriate treatment.

Intrathecal medication dosing recommendations were made including initial dose, bolus dose, maximum recommended dose, and maximum concentration. Table 56.3 includes recommendations for intrathecal opioids, while Table 56.4 includes recommendations for intrathecal non-opioids. There were no specific guidelines made to define the best rate to deliver medication, although it was noted that there was a theoretical increased risk of developing an inflammatory mass at the catheter tip with higher concentrations of drug, even though this has not been proven clinically. It was suggested that programmed bolus doses be set no more than 5–20% of daily continuous infusion, given the risk of cumulative side effects including hypotension and motor weakness. It is expected that early on in the initiation of IDD, many changes to the treatment regimen will be required to achieve optimal symptom management with the least side effects.

Suggested Reading

1. Deer TR, Prager J, Levy R, Rathmell J, Buchser E, Burton A, et al. Polyanalgesic consensus conference 2012: recommendations for the management of pain by intrathecal (intraspinal) drug delivery: report of an interdisciplinary expert panel. Neuromodulation (Technology at the Neural Interface). 2012;15(5):436–66.

A.C. Wong, MD, MPH (✉)
University Hospitals Case Medical Center, Department of Anesthesiology, Division of Pain Management, 11100 Euclid Ave, Cleveland, OH 44106, USA
e-mail: andrea.wong@uhhospitals.org

J.E. Pope, T.R. Deer (eds.), *Treatment of Chronic Pain Conditions*, DOI 10.1007/978-1-4939-6976-0_56

Table 56.1 2012 Polyanalgesic algorithm for intrathecal therapy directed at neuropathic pain

Line 1	Morphine	Ziconotide	Morphine + bupivacaine	
Line 2	Hydromorphone	Hydromorphone + bupivacaine or hydromorphone + clonidine	Morphine + clonidine	
Line 3	Clonidine	Ziconotide + opioid	Fentanyl	Fentanyl + bupivacaine or fentanyl + clonidine
Line 4	Opioid + clonidine + bupivacaine		Bupivacaine + clonidine	
Line 5	Baclofen			

Table 56.2 2012 Polyanalgesic algorithm for intrathecal therapy directed at nociceptive pain

Line 1	Morphine	Hydromorphone	Ziconotide	Fentanyl
Line 2	Morphine + bupivacaine	Ziconotide + opioid	Hydromorphone + bupivacaine	Fentanyl + bupivacaine
Line 3	Opioid + clonidine		Sufentanil	
Line 4	Opioid + clonidine + bupivacaine		Sufentanil + bupivacaine or clonidine	
Line 5	Sufentanil + bupivacaine + clonidine			

Table 56.3 Recommended dosing of intrathecal opioids

IT opioid	Initial dose	Bolus	Maximum recommended dose	Maximum concentration
Morphine	0.1–0.5 mg/day	0.2–1.0 mg	15 mg	20 mg/mL
Hydromorphone	0.02–0.5 mg/day	0.04–0.2 mg	10 mg	15 mg/mL
Fentanyl	25–75 mcg/day	25–75 mcg	No known upper limit	10 mg/mL
Sufentanil	10–20 mcg/day	5–20 mcg	No known upper limit	5 mg/mL

Table 56.4 Recommended dosing of intrathecal non-opioids

IT non-opioid	Initial dose	Bolus	Daily maximum recommended dose	Maximum concentration
Ziconotide	0.5–2.4 mcg/day	1–5 mcg	19.2 mcg	100 mcg/mL
Bupivacaine	1–4 mg/day	0.5–2.5 mg	10 mg	30 mg/mL
Clonidine	40–100 mcg/day	5–20 mcg	40–600 mcg	1000 mcg/mL

Part IX

Advanced Pain Care Therapies: IX. Spinal Cord Stimulation

Spinal Cord Stimulation Indications

57

Michael I. Yang

Key Concepts

- In the newer algorithm for treatment of chronic pain, spinal cord stimulation therapy is moving away from its position as an advanced treatment option and moving to one earlier in the pain care algorithm.
- Spinal cord stimulation therapy has increasingly better pain-control outcomes than reoperation of the spine.

Introduction

Previously, spinal cord stimulation therapy has been thought of as an advanced therapy option in the pain treatment algorithm. With newer technology and better understanding of the drawbacks of oral medication treatment, spinal cord stimulation therapy has moved forward to be considered earlier in the pain treatment algorithm. Spinal cord stimulation therapy allows the delivery of small, precise dosages of electricity directly to targeted nerve sites. The idea of using small doses of electricity in the epidural space to targeted nerve sites has many benefits: lowering systemic drug use, lowering dose-related side effects, and targeting stimulation to specific anatomical regions and pain.

Background

One of the earliest uses of electricity was in medicine for the treatment of pain. Starting in 15 A.D., torpedo fish were used to deliver an electrical shock to patients to relieve pain. Spinal cord stimulation (SCS) was first used by Norman Shealy in 1967, and since then, dorsal column stimulation has continued to improve, based on lead innovations and consistent improvements in technology of the implantable battery. These improvements provide better coverage for targeted pain areas and to deliver an alternative to oral and injected medications or nerve ablation therapies.

Candidacy

Indications for spinal cord stimulator therapy include chronic moderate to severe axial back pain and neuropathic limb pain uncontrolled by more conservative measures. The chronic pain population, where opioid analgesics and other oral medications provide pain reduction but complicated by side effect (including constipation or altered mentation), are excellent candidates.

Indications

See Table 57.1.

Physical Screening

- Diagnosis established/confirmed.
- Pain is neuropathic in origin.
- Pain in the trunk or extremities, unilateral or bilateral.
- Conservative therapies have not provided sufficient relief.
- Multidisciplinary screening, including psychological examination, completed.
- No contraindications to implantation exist.
- Patients should be medically compliant.
- Patients should undergo a psychological screen to determine psychological fitness to proceed with implanted therapies.
- The patient should be medically stable and have no systemic infection, untoward bleeding risks, nor local skin infections at the site of the proposed implant.

M.I. Yang, MD (✉)
Summit Pain Alliance Inc., Interventional Pain Management,
392 Tesconi Ct, Santa Rosa, CA 95401, USA
e-mail: Michael.i.yang@gmail.com

J.E. Pope, T.R. Deer (eds.), *Treatment of Chronic Pain Conditions*, DOI 10.1007/978-1-4939-6976-0_57

Table 57.1 Indications

Axial back pain Multiple compression fractures Arthritis pain Spinal stenosis Multilevel degenerative disc disease Foraminal stenosis
Radicular limb pain
Complex regional pain syndrome
Abdominal pain
Failed back surgery syndrome
Peripheral ischemia
Diabetic foot neuropathy
Post-chemotherapy neuropathy
Postherpetic neuralgia
Noncardiac chest pain

- The patient should have the intellectual capacity to manage the therapy.

As evident by above, there are many areas of the body that can be covered by the stimulation of the spinal cord.

Suggested Reading

1. Kumar K, Taylor RS, Jacques L, et al. The effects of spinal cord stimulation in neuropathic pain are sustained: a 24-month follow-up of the prospective randomized controlled multicenter trial of the effectiveness of spinal cord stimulation. Neurosurgery. 2008;63(4):762–70.
2. North R, Shipley J, Prager J, et al. Practice parameters for the use of spinal cord stimulation in the treatment of chronic neuropathic pain. Pain Med. 2007;8(S4):S200–75.
3. Poree L, Krames E, Pope J, et al. Spinal cord stimulation as treatment for complex regional pain syndrome should be considered earlier than last resort therapy. Neuromodulation. 2013;16(2):125–41.
4. Tiede J, Brown L, Gekht G, et al. Novel spinal cord stimulation parameters in patients with predominant back pain. Neuromodulation. 2013;16(4):370–5.

58 Anatomy for Traditional Spinal Cord Stimulation and Barolat Map

Michael I. Yang

Key Concepts

- Stimulation of the dorsal elements of the spinal cord directly corresponds to the dermatomal distribution of the body areas.
- A distinct map of the various body areas available for stimulation can be created using the large body of evidence from studies that correlate electrode placement with spinal cord levels using paresthesia elicited by stimulation of the dorsal neural elements.

Introduction

As vertebrate animals, our spine is segmented into bands, or dermatomes, of enervation by the nervous system. Spinal cord stimulation of the various dermatomal segments via the dorsal roots, dorsal horns, and dorsal/lateral column has been well documented. There is a large body of evidence that demonstrate the direct correlation between the dermatomal distribution of paresthesia elicited from cathodal stimulation and placement within the posterior epidural space overlying the spinal cord. The electricity follows Ohm's law, and therefore electricity needs to penetrate the epidural space, the CSF, and the meninges, with the target of the dorsal columns. With the need for paresthesia overlap for pain relief, placement of the leads to offer a high likelihood of paresthesia overlap is critical.

Barolat Map

In 1993, Dr. Barolat and colleagues gathered data from 106 patients who underwent spinal cord stimulator implantation. From these data points, they were able to formulate a map to correlate the region of the body most likely to be stimulated by placement of the electrode at specific spinal cord levels. This led to the development of the "Barolat Map" (Fig. 58.1).

It can be deduced that these are the most common lead placements for producing the paresthesia at the specific body region; however, it must be noted that individual anatomy may vary. Different pathologies such as scoliosis and/or rotoscoliosis, etc. may also contribute to variations in anatomical positioning of the dorsal neural elements.

Suggested Reading

1. Barolat G, et al. Mapping of sensory responses to epidural stimulation of the intraspinal neural structures in man. J Neurosurg. 1993;78:233–9.
2. Compton AK, et al. Spinal cord stimulation: a review. Curr Pain Headache Rep. 2012;16(1):35–42.
3. Fierabend H, et al. Morphometry of human superficial dorsal and dorsolateral column fibres: significance to spinal cord stimulation. Brain. 2002;125:1137–49.
4. Holsheimer J, den Boer JA, Struijk JJ, et al. MR assessment of the normal position of the spinal cord in the spinal canal. Am J Neuroradiol. 1994;15:951–9.

M.I. Yang, MD (✉)
Summit Pain Alliance Inc., Interventional Pain Management,
392 Tesconi Ct, Santa Rosa, CA 95401, USA
e-mail: Michael.i.yang@gmail.com

J.E. Pope, T.R. Deer (eds.), *Treatment of Chronic Pain Conditions*, DOI 10.1007/978-1-4939-6976-0_58

Fig. 58.1 Barolat map

Electrode positioning suggestions for Spinal Cord Stimulation

Pain Location (dermatome)	Vertebral Level (center bipole placement)	Pain Location (dermatome)	Vertebral Level (center bipole placement)
Anterior Shoulder (C4-5 fibers)	C3 (range C3-5)	Buttock through LE (L2-S1 fibers)	T9-T10 (range T11-L1)
External Arm (C5 fibers)	C4 (range C2-T3)	Low back (T9-L1 fibers)	T8 (range T7-10)
Radial Forearm (C6 fibers)	C5 (range C2-T3)	Abdomen (T9-L1 fibers)	T6 (range T4-T11)
Median Hands (C6-7 fibers)	C6 (range C2-T3)	Anterior thigh (L2-L3 fibers)	T11 (range T11-T12)
Ulnar Hand (C8 fibers)	C7 (range C2-T2)	Anterior Leg (L4-5 fibers)	T12 (range T12-L1)
Ulnar forearm (T1 fibers)	C7 (range C4-T3)	Posterior Leg (S1-S2 fibers)	L1 (range T11-L1)
Internal Arm (T2 fibers)	T1 (range C5-T3)	Posterior thigh (S1-S2 fibers)	L1 (range T11-L1)
Chest (T2-6 fibers)	T2 (range T1-T7)	Foot (L5-S1 fibers)	L1 (range T11-L1)

Spinal Cord Stimulation Trial

59

Michael I. Yang

Key Concepts

- There are very few procedures where the patient is able to trial the procedure prior to deciding whether he/she would like to proceed with the actual permanent procedure.
- A trial not only determines whether the patient will have adequate coverage of the pain but also can demonstrate whether the patient will have any undesirable stimulation.
- The spinal cord stimulation trial is required by most insurance companies prior to permanent implant.
- It is extremely important that the patient is medically compliant and psychologically fit to proceed with the trial procedure.
- Though it is not required, most insurance companies want the patients to have psychological clearance to proceed with the spinal cord stimulator trial.
- As with all epidural procedures, the patient cannot be anticoagulated at the time of the procedure, and care must be taken to decrease the chance of epidural hematomas.
- As with all procedures, informed consent must be obtained. The patient should know the risks and benefits, dangers, and possible side effects to the procedure.

Introduction

There are very few procedures where the patient is able to trial the procedure prior to deciding whether he/she would like to proceed with the actual permanent procedure. With spinal cord stimulation, most insurance companies require a trial of the procedure prior to permanent implant to ensure high success rate of the implant procedure.

Pretrial Preparation

- The MRI of the thoracic spine should be reviewed for any anatomical anomalies and to verify whether implantation of the leads would further compromise the caliber of the spinal canal.
- The spine should be checked for stability; should there be instability, the patient should undergo stabilization prior to stimulator implant.
- A thorough physical exam is necessary to document the areas of the body with pain.

Trial Lead Implant

One of the keys to a safe and successful spinal cord stimulator trial is the positioning and entry point of the Tuohy needle for insertion of the stimulator lead. For cervical trials, the entry point is usually at T1/2 intervertebral level; for thoracic lead placement, entry point is usually at L1/2 intervertebral level. The entry angle for the Tuohy needle is preferably approximately 30° from the skin, angling toward anatomical midline. As the leads are fed through the needle, it is important to try to keep the leads as close to midline as possible so as to avoid hitting the lateral nerve roots or having the leads move to the ventral aspect of the spinal cord.

Troubleshooting

A few of the more common problems one can encounter during a trial procedure are:

- Difficulty driving the lead wire – rotate the stylette in small, quarter-turns while feeding the wire into the Tuohy needle with consistent pressure.
- Lead tip hitting obstructions – obstructions such as adhesions, scar tissue, and or septated dura. Sometimes the tip

M.I. Yang, MD (✉)
Summit Pain Alliance Inc., Interventional Pain Management, 392 Tesconi Ct, Santa Rosa, CA 95401, USA
e-mail: Michael.i.yang@gmail.com

J.E. Pope, T.R. Deer (eds.), *Treatment of Chronic Pain Conditions*, DOI 10.1007/978-1-4939-6976-0_59

is directed dorsally and is hitting against the ligamentum flavum.
- Dural puncture – immediately remove the Tuohy needle and attempt at a superior level or the contralateral side.

Post-implant

The patient should attempt the usual activities of daily living so as to test the efficacy of the spinal cord stimulator system. The trial system remains in place from 3 to 10 days, and some physicians will leave the system in for even longer than 10 days. During that time, the patient should decide whether he/she has greater than 50% pain relief and, if so, proceed with the permanent stimulator implant.

Suggested Reading

1. North R, Shipley J, Prager J, et al. Practice parameters for the use of spinal cord stimulation in the treatment of chronic neuropathic pain. Pain Med. 2007;8(S4):S200–75.

Spinal Cord Stimulation Permanent Implant

60

Michael I. Yang and Nomen Azeem

Key Concepts

- Spinal cord stimulation can be placed surgically with many techniques and include percutaneous or paddle lead arrays.
- A successful spinal cord stimulation trial that merits candidacy for permanent placement of the device is typically defined as greater than 50% relief of the target painful location and an improvement in function.
- Vigilance with preoperative preparation, intraoperative management, and postoperative care is crucial for a successful outcome.

Introduction

After a successful spinal cord stimulator trial, the patient would be scheduled for the permanent implant. Based on the patient's MRI as well as how smoothly the trial procedure carried out, the surgeon and the patient would decide whether to proceed with the cylindrical implants versus the paddle lead implant.

Cylindrical Lead Implantation

After appropriate surgical preparation with an antimicrobial skin cleaning solution and appropriate draping including a full body lap and ¾ side drape, a C-arm is utilized to identify the target location and the planned skin incisions. Some surgeons elect to place the needles within the epidural space and then perform the surgical direction in the paraspinal area around the leads. Others perform the surgical dissection first. The latter is described here. A superficial incision is made down to the level of the lumbodorsal fascia. The dissection is carried through the skin, adipose tissue, superficial fascia, adipose, and then to lumbodorsal fascia. The lumbodorsal fascia is easily identified as a pearly white connective tissue. A wet lap is then placed within the incision. Attention is then redirected to the paraspinal incision. Using fluoroscopic guidance, the inferior end plate of the T12 vertebral body is squared off. This opens the T12-L1 interlaminar space and is typically achieved by a caudal tilt with the intensifier of the C-arm. A 14-gauge Tuohy needle is then advanced to the epidural space using a loss of resistance technique. The second needle is advanced ipsilaterally within the same epidural space and cephalad to the existing needle. The cylindrical leads are introduced in the posterior epidural space, and live or intermittent fluoroscopy is used to navigate the leads to the desired spinal level. Testing is performed to ensure appropriate lead placement. The Tuohy needles are then removed, and the leads are anchored to the lumbodorsal fascia. Stress relief loops are created, and the leads are then tunneled to the battery location, typically in the left flank, and the leads are secured in the IPG with a hex wrench. Copious irrigation is performed and the incisions are closed with 3-O Vicryl and 4-O monocryl. Sterile dressings are applied and an abdominal binder is recommended.

Paddle Lead Implantation

A superficial incision is made down to the level of the lamina near the desired paddle location. A partial laminectomy is performed and the paddle lead inserted into the epidural space, under direct vision. The paddle lead can be secured. The pocketing and lead closure is the same.

M.I. Yang, MD (✉)
Summit Pain Alliance Inc., Interventional Pain Management, 392 Tesconi Ct, Santa Rosa, CA 95401, USA
e-mail: Michael.i.yang@gmail.com

N. Azeem, MD
Sarasota Orthopedic Associates, Sarasota, FL, USA

J.E. Pope, T.R. Deer (eds.), *Treatment of Chronic Pain Conditions*, DOI 10.1007/978-1-4939-6976-0_60

Intraoperative Troubleshooting

A few of the more common problems that can occur with the permanent implant are:

- There is typically hesitancy when beginning the surgical dissection to the lumbodorsal fascia, and a common mistake is to misidentify the superficial fascia as the lumbodorsal fascia.
- The anchor "noses" need to be placed underneath the lumbodorsal fascia.
- Correct tissue management is needed and closure of dead space is encouraged. An abdominal binder is helpful in this regard.
- When placing the second needle into the same laminar epidural space, it is helpful to caudally tilt the intensifier to the gain a "gun barrel" view of the needle, which will identify the interlaminar epidural space above and below the existing needle.
- The caudal end of the paraspinal incision for the anchors and the leads should coincide with the needle skin entry site for a percutaneous placement with cephalad placement to accommodate visualization of the lumbodorsal fascia.
- Two-layer closure is recommended to mitigate wound dehiscence.

Post-implant

The immediate postoperative phase is accompanied by recommendations of maintaining dryness of the incisions and the dressing, avoiding hot tubs, pools baths, or showers, keeping an occlusive dressing for at least 48 h. An abdominal binder is placed to apply gentle pressure on the incision site to reduce dead space around the battery site. The patient should refrain from participating in rigorous activities for approximately up to 4 weeks postoperatively. This will ensure the body to scar around the leads and decrease the chances of lead migration and/or breakage. Some physicians also put patients on a week of prophylactic antibiotics to decrease the chances of infection, although no data supports this practice.

Suggested Reading

1. Oakley J, Prager J. Spinal cord stimulation: mechanism of action. Spine. 2002;27(22):2574–83.
2. Deer T, Skaribas I, Nelson C. Results From the Partnership for Advancement in Neuromodulation Registry: A 24-Month Follow-Up. Neuromodulation. 2016 Feb;19(2):179–87. doi:10.1111/ner.12378.
3. Deer TR, Mekhail N, Provenzano D, et al. The appropriate use of neurostimulation of the spinal cord and peripheral nervous system for the treatment of chronic pain and ischemic diseases: the neuromodulation appropriateness consensus committee. Neuromodulation. 2014;17(6):515–50.
4. Tiede J, Brown L, Gekht G, et al. Novel spinal cord stimulation parameters in patients with predominant back pain. Neuromodulation. 2013;16(4):370–5.
5. de Vos CC, Dijkstra C, Lenders MW, et al. Spinal cord stimulation with hybrid lead relieves pain in low back and legs. Neuromodulation. 2012;15(2):118–23.

Spinal Cord Stimulation Maintenance

61

Kasra Amirdelfan and Jason E. Pope

Key Concepts

- Spinal cord stimulation is a therapy that is indicated for refractory neuropathic pain of the trunk and limb.
- Nearly 30% of patients with spinal cord stimulation develop tolerance to the pain-relieving effects.
- Rechargeability has been reported to be somewhat troublesome for tonic stimulation therapy.
- Explant data suggests the reason may have been related to loss of therapeutic effect in nearly 20%.
- New neuromodulation strategies may be helpful in mitigating these therapeutic losses.

Introduction

Neuromodulation is one of the fundamental tools among the armamentarium of treatment choices in pain management. The International Neuromodulation Society defines neuromodulation as the alteration of nerve activity through the delivery of electrical stimulation and/or chemical agents to targeted sites in the body [1–4]. The field of neuromodulation is on an exciting trajectory of growth and development beyond pain control. SCS is the only modality in chronic pain management which has not only shown to provide long-term pain relief [5], but it has also been proven effective in reduction of medications [6] and return to work in the chronic pain patient population. Maintenance of the benefit of these therapies are essential, as cost-effectiveness and sustained relief deserve special comment.

K. Amirdelfan, MD
IPM Medical Group, Inc., Department of Interventional Pain Management, Walnut Creek, CA, USA

J.E. Pope, MD (✉)
Summit Pain Alliance,
392 Tesconi Ct, Santa Rosa, CA 95401, USA
e-mail: popeje@me.com

Sustainability

The importance of a maintained therapy is critical for patient care and the future of the therapy. Maintenance of therapy centers on troubleshooting the device and management of the patient-device interface. We will explore each individual section; however, it would be remiss to not comment on cost-effectiveness. In a historical retrospective review performed by Kumar, the cost-effectiveness of SCS, as compared to medical management, is 2.5 years. Further, Lad et al. discussed cost savings when SCS is offered earlier in the treatment strategy, as compared to other conservative measures. These points are critical, in that over a third of the patients explanted within a year of implant. Of the reasons cited for explant, the most common was loss of therapeutic effect. Interestingly, approximately half of his implanted patients could expect a return visit to the operating room.

Troubleshooting the Device

Reprogramming

Most commonly, patients need to be informed that the device is one that requires refinement. Reprogramming is performed in an effort to better capture and minimizes the pain complaint. In a paresthesia-inducing stimulation strategy, this can be performed by reorienting the cathodal stimulation electrodes (Figs. 61.1, 61.2, 61.3 and 61.4) and guarding anodes, by adjusting the frequency and the amplitude. This is recommended to be performed in the office for patient feedback. For HF10, this is perfumed by adjustment of the amplitude and the lead cathode configuration. If the response to reprogramming is successful, then the patient can follow-up as needed, with recommendations to have the device optimized every 3–4 months. However, if the paresthesia field is markedly different, as compared to when it was originally programmed, or fails to cover the intended target, one should consider migration of the leads.

J.E. Pope, T.R. Deer (eds.), *Treatment of Chronic Pain Conditions*, DOI 10.1007/978-1-4939-6976-0_61

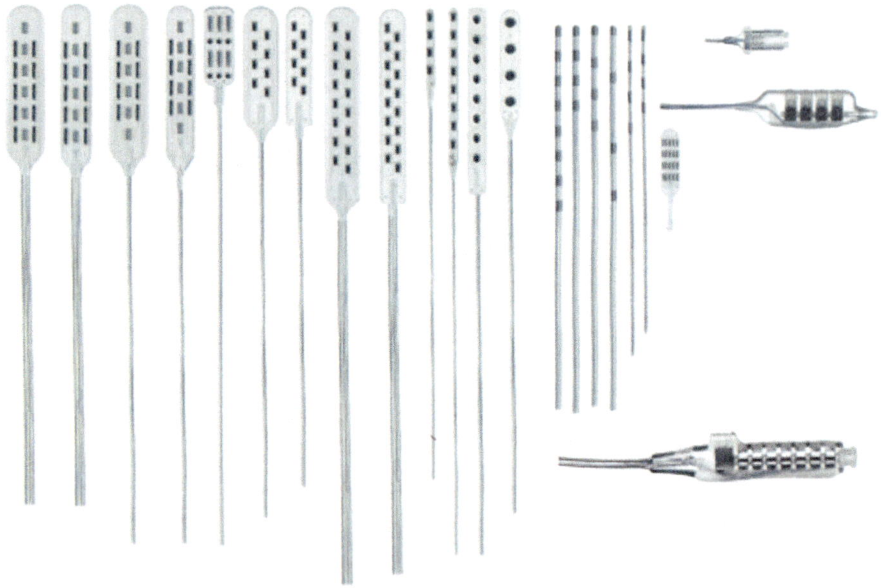

Fig. 61.1 Example of percutaneous and paddle leads (Courtesy of St. Jude Medical, with permission)

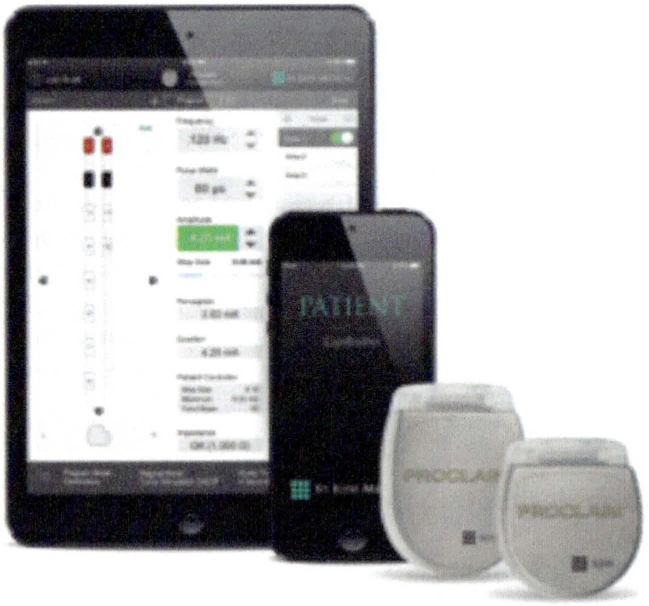

Fig. 61.2 Primary cell and rechargeable IPGs (Courtesy of St. Jude, with permission)

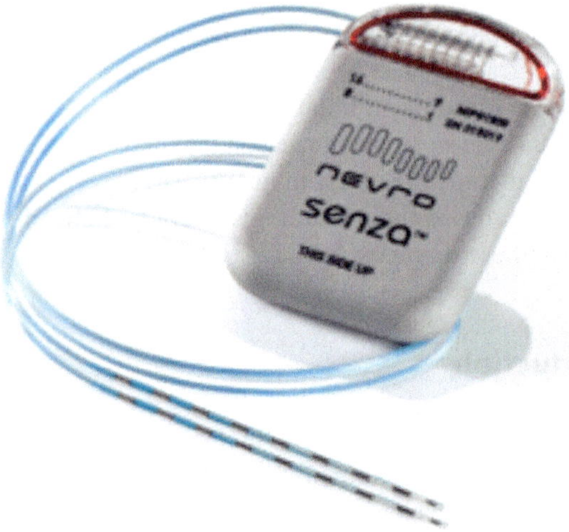

Fig. 61.3 Senza IPG and leads capable of HF10 therapy (Courtesy of Nevro, with permission)

There is a growing interest to have centers for programming through data acquisition and remote programming from the clinic. Further ease of programming has been created through innovative computerized programming strategies.

Migration

Migration, or movement of the leads from the original placement, can interfere with the delivery of the stimulation to the intended target, resulting in a suboptimal outcome. If this is discovered, which most commonly is related to failure of the anchor, the patient needs to be revised with a reoperation and replacement of the leads.

Infection

With any surgical procedure, surgical site infection is a concern. These are commonly identified within 3 months of the permanent therapy. Most commonly, this is related to the IPG location. Once identified, infection needs to be managed aggressively. If only very subcutaneous infection is surrounding the incision site, wound care can be attempted with careful monitoring. If any systemic signs of illness occur, the device needs to be removed, the wound

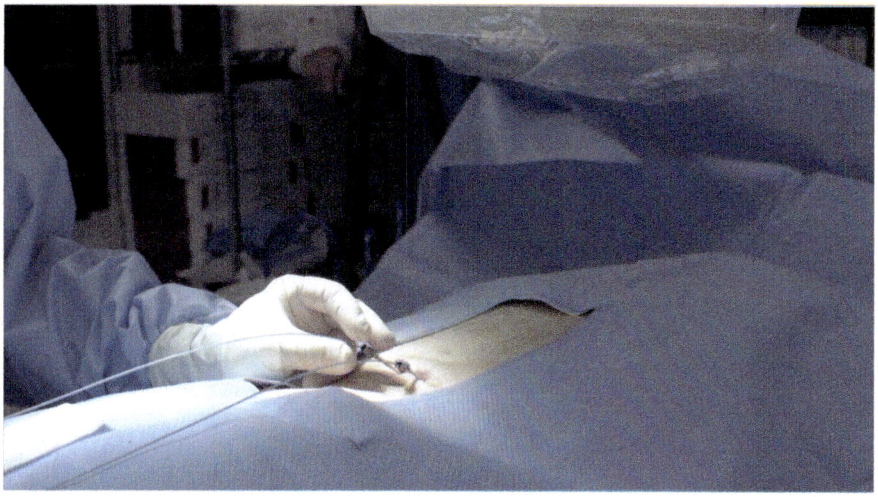

Fig. 61.4 Trial lead placement

cultured, a neuraxial MRI with and without contrast performed, and antibiotics initiated with recommendations from an infectious disease specialist.

Habituation/Tolerance

Hayek et al. reported on an 8-year retrospective review within his center experience demonstrating a failure rate of near 25% ending in explant, with 41% of those related to loss of therapeutic effect. This demonstration of habituation (or tolerance) has been reported with traditional stimulation nearing 30%. New waveforms have demonstrated success with returning these patients to a state of improved pain care, both for HF10 and Burst DR.

Patient Device Interface

Recharging

Spinal cord stimulation therapies are largely powered by two types of implantable batteries – primary (non-rechargeable) or rechargeable (Fig. 61.2 and 61.3). The described benefits from the rechargeable system are often described as being of longer duration and smaller profile. For traditional, paresthesia-inducing stimulation strategies, the recharging burden is approximately once a week for 30–40 min. Some data suggests that oftentimes the recharging episodes and frequency are less efficient, with charging episodes 5.2 times per month with charging episodes up to 2.3 h.

For HF10 therapy, with a higher energy requirement, the recharging strategy is usually daily for 30–40 min. A prospective study was performed suggesting that reliable recharging did not impact fatigue with the device. A retrospective review of devices that ended in explant suggested a faster explant rat with rechargeable systems as compared to primary cell therapies.

Patient-Controlled Programming

As device innovation continues, so too does the patient programming of their therapy. For paresthesia-inducing strategies, positional changes need to be accommodated by commonly adjusting the amplitude of the therapy. RF and Bluetooth technology now make it easier to program.

Conclusion

The future of spinal cord stimulation is dependent on sustain treatment success. With a mindful approach to maintain and troubleshooting the therapy, clinicians enable the device and the patient the best chance for success.

References

1. Shealy CN, Mortimer JT, Becker DP. Electrical inhibition of pain by stimulation of the dorsal columns: preliminary clinical report. Anesth Analg. 1967;46(4):489–91.
2. Mekhail N, Matthews M, Nageeb F, Guiguis M, Mekhail M, Cheng J. Retrospective review of 707 cases of spinal cord stimulation: indications and complications. Pain Pract. 2011;11(2):148–53.
3. North RB, Kidd D, Shipley J, Taylor RS. Spinal cord stimulation versus reoperation for failed back surgery syndrome: a cost effective

and cost utility analysis based on a randomized, controlled trial. Neurosurgery. 2007;61(2):361–8.
4. Poree L, Krames ES, Pope J, Deer TR, Levy R, Schultz L. Spinal cord stimulation as treatment for complex regional pain syndrome should be considered earlier then last resort therapy. Neuromoduelation. 2013;16(2):125–41.
5. Kumar K, Hunter G, Demeria DD. Treatment of chronic pain by using intrathecal drug therapy compared with conventional pain therapies: a cost effectiveness analysis. J Neurosurg. 2002;97(4):803–10.
6. Pope JE, Deer TR, Kramer J. A systematic review: current and future directions of dorsal root ganglion therapeutics to treat chronic pain. Pain Med. 2013;14(10):1477–96.

Suggested Reading

1. Al-Kaisy A, et al. Sustained efficacy of 10 KHz high frequency stimulation for patients with chronic low back pain: 24 month results of a prospective multicenter study. Pain Med. 2014; 15(3):354–7.
2. Deer T. Atlas of implantable therapies for pain management. New York: Springer; 2011.
3. Mekhail N, Matthews M, Nageeb F, Guiguis M, Mekhail M, Cheng J. Retrospective review of 707 cases of spinal cord stimulation: indications and complications. Pain Pract. 2011; 11(2):148–53.

Spinal Cord Stimulation Surgical Paddle Placement

62

Steven M. Falowski

Key Concepts

- Spinal cord stimulation (SCS) has Class I evidence of its superiority when placed against conventional medical management and against repeat spinal.
- Published literature describes the advantages with laminectomy electrode placement, although more invasive than percutaneous placement.
- Electrode implantation via laminectomy can be performed either under local anesthetic with intravenous sedation or under general anesthesia utilizing neuromonitoring.
- The advent of paddle electrodes has expanded treatment options and has inherent benefits such as broader stimulation patterns and lower stimulation requirements.

Stimulation

Spinal cord stimulation (SCS) is an adjustable, nondestructive, neuromodulatory procedure that delivers therapeutic doses of electrical current to the spinal cord for the management of neuropathic pain. The most common indications are failed back surgery syndrome (FBSS) and complex regional pain syndrome (CRPS), but may also include ischemic limb pain and angina. There are scattered reports regarding the treatment of intractable pain due to other causes including visceral/abdominal pain, cervical neuritis pain, spinal cord injury pain, postherpetic neuralgia, and neurogenic thoracic outlet syndrome. Experience suggests that, in selected patients, SCS can produce at least 50% pain relief in 50–60% of the implanted patients. Interestingly, with the proper follow-up care, these results can be maintained over several years.

S.M. Falowski, MD (✉)
St. Lukes University Health Network, Department of Neurosurgery, 701 Ostrum St, Ste 302, Bethlehem, PA 18017, USA
e-mail: SFALOWSKI@GMAIL.COM

Peripheral nerve stimulation (PNS) has been coming in favor of treating neuropathic pain of the back, trunk, and neck, as well as with occipital nerve stimulation for the treatment of various headache syndromes and occipital neuralgia.

Early stimulating systems were only radiofrequency (RF)-driven passive receivers coupled with unipolar electrodes. This has now been followed by implantable pulse generators powered by a lithium battery that have options such as rechargeable generators (Fig. 62.1). These are then coupled with many different types of percutaneous and paddle-type arrays (Fig. 62.2). This has led to the advent of surgical leads and implants.

It is paramount that spinal cord stimulation be a part of every spine surgeon's armamentarium. Multiple randomized controlled trials have demonstrated the superiority of spinal cord stimulation to reoperation in the spine. It is crucial that these options be available to patients from both their surgeons and pain management physicians to adequately and completely treat their patients with all available options.

Relevant Anatomy

Understanding the somatotopy of the spinal cord is paramount to knowing the technical aspects of implantation. A basic tenet of SCS is to create an overlapping of paresthesia and pain region. In order to do this, correlation of the somatotopy and the level of the spinal cord are necessary.

High cervical regions such as C2 can cover the posterior occipital region and occasionally the lower jaw. C2–C4 stimulation will provide coverage of the shoulder, while stimulation in the lower cervical region such as C5–C6 will provide for the entire hand. To cover the anterior chest wall or the axilla, an electrode toward C7 will be necessary.

More commonly, an implanter will seek cover the lower extremities. Lateral placement at T11–T12 will cover the anterior thigh, while placement at T11–L1 can cover the posterior thigh. Coverage off the foot as a whole can be achieved along these same areas, but it becomes more difficult to

J.E. Pope, T.R. Deer (eds.), *Treatment of Chronic Pain Conditions*, DOI 10.1007/978-1-4939-6976-0_62

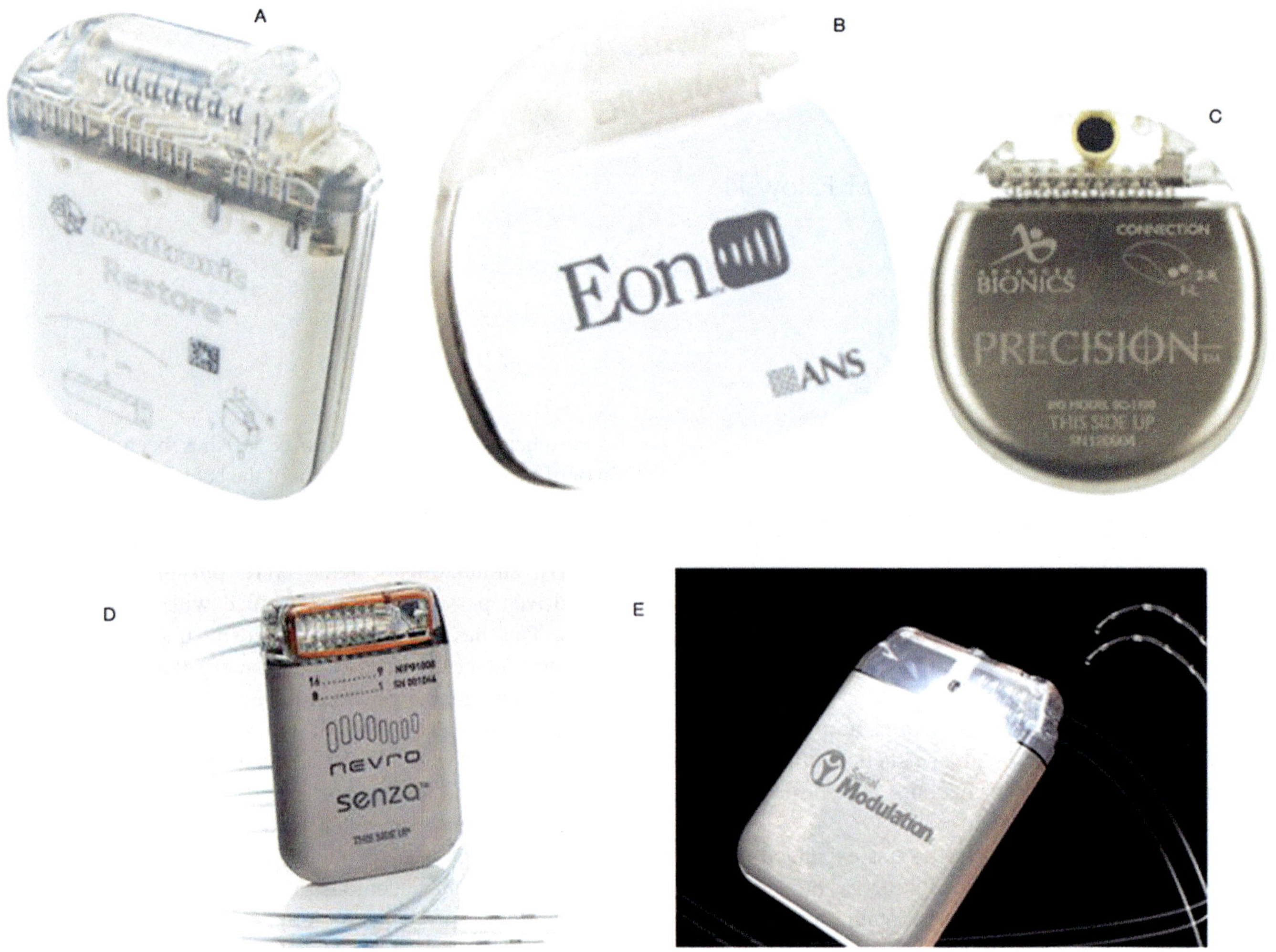

Fig. 62.1 Internal pulse generators. (**a**) Medtronic. (**b**) St. Jude Medical, Inc. (**c**) Boston Scientific. (**d**) Nevro. (**e**) Spinal modulation

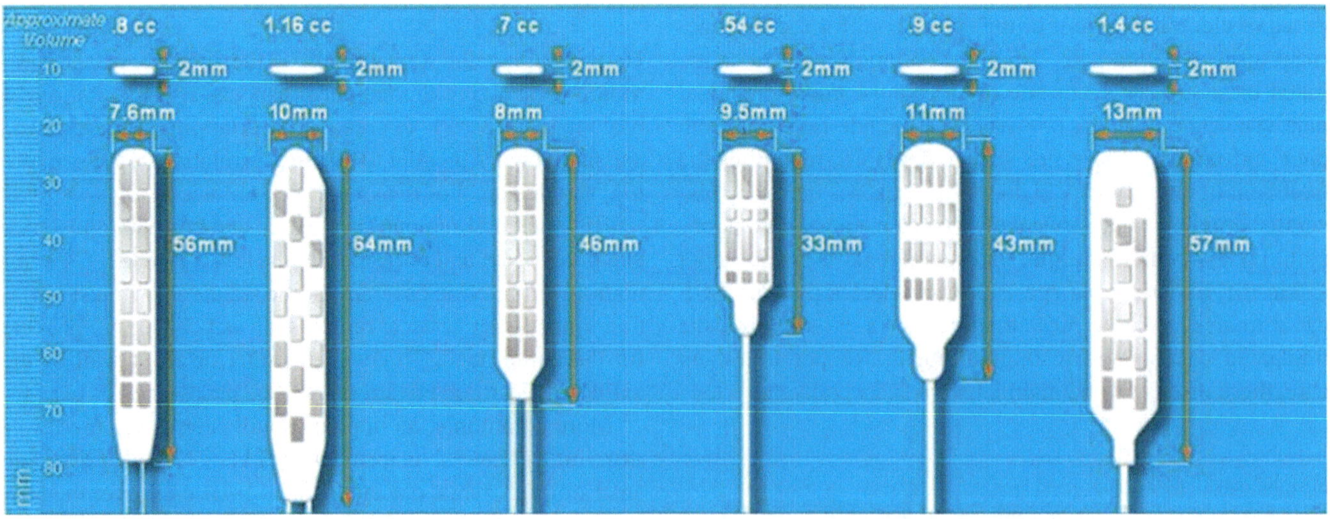

Fig. 62.2 Paddle electrodes

cover the sole of the foot. Alternatively for coverage of the sole of the foot, a patient may require insertion on the lumbar L5 or S1 nerve roots. Low back pain is very difficult to cover because mid-thoracic stimulation can affect the chest and abdominal wall. The best localization for low back coverage is with midline placement at T8–T9. Paddle electrodes can vary in width and length covering from one to three vertebral bodies, as well as vary in contact configuration. The surgeon will need to make decisions for which electrode is based on patient's pain etiology, pain pattern, and intended coverage.

Stimulation of the dorsal spinal cord likely affects large afferent myelinated fibers that can include the dorsal columns, dorsal roots, dorsal root entry zone, and the dorsal horn. It becomes increasingly difficult to distinguish stimulation patterns secondary to the overlap with simultaneous stimulation of more than one structure. Midline versus lateral placement would also affect desired outcome. Most patients prefer stimulation of the dorsal column from electrodes closer to the midline. Laterally, placed thoracic electrodes are more likely to stimulate the thoracic nerve roots and result in painful stimulation.

Screening Trial

Most physicians will utilize a screening trial prior to permanent implantation of the system. Several methods have been utilized to implement a trial. A patient may have a temporary percutaneous electrode implantation where the leads are externalized allowing the patients to return home and determine efficacy. Another method is to surgically implant the electrodes and leave them externalized allowing the patient to assess the efficacy while being observed in either a hospital setting or return home. Finally, an intraoperative trial can be utilized where the patient is awakened during surgery and allowed to determine the degree of pain relief.

All of these screening trial methods can be followed by permanent implantation or removal of the system. Although each can be effective, it is largely determined on a single-patient basis. Each method has pros and cons and must be tailored to each individual patient. Most authors would agree that a screening trial with 50% pain relief would warrant permanent implantation.

Recording the results of the trial, position of the electrode, definition of the paresthesia experienced by the patient, and accurate management of expectations are paramount for the implanting surgeon.

Advantages and Disadvantages of Surgical Lead Implants

Percutaneous electrodes can be inserted without much dissection and offers a substantial advantage when one performs a trial to assess candidacy for a permanent implant. After the trial period, the temporary percutaneous electrode can easily be removed in the implanting physician's office. During implantation, these electrodes can be advanced over several segments in the epidural space, allowing testing of several spinal cord levels to assess for optimal electrode position.

A major disadvantage that has been cited with percutaneous electrodes is their tendency to migrate. This is related to their inherent flexibility, which is necessary for their insertion through a Touhy needle, and to their cylindrical shape, which does not prevent migration even months after implantation. Also, percutaneous electrodes are less energy efficient than paddle electrodes. The electrical current is distributed circumferentially around the electrode and is expected to result in greater shunting of current. In addition, patients with percutaneous leads may also describe a greater positional variance in their paresthesia.

Paddle electrodes require a surgical laminotomy and implantation under direct vision. Implantation under direct vision may be safer in the upper thoracic and cervical areas, where there is a risk of damaging the spinal cord with the large-bore Touhy needle. Most implants can be done through a small skin incision. The amount of bony removal is usually minimal.

Multiple arrays or different electrode configurations can be also constructed with plate electrodes. The main advantage of plate electrodes resides in their more inherent stability in the dorsal epidural space and lesser propensity to migrate. In addition, direct visualization and implantation of a surgeon can lead to improved patient paresthesia coverage with electrode positioning, better anchoring methods, and access to additional technology not available with percutaneous implants. Paddle electrodes have broader stimulation patterns and lower stimulation requirements. Plate electrodes are more energy efficient in delivering electrical stimulation. Another advantage is the ease in current steering, as well as current shielding which leads to increased fiber selectivity and more focused pain control. Long-term efficacy with paddle electrodes is inherent given the ability for various programming adjustments and configurations. Published literature describes the advantages with laminectomy electrode placement, although more invasive than percutaneous placement, yielded significantly better clinical results in patients with failed back surgery syndrome with long-term follow-up.

A long-term issue has been the inability of patients to get an MRI with these systems. Presently, there are specific Medtronic and Boston Scientific stimulator systems that have a MRI conditional scenario for a brain MRI that includes both percutaneous and surgical implanted systems. More recently, Medtronic has released a fully MRI conditional system that only includes percutaneous implants with cylinder leads.

Surgical Implantation Techniques

Electrode implantation can be performed either under local anesthetic with intravenous sedation or under general anesthesia. With modern anesthetic techniques, testing an awake patient yields immediate feedback regarding the stimulation-induced paresthesia. When the procedure is performed with the patient under general anesthesia, one relies on the radiographical position and on evoked motor or sensory responses to assure proper electrode positioning.

In the awake placement, the anesthetic management during the procedures performed is of crucial importance to the success of the procedure. A patient awakening from anesthesia may be very uncooperative and disoriented, while a patient who is too sedated would not be able to answer questions during the testing. Either would result in complete failure of the procedure or, even worse, in accidental neural injury. Most patients undergoing implantation are positioned in a lateral decubitus position or prone position, and the anesthesiologist places a laryngeal mask airway (LMA). With the LMA, the anesthesiologist can maintain the airway while simultaneously keeping the patient deeply sedate. As the patient emerges from the anesthesia, the LMA is removed, and conversation may be held with the patient.

The more recent trend is toward implantation under general anesthesia secondary to a number of reasons why implantation under general anesthesia may be desirable. The awake operation is often performed while the patient is under local anesthesia, which is very stressful for the patient, and predisposes them to movement. This can lead to decreased patient satisfaction, equipment migration, undesired stimulation effects, and treatment failure. These factors lead to the implanting surgeon having a preference for non-awake placement. Additionally, personal experience for most implanting physicians reveals that intraoperative wake-up is not always desirable. Some patients are severely disoriented, and others are agitated, which interferes with reliable communication with the surgeon. Further, the preoperative narcotic medication doses frequently required for these patients with chronic severe pain often make pain control during the wake-up very difficult even with generous local anesthetic. Finally, x-ray identification of the midline is oftentimes not possible in the lateral decubitus position.

The use of EMG/SSEP during implantation allows a stimulation lead to be positioned relative to a physiologic midline and/or positioned along the dorsal column in a longitudinal direction. The availability of multiple channel arrays and implantable pulse generators that can function with multiple electrodes now allows for generous implantation of extra electrodes as well as larger paddle electrodes. Some recent studies have conclusions reporting that implantation performed under general anesthesia utilizing monitoring techniques was associated with fewer failure rates and fewer reoperations. It is becoming accepted as a safe and efficacious alternative to awake surgery.

Conclusions

The treatment of chronic pain remains challenging. Spinal cord stimulation has been performed for over 30 years, and advances have been made making it a more reliable and safe modality. When compared to most of the other chronic pain treatment modalities, the magnitude of its long-term results are not easily matched with very few other invasive modalities claiming this success rate with a few years of follow-up. It is important to remember that the goal of neurostimulation is to reduce pain, rather than to eliminate pain and should be used as a treatment adjunct. The advent of tripole and pentad paddle electrodes has expanded treatment options and has earned an established and firm role in contemporary chronic pain management.

Suggested Reading

1. Barolat G, Massaro F, He J, Zeme S, Ketcik B. Mapping of sensory responses to epidural stimulation of the intraspinal neural structures in man. J Neurosurg. 1993;78:233–9.
2. Falowski S, Sharan A. A review on spinal cord stimulation. J Neurosurg Sci. 2012;56(4):287–98.
3. Falowski SM, Celii A, Sestokas AK, Schwartz DM, Matsumoto C, Sharan A. Awake vs. asleep placement of spinal cord stimulators: a cohort analysis of complications associated with placement. Neuromodulation. 2011;14(2):130–4; discussion 134–5.
4. North RB, Kidd DH, Farrokhi F, Piantadosi SA. Spinal cord stimulation versus repeated lumbosacral spine surgery for chronic pain: a randomized, controlled trial. Neurosurgery. 2005;56:98–106; discussion 106–107.

63 Innovative Central Neuromodulation Targets for Pain

Timothy R. Deer and Jason E. Pope

Key Concepts

- The dorsal root ganglion represents well-defined structure that lends itself to stimulation therapy.
- Robust clinical data defines patient safety and efficacy in the largest randomized, controlled study on CRPS.
- Patients have greater than 85% success at 1 year following implantation.

Introduction

Neuromodulation continues to evolve, with a focus on novel targets and expanding indications. This expansion often times brings novel strategies to treat traditionally challenging chronic pain conditions. Dorsal root ganglion (DRG) stimulation provides a predicate strategy for revisiting old targets and the development of a space changing therapy. DRG therapy, with recent approval by the Food and Drug Administration (FDA) in February of 2016, now makes it possible to treat CRPS or peripheral causalgia of the lower extremity (defined as the iliac crest to the foot).

Science

The DRG is a paired structure with the spinal canal, accessible via the epidural space, just caudal to the pedicles, and encased by a dural layer. It is termed a pseudo-unipolar structure that has axons that extend from the periphery and travel to the dorsal horn of the spinal cord, with extension to adjacent vertebral segments. This redundancy describes the failures of ablative or excisional therapies to the DRG.

Chronic pain creates an environment that raises the firing threshold of these abnormal fibers, as compared to normal physiologic fibers, with preferential activation. This creates a stimulation therapeutic window, allowing for preferential selection of the abnormal fibers. Important to the transmission of the action potential is the T-junction, which serves as a low-pass filter. Stimulation increases this effect, with the resultant reduction of action potential generation to the dorsal horn.

The Device

Equipment designed for the placement of the newly developed lead is required for safe and accurate deployment. The introduction system includes a sheath (big curve and small curve), a guide-wire, a lead, and a stylette. The lead is more pliable, with a smaller diameter, than the traditional SCS lead and has four contacts.

The Targets

- Ilioinguinal: T12, L1, L2
- Genitofemoral L1, L2
- Hip L3
- Knee L3
- Foot L5, L4, S1

The Procedure

Patients are placed in the prone position, similar to SCS. The FDA has approved the device placement for T10 to S2. Needle placement is contralateral trajectory with entry into the interlaminar epidural space of the target DRG. It is advocated that skin entry is two vertebral bodies below and con-

T.R. Deer, MD
The Spine and Nerve Center of The Virginias, Charleston, WV, USA

J.E. Pope, MD (✉)
Summit Pain Alliance, 392 Tesconi Ct, Santa Rosa, CA 95401, USA
e-mail: popeje@me.com

J.E. Pope, T.R. Deer (eds.), *Treatment of Chronic Pain Conditions*, DOI 10.1007/978-1-4939-6976-0_63

tralateral to the target DRG, for a normal body habitus. Once the needle is placed in the optimal location, the big curve sheath and guide-wire system are steered under fluoroscopy to the target DRG, with care to place the system in the superior and posterior portion of the foramen, with the distal end of the sheath at the location where the distal contact is to be placed. The placement is then confirmed in the lateral view, the guide-wire removed, and the styletted lead introduced. The sheath is withdrawn, the superior stress relief loop is placed, then the inferior stress relief loop is created, and then the sheath, stylette, and needle are removed. When multiple levels are placed, the superior location is placed first.

The Evidence

DRG stimulation is statistically superior to SCS for treatment of the CRPS or peripheral causalgia of the lower extremity. 86% of patients received >50% at 1 year of those that receive the implant. Equally impressive, 75% of patients of those that were offered and completed the trial had greater than 50% at 1 year. This fundamentally changes the approach to the therapy. 67% of patients had greater than 80% relief at 1 year. Migration rate of the device was less than 1%, as compared to the published SCS experience of near 18%.

Precision of the perceived paresthesia overlying the painful extremity was markedly improved, with 95% accuracy, while the need for paresthesia to promote pain reduction was less dependent than SCS. Since commercialization in April of 2016, the programming suggests pain relief with subthreshold stimulation.

Conclusion

DRG therapy is a revolutionary strategy to treat a historically difficult chronic pain disease. With success that rivals the benefits of antibiotics for pneumonia, this therapy will change the landscape of the pain care algorithm for CRPS.

Suggested Reading

1. Deer TR, Levy R. A prospective, randomized, multicenter, controller clinical trial to assess the safety and efficacy of the spinal modulation axium neurostimulator system in the treatment of chronic pain. 19th Annual NANS meeting. December 11, 2015. Plenary Session. Las Vegas.
2. Hayek SM, Veizi E, Hanes M. Treatment-limiting complications of percutaneous spinal cord stimulator implants: a review of eight years of experience from an academic center database. Neuromodulation. 2015;18(7):603–8. doi:10.1111/ner.12312. discussion 608–9. Epub 2015 Jun 5
3. Mailis-Gagnon A, Lakha SF, Allen MD. Characteristics of complex regional pain syndrome in patients referred to a tertiary pain clinic by community physicians, assessed by the Budapest clinical diagnostic criteria. Pain Med. 2014;15(11):1965–74. doi:10.1111/pme.12584. Epub 2014 Oct 23
4. Pope JE, Deer TR, Kramer J. A systematic review: current and future directions of dorsal root ganglion therapeutics to treat chronic pain. Pain Med. 2013. Jun 26;14(10):1477–96. doi:10.1111/pme.12171.

Part X

Advanced Pain Care Therapies: X. Peripheral Nerve Stimulation

Peripheral Nerve Stimulation (PNS): Indications

64

Alexios G. Carayannopoulos

Key Concepts

- Peripheral nerve stimulation (PNS), which requires implantation of stimulating electrode leads over the affected injured peripheral nerve
- Percutaneous PNS, which involves percutaneous insertion of stimulating electrode leads in the vicinity of an affected injured nerve, with proper guidance
- Peripheral nerve field stimulation (PNFS), which stimulates smaller nerves in the generalized region of pain

Introduction

PNS is defined as electrical stimulation, which is performed on the peripheral nervous system and applied over or near a specific nerve or region of pain. Electrical current can be delivered to nerves transcutaneously (transcutaneous electrical nerve stimulation, TENS), percutaneously with a temporary electrode (so-called percutaneous electrical nerve stimulation, PENS), and with the help of surgically or percutaneously implanted electrodes (PNS).

Background

Historically, the first published report of PNS for treatment of neuropathic pain described a procedure performed on October 9, 1965 when Drs. Wall and Sweet implanted electrodes around the median and ulnar nerves of a 26-year-old woman with a clinical presentation consistent with complex regional pain syndrome (CRPS). Electrical stimulation of the median nerve provoked pleasant paresthesias and modulated pain in the medial three fingers. Subsequently, Drs. Melzack and Wall published the "gate control" theory of pain in their article in *Science*, which hypothesized that innocuous stimulation of the sensory nervous system might modulate or suppress the transmission of pain. This paved the way for the development of a new treatment modality, which was called "neuromodulation."

Soon thereafter, *Pain and the Neurosurgeon* by White and Sweet was published in 1969 and detailed a radiographic image of a PNS device implanted on the ulnar nerve of a patient with post-traumatic neural impingement. Subsequently, there were dozens of clinical reports, which explored various aspects of PNS through the 1990s. Since that time, PNS has remained relatively consistent, such that the target nerve was exposed, and a paddle-type electrode lead was placed in direct contact with the injured nerve trunk.

Introduction of a percutaneous PNS insertion technique in the late 1990s then revolutionized the PNS field. This approach was initially applied to craniofacial stimulation, but was then later expanded to include other parts of the body, including the neck, chest wall, abdomen, pelvic, lower back, groin, and extremity regions. Next, there was development of peripheral nerve field stimulation (PNFS), which targets more distal nerve structures, including unnamed branches and subcutaneous nerve endings, in a generalized region of pain.

More recently, PNS was advanced by addition of ultrasound guidance, helping in more accurate visualization of peripheral nerves during percutaneous lead insertion. Finally, technical innovations were made, which were specific to PNS applications.

Candidacy

PNS is indicated for cases of chronic, severe, disabling pain of neuropathic origin, which has not responded to more conservative measures including medical treatments, which is associated with a clear diagnosis, and which occurs in the

A.G. Carayannopoulos, DO, MPH (✉)
Comprehensive Spine Center, Pain and Rehabilitation Medicine, Rhode Island Hospital, Neurosurgery Department, 593 Eddy St, Providence, RI 02903, USA
e-mail: acarayannopoulos@lifespan.org

J.E. Pope, T.R. Deer (eds.), *Treatment of Chronic Pain Conditions*, DOI 10.1007/978-1-4939-6976-0_64

absence of correctable pathology. Candidates are expected to be familiar with the modality and should be willing to use the system. Furthermore, candidates should have a favorable neuropsychological profile and should respond positively to a trial of PNS before the permanent device is implanted, with both subjective pain and objective functional improvement. The usual contraindications, such as short life expectancy, active infection, uncorrectable coagulation disorder, and poorly controlled medical comorbidities, which would preclude patients from undergoing elective surgery and/or anesthesia, should be considered.

Indications

The most common indications for PNS are chronic pain, which is subsequent to peripheral nerve injury, persistent pain from compressive neuropathy (following adequate decompression), complex regional pain syndromes (CRPS) type 1 (formerly known as reflex sympathetic dystrophy) and type 2 (formerly known as causalgia), and painful peripheral neuropathy. For PNS (or PNFS) of the chest wall, abdomen, neck, upper and lower back, groin, and other parts of the trunk, the most common indications are postsurgical neuropathic pain, post-infectious (particularly postherpetic) pain, and post-traumatic neuropathy. Newer indications include headache, tinnitus, fibromyalgia, and peripheral pain.

Suggested Reading

1. Abejon D, Perez-Cajaraville J. Peripheral nerve stimulation: definition. Prog Neurol Surg. 2011;24:203–9.
2. Huntoon MA, Burgher AH. Ultrasound-guided permanent implantation of peripheral nerve stimulation (PNS) system for neuropathic pain of the extremities: original cases and outcomes. Pain Med. 2009;10:1369–77.
3. Melzack RA, Wall PD. Pain mechanisms: a new theory. Science. 1965;150:971–9.
4. Slavin KV. History of peripheral nerve stimulation. Prog Neurol Surg. 2011;24:1–15.
5. Weiner RL, Reed KL. Peripheral neurostimulation for control of intractable occipital neuralgia. Neuromodulation. 1999;2:217–21.
6. White JC, Sweet WH. Pain and the neurosurgeon. A forty-year experience. Springfield: Thomas; 1969. p. 894–9.

Peripheral Nerve Stimulation (PNS): Trial

65

Alexios G. Carayannopoulos

Key Concepts

- PNS therapy, like spinal cord stimulation (SCS) therapy, includes a trial or test phase, as well as an implant phase.
- This staged treatment should only be offered to appropriate candidates, who are appropriately screened, and only after careful setting of realistic goals and expectations for pain and functional improvement.

Introduction

Implantation of a peripheral nerve stimulator is performed in two stages, which are similar to the two stages of spinal cord stimulation. During the first stage, an electrode lead is inserted via the percutaneous or surgical approach directly over a targeted nerve, in the vicinity of a targeted nerve or branch, or in a generalized region of pain. The trial of stimulation lasts several days or weeks. Three PNS techniques are used by neuromodulators for various types of neuropathic pain: (1) PNS, in which leads are implanted in subcutaneous tissue, over a specific sensory nerve, which correlates with the painful area; (2) Percutaneous PNS, in which leads are implanted subcutaneously in the region of a sensory nerve territory; (3) PNFS, in which leads are implanted within a perceived or generalized area of pain.

The goal of PNS or percutaneous PNS is to produce tingling paresthesias along the territory of a specific stimulated nerve. The goal of PNFS is to distribute paresthesias in an electrical field around the lead's active electrodes, without achieving a clearly defined nerve distribution, which results in a concentric stimulation-induced sensation/paresthesia in a specific area of precise zone of pain, without radiation, and without following a specific named nerve target.

Candidacy

Patients with extremity pain, which is limited to the distribution of a single nerve, are better candidates for PNS. Patients with pain in the trunk, chest, and abdomen are better candidates for PNFS. Pure sensory nerves are generally better targets for PNS than mixed motor/sensory or pure motor nerves, whereby stimulation may also provoke unwanted motor stimulation. Patients should have documented 50% or greater improvement in pain and level of function during a trial of stimulation. Standardized pain rating scales, as well as functional assessment tools, can be used before trial, at the end of trial before lead removal, and again at baseline, after lead removal to more accurately gauge response to trial stimulation. Patients and providers should have a candid discussion to review this trial information before deciding whether it is appropriate to proceed with implant. Decision to move to implant should not be rushed.

Suggested Reading

1. Levy RM. Differentiating the leaves from the branches in the tree of neuromodulation: the state of peripheral nerve field stimulation. Neuromodulation. 2011;14:201–5.
2. Nashold Jr BS, Goldner JL, Mullen JB, Bright DS. Long-term pain control by direct peripheral-nerve stimulation. J Bone Joint Surg Am. 1982;64:1–10.

A.G. Carayannopoulos, MD (✉)
Comprehensive Spine Center, Pain and Rehabilitation Medicine, Rhode Island Hospital, Neurosurgery Department, 593 Eddy St, Providence, RI 02903, USA
e-mail: acarayannopoulos@lifespan.org

J.E. Pope, T.R. Deer (eds.), *Treatment of Chronic Pain Conditions*, DOI 10.1007/978-1-4939-6976-0_65

Peripheral Nerve Stimulation (PNS): Permanent

66

Alexios G. Carayannopoulos

Key Concepts

- Implantation after a successful trial, like SCS, can be performed in either a percutaneous or surgical fashion.
- There are advantages to each approach, which should be considered carefully in light of the specific clinical scenario and should be reviewed with the candidate.

Introduction

If the trial is successful, the second stage involves insertion of a permanent electrode. This electrode is anchored in place, usually to the underlying fascia. Subsequently, the electrode lead or an appropriate extension cable is connected to an implantable pulse generator (IPG)/battery via a tunneling procedure.

Percutaneous

Historically, PNS electrode leads were implanted surgically via an open technique to better visualize deeper anatomical structures, such as nerves and blood vessels, proximate to the more superficial nerves being treated. However risks, such as perineural scarring, made the open approach problematic historically. More recently, introduction of ultrasound guidance has gained favor, allowing minimally invasive access for accurate percutaneous electrode insertion. Because of the variable course and depth of the nerves to be stimulated, as well as the proximity of nerves to blood vessels, ultrasound guidance has become very helpful to differentiate pertinent structures and to allow for safe placement of electrodes.

Currently, percutaneous electrode leads are usually selected for several reasons: (1) when the nerve of interest is to be found in a predictable anatomical area, whereby stimulation is deliverable without direct contact with the nerve, and (2) when the painful area may require coverage with multiple leads, whereby stimulating paresthesias are concordant with the pain distribution. Generally, percutaneous placement dominates the field of PNS.

Surgical

Some neuromodulators still use surgically placed paddle leads for PNS because of several important benefits:

1. Paddle electrodes have several rows of electrode contacts separated by a preset distance, which allows for multiple stimulation paradigms in the longitudinal, transverse, and oblique directions. Thus, electrode contact configuration parallels the course of sensory fibers inside the nerve trunk and allows for more precise targeting and programming.
2. Paddle electrodes are flat and offer unidirectional stimulation, directing electrical energy toward the nerve while shielding the surrounding tissue via insulation of the paddle's backing, leading to more efficient use of energy, which maintains battery life of the IPG.
3. Paddle electrodes are more stable over time and are associated with lower migration rates.

The most important requirement in selecting the surgical approach over percutaneous approach is the need for highly refined surgical skills, which allows better exposure of peripheral nerves, since multiple reports of perineural fibrosis following long-term PNS therapy with paddle leads have raised concerns about their safety and appropriateness of this approach in future applications.

A.G. Carayannopoulos, MD (✉)
Comprehensive Spine Center, Pain and Rehabilitation Medicine, Rhode Island Hospital, Neurosurgery Department, 593 Eddy St, Providence, RI 02903, USA
e-mail: acarayannopoulos@lifespan.org

J.E. Pope, T.R. Deer (eds.), *Treatment of Chronic Pain Conditions*, DOI 10.1007/978-1-4939-6976-0_66

Suggested Reading

1. Bouche B, Eisenberg E, Meigner M, Durand S, Papaniaou M, Suarez A, Verlysen M, Lemarie J. Facilitation of diagnostic and percutaneous trial lead placement with ultrasound guidance for peripheral subcutaneous field stimulation on infra-patellar branches of saphenous nerve. Neuromodulation. 2011;14:564.
2. Hassenbusch SJ, Stanton-Hicks M, Schoppa D, Walsh JG, Covington EC. Long-term results of peripheral nerve stimulation for reflex sympathetic dystrophy. J Neurosurg. 1996;84:415–23.
3. Kent M, Upp J, Spevak C, Shanon C, Buckenmaier C. Ultrasound-guided peripheral nerve stimulator placement in two soldiers with acute battlefield neuropathic pain. Anesth Analg. 2012;114:875–8.
4. Mobbs RJ, Nair S, Blum P. Peripheral nerve stimulation for the treatment of chronic pain. J Clin Neurosci. 2007;14:216–21.

Peripheral Nerve Stimulation (PNS): Maintenance

67

Alexios G. Carayannopoulos

Key Concepts

- Maintenance of PNS, like SCS, refers to procedural and management considerations, which promote successful PNS treatment longitudinally.
- Reprogramming to maintain appropriate stimulating paresthesias.
- Monitoring for adverse events/complications during trial, implant, and postoperative phases.
- Ongoing monitoring of pain management with frequent reassessment of function, quality of life (QOL), and patient satisfaction.

Introduction

After following the appropriate indications for therapy and candidate selection, and after setting realistic goals and expectations, maintenance of therapy involves three general considerations, which should be carefully monitored and documented to sustain the life of PNS therapy treatment. These include the following:

Managing Therapy Through Reprogramming

Patients undergoing PNS therapy will need ongoing adjustments to stimulation to maintain stimulating paresthesias in areas of pain, which may evolve over time. Re-programming should always follow a focused re-assessment of pain to assess for change in quality, location, or intensity of pain, as well as diurnal variation or relation of pain to activity level. Reprogramming should always be accompanied by patient education to promote understanding of how individualized programming can achieve pain control and improve function.

Monitoring for Adverse Events/ Complications

This includes avoidance of complications during the trial, implant, postoperative, and maintenance phases. Potential complications include infection, hemorrhage, injury to nervous tissue, placement of electrode/device in the wrong compartment, hardware migration, erosion, and device malfunction, which includes lead fracture and disconnection. Overall, most PNS complications are minor and rarely, if ever, require hospitalization. Because of recent technological advancements, many early PNS complications are rarely seen today, while others remain static. One reason for the unchanged rate of some complications is that peripheral nerve stimulation is still mostly performed using devices developed and marketed for spinal cord stimulation applications. As the anatomy of peripheral nerves and surrounding soft tissues is very different from the epidural spinal space, where SCS electrodes are generally placed, PNS complications persist from adapting technology to the peripheral nervous system.

Fortunately, morbidity associated with PNS and percutaneous PNS is low, and most issues may be resolved with simple outpatient revision surgeries. Reduction in the complication rate is expected to occur when the hardware used in PNS procedures is appropriately adapted and designed for PNS applications. Introduction of dedicated PNS/PNFS devices will reduce complication rates and will improve reliability and sustainability of the therapy. Morbidity of the more recently introduced PNFS technique is still generally unknown, but will become more available as the use of this technique increases.

A.G. Carayannopoulos, MD (✉)
Comprehensive Spine Center, Pain and Rehabilitation Medicine, Rhode Island Hospital, Neurosurgery Department, 593 Eddy St, Providence, RI 02903, USA
e-mail: acarayannopoulos@lifespan.org

J.E. Pope, T.R. Deer (eds.), *Treatment of Chronic Pain Conditions*, DOI 10.1007/978-1-4939-6976-0_67

Monitoring of Pain, Function, QOL, and Patient Satisfaction

Maintenance of therapy also involves maintaining pain reduction and level of function, which in turn maintains patient satisfaction.The use of validated pain scales and functional assessment tools is pivotal in documenting clinical status and can be used as an educational tool in counseling patients on overall progress of therapy. Finally, maintenance of therapy includes ongoing enhancement of technology to improve accuracy, efficiency, and sustainability of therapy.

Suggested Reading

1. Slavin KV. Placing neuromodulation in the human body: limiting morbidity. In: Arle JA, Shils JL, editors. Essential neuromodulation. Philadelphia: Elsevier; 2011. p. 301–20.

Peripheral Nerve Stimulation (PNS): New Therapies

68

Alexios G. Carayannopoulos

Key Concepts

- New therapies include C2-C3 nerve stimulation and chronic neuropathic pain, both of which have widespread applications, with several proposed but unproven mechanisms of action.

Introduction

Peripheral nerve stimulation of the occipital branch of the C2 nerve for occipital neuralgia, intractable chronic migraine, transformed migraine, chronic cluster headache, hemicrania continua, facial pain, fibromyalgia, peripheral pain, and tinnitus represents new applications. Electrical stimulation of the occipital branch of the C2 nerve takes a special place in PNFS, because of its seemingly widespread effects, which are not fully explained. Hypotheses have been proposed including:

1. The reduction of the activity of nociceptive fibers, providing pain relief according to the "gate control" theory promulgated by Melzack and Wall
2. The reduction of peripheral nerve excitability by electrical stimulation, thereby reducing pain
3. The central effect on thalamic structures, which alleviates pain via the trigemino-cervical complex

New Targets

Peripheral nerve stimulation has also been found to be an appropriate therapeutic tool for refractory neuropathic pain (such as intractable chronic headache, pelvic pain, testicular pain, abdominal pain, low back pain), when placed over the affected nerve or plexus, when other less invasive modalities have failed. Specifically, PNS has been shown to be effective in treating severe neuropathic and intractable pain after multiple joint surgeries complicated by causalgia-type pain. This treatment approach is generally successful as long as there is some level of preserved sensation in the painful area. Evidence for efficacy is not strongly conclusive, and long-term controlled studies have not been conducted.

Peripheral nerve stimulation has been found to be a safe and effective short-term treatment option in poststroke patients with hemiplegic shoulder pain (HSP) by stimulating the peripheral nerves in a percutaneous approach, which affect the trapezius, supraspinatus, and medial and posterior deltoids.

New technology includes wireless electrical nerve stimulations (WENS), which uses an external power source, subsequently reducing the need for an internal battery or implanted pulse generator (IPG). This approach could increase long-term viability and efficacy of PNS technology in vivo.

New applications include the use of peripheral nerve field stimulation (PNFS) or subcutaneous peripheral nerve stimulation (SQ PNS). Although the mechanism by which PNFS provides pain relief is poorly understood and probably involves a number of interrelated mechanisms, it involves placement of subcutaneous leads over a painful area to stimulate nerve endings and dermal receptors, eventually traveling through the dorsal roots to reach the spinal cord. This treatment has been used to treat both neuropathic as well as nociceptive pain related to intractable failed back surgery syndrome (FBSS) and sacroiliac pain. PNFS used in conjunction with spinal cord stimulation has also been widely documented and has successfully treated conditions including intractable low back pain in patients with FBSS, as well as post-herniorrhaphy pain. In fact, combination therapy has been shown to be more affective than SCS alone or intrathecal opioid therapy for the subset of patients who have axial greater than radicular pain or in patients with persistent inguinal pain after hernia repair surgery.

A.G. Carayannopoulos, MD (✉)
Comprehensive Spine Center, Pain and Rehabilitation Medicine, Rhode Island Hospital, Neurosurgery Department, 593 Eddy St, Providence, RI 02903, USA
e-mail: acarayannopoulos@lifespan.org

J.E. Pope, T.R. Deer (eds.), *Treatment of Chronic Pain Conditions*, DOI 10.1007/978-1-4939-6976-0_68

Further exploration of using ultrasound guidance for peripheral nerve stimulation among neuromodulators will undoubtedly help to advance generalizability of this treatment and increase clinical applications.

Suggested Reading

1. Lepsli G, et al. Combined spinal cord and peripheral nerve field stimulation for persistent post-herniorrhaphy pain. Neuromodulation. 2013;16:84–9.
2. Mironer E, et al. Prospective, two-part study of the interaction between spinal cord stimulation and peripheral nerve field stimulation in patients with low back pain: development of a new spinal–peripheral neurostimulation method. Neuromodulation. 2011;14:151–5.
3. Patil A, et al. Letter to the editor: peripheral nerve field stimulation for sacroiliac pain. Neuromodulation. 2014;17:98–101.
4. Plazier M, et al. Peripheral nerve stimulation for fibromyalgia. Prog Neurol Surg. 2011;24:133–46.
5. Reverberi C, et al. Using peripheral nerve stimulation (PNS) to treat neuropathic pain: a clinical series. Neuromodulation. 2014;17(8):777–83.
6. Rosellini W, et al. Wireless peripheral nerve stimulation increases pain threshold in two neuropathic rat models. Exp Neurol. 2012;235:621–6.
7. Serra G, Marchioretto F. Occipital nerve stimulation for chronic migraine, a randomized trial. Pain Physician. 2012;15:245–53.
8. Wilson R, et al. Peripheral nerve stimulation vs. usual care for pain relief of hemiplegic shoulder pain. Am J Phys Med Rehab. 2014;93:17–27.
9. Yakovlev A, et al. Peripheral nerve field stimulation in the treatment of postlaminectomy after multilevel spinal surgeries. Neuromodulation. 2011;14:534–8.

Part XI

Advanced Pain Care Therapies: XI. Minimally Spinal Stenosis Treatments

Percutaneous Image-Guided Lumbar Decompression (PILD) Indications

69

W. Porter McRoberts and Paul Wu

Key Concepts

- PILD allows access to the posterior central canal via ultra-minimally invasive approaches without the need for general anesthesia.
- Three critical criteria for patient selection portend success: (1) the patient has neurogenic claudication and leg pain with walking or standing, (2) the patient has central canal lumbar spinal stenosis which is a function of ligamentum flavum hypertrophy, and (3) there exists no other rational cause of the patient's pain, e.g., far lateral recess stenosis, foraminal stenosis, or vascular claudication.
- PILD has been demonstrated by multiple prospective studies to be both safe and effective.

Introduction

Lumbar spinal stenosis (LSS) is a common progressive condition affecting predominantly older populations. Symptoms of LSS are manifested by low back pain and leg pain upon standing or walking or both, and symptoms cease with resting, termed neurogenic intermittent claudication (NIC). Treatments for symptomatic LSS depend on severity, ranging from conservative approaches such as physical therapy with or without epidural steroid injection in mild cases to open spinal surgical decompressive approaches such as laminectomy with and without complex fusion. For symptomatic patients with mild-moderate and moderate-severe degree of LSS, or those with high surgical risk, or those unwilling to have open surgery, PILD is poised as an effective and attractive minimally invasive treatment alternative to traditional approaches.

Background (for LSS Definition and Diagnosis, LSS Types, and Treatment Effectiveness)

LSS has three main subclassifications or components: lateral stenosis (LS), canal stenosis (CS), and spondylolisthesis. Frequently, canal stenosis occurs in combination with either of the other two or both. PILD addresses specifically central canal stenosis, which refers to decreased AP or transverse diameter of the canal and/or decreased cross-sectional area of central spinal canal. The most commonly accepted radiological criteria for diagnosis of CS in lumbar region are an AP diameter of 10 mm or less and cross-sectional area less than 70 mm^2, although there is no consensus. Etiologies of LSS can be classified as congenital/developmental or acquired/degenerative in nature. The distinction is important for treatment. In the former case, the LSS usually is the result of congenital bone structural constriction of the canal and naturally small thecal sac, whereas in the latter the narrowing is due to ligamentum flavum hypertrophy (LFH) resulting from disc degeneration and movement, weight-bearing facet joints, and spinal instability. Spondylolisthesis in itself can also cause spinal stenosis in either spondylolytic or degenerative type. Furthermore, foraminal stenosis (FS) and disc herniation (DH) can also contribute to the formation and symptoms of LSS. Maximal efficacy of PILD relies heavily on knowing components and etiology of LSS.

Candidacy

The main indication of PILD is symptomatic LSS of the degenerative CS associated with LFH. Additionally, imaging finding should have minimal LS, FS, or potential symptomatic disc herniation. LSS symptoms are described as

W. Porter McRoberts, MD (✉)
Interventional Spine, Pain and Neurosurgery, Holy Cross Hospital, 3111 NE 44th St, Fort Lauderdale, FL 33308, USA
e-mail: portermcroberts@gmail.com

P. Wu, MD
Holy Cross Hospital, Holy Cross Orthopedic/Neuroscience Institutes, Fort Lauderdale, FL, USA

J.E. Pope, T.R. Deer (eds.), *Treatment of Chronic Pain Conditions*, DOI 10.1007/978-1-4939-6976-0_69

neurogenic intermittent claudication (NIC). NIC is defined as discomfort distributed in unilateral or bilateral buttock/groin/leg, described as pain, heaviness, or paresthesia (numbness, tinging, burning), worsened with standing and walking but relieved by flexion (sitting or bending, e.g., over a shopping cart). Frequently, LSS also presents with low back pain in conjunction with NIC, in a similar exacerbating symptoms by standing and walking and alleviation by flexion. Radiological findings of LSS which favors the use of PILD include:

1. Stenosis limited to one or two levels.
2. NIC symptoms should be attributed predominantly to canal stenosis, not lateral or foraminal stenosis or disc herniation.
3. Absence of significant instability on flexion/extension x-ray if spondylolisthesis presents.
4. Anterior listhesis <5 mm.
5. Ligamentum flavum hypertrophy >2.5 mm.
6. No prior fusion or bone removal surgery at index level.

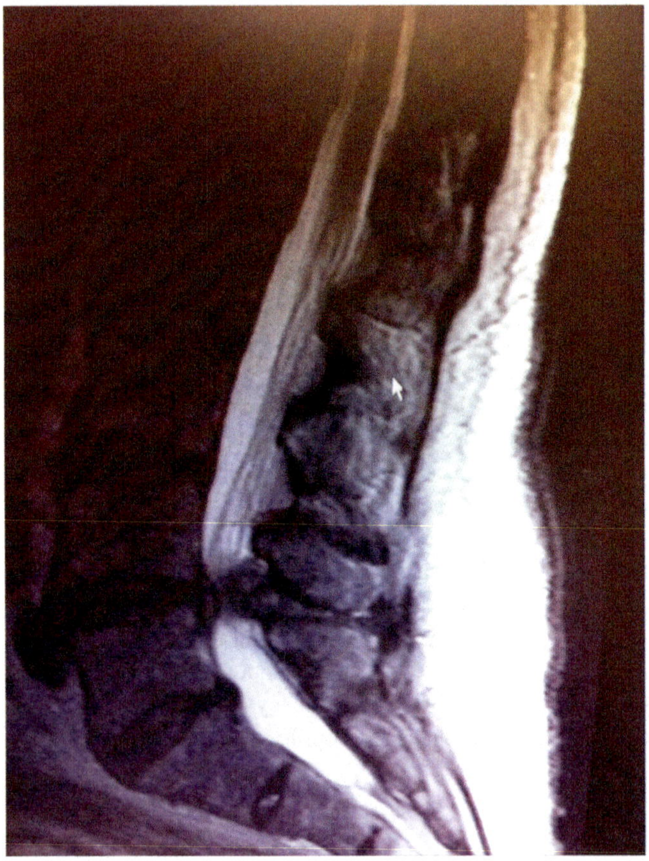

Fig. 69.1 Central canal stenosis as a function of ligamentum flavum hypertrophy

Both appropriate LSS clinical and radiological criteria should be combined to identify the ideal candidate to ensure the likelihood of good outcome. Typical candidates might have sagittal MRI findings as seen in Figs. 69.1 and 69.2. Readers should also know that the selecting standards for the right PILD patient will likely continue to evolve, and aforementioned measures should serve as general guideline (Tables 69.1 and 69.2).

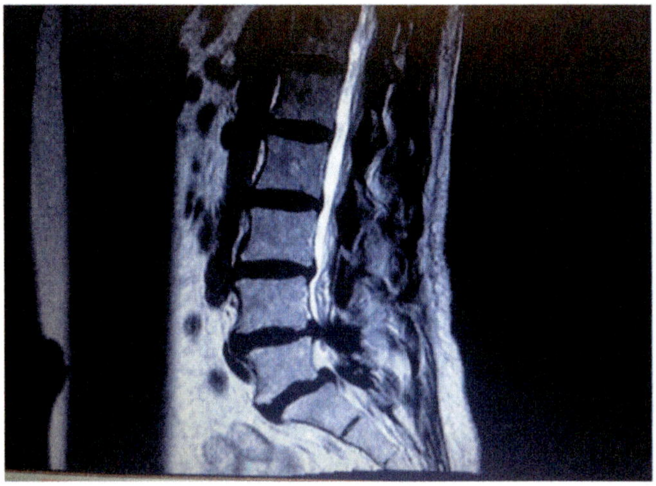

Fig. 69.2 Ligamentum flavum hypertrophy contributing to LSS. Note anteriorly, disc bulge also contributes, but not significantly minus the LH

Table 69.1 Patient inclusion criteria

Symptomatic LSS primarily caused by dorsal element hypertrophy
>6 months of NIC
Prior failure of conservative therapy
Radiologic evidence of LSS
LFH > 2.5 mm
Central canal sectional area ≤100 square mm
Anterior listhesis ≤5.0 mm
Ability to walk at least 10 feet unaided before being limited by pain

Table 69.2 Patient exclusion criteria

Prior surgery at the intended treatment level
History of recent spinal fractures with concurrent pain symptoms
Disabling back or leg pain from causes other than LSS
Significant/symptomatic disc protrusion or osteophyte formation
Excessive/symptomatic facet hypertrophy
Spinal stenosis with minimal or no LFH [4]

LFH Ligamentum flavum hypertrophy [2]

Summary

PILD is a minimally invasive, percutaneous option for those suffering from LSS. Compared with open surgical resection, it presents as arguably a vastly less risky alternative. Open surgical series report dural tears from 6.8% to 15.6% of cases [2]. The rate of blood transfusion in surgical patients ranges from 9.9% in the Maine Lumbar Spine Study [3] to 14.2% in the SPORT Lumbar Spinal Stenosis Study [1]. Total complications in open surgical series range from 13.8% to 27.2%. Deer and Kapural in their initial study of 90 patients reported no complication. Persons wishing to avoid this exposure to surgical risk may consider this arguably safer option.

Suggested Reading

1. Atlas SJ, Deyo RA, Keller RB, Chapin AM, Patrick DL, Long JM, Singer DE. The Maine lumbar spine study, part III:1-year outcomes of surgical and nonsurgical management of lumbar spinal stenosis. Spine. 1996;21:1787–94.
2. Chopko B, Caraway DL. MiDAS I (mild® Decompression Alternative to Open Surgery): a preliminary report of a prospective, multi-center clinical study. Pain Physician. 2010;13:369–37.
3. Deer TR, Kapural L. New image-guided, ultra-minimally invasive lumbar decompression method: the mild procedure. Pain Physician. 2010;13:35–41.
4. Weinstein JN, Tosteson TD, Lurie JD, Tosteson AN, Blood E, Hanscom B, Herkowitz H, Cammisa F, Albert T, Boden SD, Hilibrand A, Goldberg H, Berven S, An H, Investigators SPORT. Surgical versus nonsurgical therapy for lumbar spinal stenosis. N Engl J Med. 2008;358:794–810.

70 Percutaneous Image-Guided Lumbar Decompression Procedure

W. Porter McRoberts and Paul Wu

Key Concepts

- PILD, at present either MILD® or Totalis®, requires familiarization with the technique and instrumentation through formal training.
- Whenever working near neural elements the risk of neural compromise or injury is correlated with the level of sedation, the more awake a patient is, the lower the risk of injury.
- Good local anesthesia to the lamina will provide comfort to the patient while preserving a wakeful state.
- Imaging and understanding of the safe working zones will allow for adequate decompression.

Introduction

Traditionally, choices for lumbar spinal stenosis (LSS) management are limited, ranging from conservative treatment to epidural steroid injection and if recalcitrant to conservative measures spinal surgery involving laminar resection. Conservative treatments include physical therapy and medications. In majority of cases, physical therapy provides either temporary or no relief for neurogenic intermittent claudication (NIC). Medications commonly used for LSS typically consist of NSAIDs, anticonvulsant, and pain medications. However, as LSS is predominantly affecting the older population, the health risk of polypharmacy needs to be considered. Epidural injection provides short-term relief and is often limited by steroid exposure in repeating injections. The effect of complementary alternative medicine is unclear for treatment of LSS. Surgery offers the ability of stenosis decompression, but may have unexpected spinal complications. Given the older population as the primary patient group, medical comorbidities present as a potential obstacle in surgical clearance. Therefore, a gap exists in the treatment of moderate to moderate-severe LSS, where surgery may not be the most appropriate option. The development of PILD fills that gap.

W. Porter McRoberts, MD (✉)
Interventional Spine, Pain and Neurosurgery, Holy Cross Hospital, 3111 NE 44th St, Fort Lauderdale, FL 33308, USA
e-mail: portermcroberts@gmail.com

P. Wu, MD
Holy Cross Hospital, Holy Cross Orthopedic/Neuroscience Institutes, Fort Lauderdale, FL, USA

Background

Decompressing neural elements while preserving spinal and connective tissue anatomy remains the goal of any surgical treatment for LSS. Both laminectomy and laminotomy require open dissection from skin to the level of lamina, with supporting muscles and fascia interrupted during the process. Incisions are usually 4–6 cm in size, possibly larger in multilevel approaches. With frank instability, or if there exists concern for instability after laminectomy, the surgeon often includes instrumented fusion. Such broad and extensive surgery causes tissue disruption and can leave patients with significant postsurgical pain, in addition to exposure to a host of neurological risk. Endoscopic decompression is less invasive, but with similarly high complication rates, mainly dural tears. PILD uses a smaller incision, causes minimal tissue disruption, and decompresses neural elements by debulking the ligamentum flavum with nominal effect to the osseous and muscular integrity of the spine. Currently, there are two PILD systems available commercially: MILD® procedure by Vertos and Totalis® procedure by Vertiflex.

MILD Procedure

Kit

The MILD kit comes with instruments needed to perform the procedure. They are (1) MILD Portal, (2) MILD Trocar and Handle, (3) MILD Portal Stabilizer, (4) MILD Depth Guide,

J.E. Pope, T.R. Deer (eds.), *Treatment of Chronic Pain Conditions*, DOI 10.1007/978-1-4939-6976-0_70

(5) MILD Bone Sculpter Rongeur, (6) MILD Tissue Sculpter, and (7) MILD Surgical Clamp.

Overview

MILD accesses the interlaminar space through posterior lumbar spine from a lateral-oblique approach. The access point starts at inferior lumbar lamina of the index level, and the skin entry point is located lateral to the inferior spinal process of the index level. The Bone Sculpter Rongeur and the Tissue Sculpter access the ligamentum flavum and lamina through the Portal. Fluoroscope is placed in cephalocaudal AP positioning, parallel to the lamina surface in order to obtain an open trajectory view for initial approach. The depth of the Tissue Sculpter insertion requires contralateral oblique fluoroscopic view, in conjunction with ipsilateral epidurography, to assess the tip position of the Sculpter relative to epidural space. Resection by the Tissue Sculpter through the Portal allows the debulking of the ligamentum flavum. A small amount of the lamina is also removed.

Procedure Detail

1. Patient placed on a radiolucent table in prone position.
2. Perform preoperative AP and contralateral fluoroscopic views to determine the path of initial approach. Patient is prepped and drapped in a sterile fashion.
3. Perform interlaminar epidurography using standard median or paramedian techniques. This identifies the border of the ligamentum flavum and epidural and dural space.
4. Administer local and deep anesthesia at the skin entry site, based on preoperative fluoroscopic planning, typically 1–1.5 vertebral segment caudal to index level. Make a small dime-sized skin incision.
5. Insert and lock the Trocar into the Portal. Advance the combination to the inferior dorsal lamina surface, lateral to the spinal process. Position the tip toward the superior margin of the inferior lamina. Remove the trocar.
6. Secure the Portal with either Portal Stabilizer or Surgical Clamp. Attach the Depth Guide.
7. Placing the Bone Sculpter Rongeur through the Portal, use clock–/counterclockwise rotation to remove small portion of lamina bone to create better access to interlaminar space. Repeat the process as needed.
8. Remove the Rongeur and use the contralateral epidurography view to deploy the Tissue Sculpter through the portal into dorsal ligamentum flavum. Adjust the Depth Guide as needed. Squeezing the trigger opens the jaws at the device tip. Releasing the device trigger allows an effective resection of the ligamentum. Remove the resected tissue and repeat until satisfactory unobstructed epidurography is obtained.
9. Remove the Portal. Repeat the steps on contralateral side and other levels.

Totalis Procedure

Kit

The Totalis Direct Decompression System comes with specialized non-sterile reusable instrumentation set and a sterile single use kit. The reusable instrument set includes sized sequential dilators and access cannulas, small blunt tip, and bunt tip reamers. The single use kit includes the Cannula Base Stabilizing Platform, the Tissue Dissector, and the Rongeur.

Overview

The Totalis accesses the interlaminar space and the posterior lumbar spine. The approach is midline and through the interspinous ligament of the index level. AP and lateral fluoroscopic views are utilized for midline and depth assessment for the instrument placement. Epidurography is recommended. The Tissue Sculpter and the Rongeur remove the ligamentum flavum and small portion of the bone from superior, inferior, and lateral aspects of the lamina.

Procedure Detail (Figs. 70.1 and 70.2)

1. Place patient on a radiolucent table in prone position. Prepped and drapped patient in a sterile fashion.
2. Perform AP and contralateral fluoroscopic views to determine the index level, depth, interspinous space width, and path of initial approach.
3. Perform interlaminar epidurography using standard median or paramedian techniques.
4. Administer local and deep anesthesia at the skin entry site, which is midline between the spinous process at the index level. Make a dime-sized midline incision.
5. Palpate the interspinous ligament through the incision. Make a longitudinal midline stab at the ligament.
6. Insert appropriate sized dilators sequentially over each other, manually or with a mallet. Use AP fluoroscopy to align the distal groove channel of the dilators with the spinous process in the groove. Use lateral fluoroscopy to advance the tip of the dilators to the dorsal aspect of the facet. Remove the inner dilator. Mark the depth.

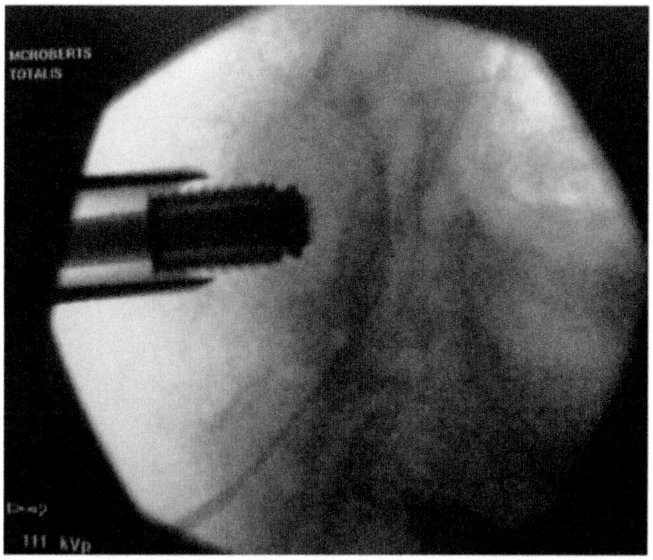

Fig. 70.1 Intraprocedural spot films of Totalis®. Tissue reamer preparing the route of the Rongeur under lateral view. Note epidural guide wire as delineation of posterior epidural space

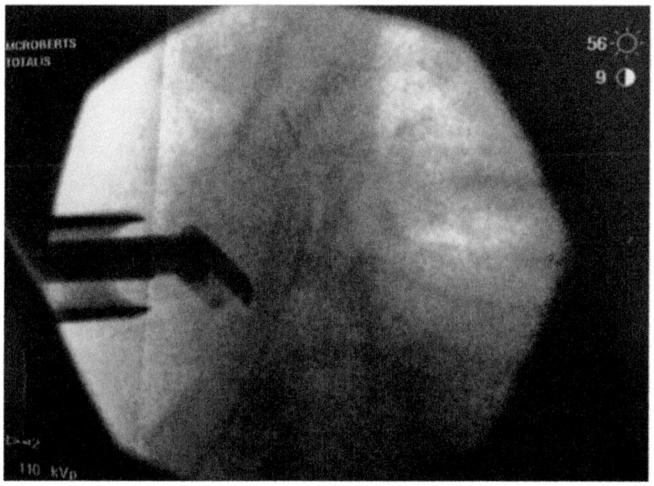

Fig. 70.2 Lateral view of Kerrison resecting inferior ligament in the interlaminar space

7. Insert appropriate sized cannula. Advance the tip of the cannula just past apexes of the spinal process with lateral fluoroscopy.
8. Place the cannula-based stabilizing platform over the proximal end of the cannula against the skin.
9. Insert the desired sized blunt tip reamer through the cannula. Advanced to the previously marked depth or desired depth with lateral fluoroscopy. Rotate clock- and counterclockwise to remove medial lamina bone and ligament tissue. Use the adjustable depth stop on the reamer for safety.
10. Remove the reamer. Advance the tissue dissector through the cannula under lateral fluoroscopic view for depth. Use tactile feedback and adjustable depth stop, and place the tip against the undersurface of the superior lamina. Use left-right sweeping motion to loosen the ligamentum from the lamina, from midline toward lateral recess. Remove the dissector.
11. Advance the Rongeur through the cannula under lateral fluoroscopy. Remove lamina bones and ligamentum flavum in different directions under lateral fluoroscopy. Use epidurography to assess adequacy of the procedure. Remove all instruments once complete .

Summary

When successful, both MILD and Totalis allow minimal disruption to the neural elements as well as bony attachments of the muscular spine. This combination of safety, efficacy, and preservation of stability has promise. Future studies will determine if these iterations will be successful enough to woo insurance coverage; otherwise, likely new variations of equipment and technique will improve on these successful ultra-minimally invasive options for lumbar spinal stenosis.

Suggested Reading

1. Carragee EJ. The increasing morbidity of elective spinal stenosis surgery: is it necessary? JAMA. 2010;303:1309–10.
2. Deer TR, Kapural L. New image-guided, ultra-minimally invasive lumbar decompression method: the mild procedure. Pain Physician. 2010;13:35–41.
3. Deer TR, Mekhail N, Lopez G, Amirdelfan K. Minimally invasive lumbar decompression for spinal stenosis. J Neursurg Rev. 2011; 1(S1):29–32.
4. Lawrence MM, Hayek SM. Minimally invasive lumbar decompression a treatment for lumber spinal stenosis. Curr Opin Anesthesiol. 2013;26:573–9.
5. Lingreen R, Grider JS. Retrospective review of patient self-report- ed improvement and post-procedure findings for mild (minimally invasive lumbar decompression). Pain Physician. 2010;13:555–60.

Percutaneous Image-Guided Lumbar Decompression (PILD): Follow-Up and Risk Management

71

W. Porter McRoberts and Paul Wu

Key Concepts

- PILD is a neurosurgical procedure with the potential for all the sequelae of open surgical laminar resection, and careful follow-up is required.
- Attention to risk reduction steps before and during the procedure will translate into safe recovery.
- Developing a protocol for follow-up will streamline the process of discharge and surveillance in the perioperative period for all patients and ensure highest level of safety.
- Despite the majority of risk being associated with, and temporally related to, the time of the procedure, several late-occurring complications need to be watched for.

Introduction

PILD involves the surgical resection of ligamentum flavum and bony lamina, and possibly facet joint as well. Although great care has been taken in the design of the instruments, they are sharp tools designed for cutting tissue and bone. Injury at the time of the procedure and introduction of foreign materials and bacteria into the spine are of primary concern.

W. Porter McRoberts, MD (✉)
Interventional Spine, Pain and Neurosurgery, Holy Cross Hospital, 3111 NE 44th St, Fort Lauderdale, FL 33308, USA
e-mail: portermcroberts@gmail.com

P. Wu, MD
Holy Cross Hospital, Holy Cross Orthopedic/Neuroscience Institutes, Fort Lauderdale, FL, USA

Preoperative Planning Steps for Risk Reduction (RR)

1. Patients bathe with Hibiclens for 3–5 days prior to surgery.
2. Patients use intranasal Mupirocin for 5 days prior to surgery.
3. Patients discuss with prescribing physician and then stop the use of anticoagulants for appropriate timeframe. See the 2014 NACC (Neuromodulation Appropriateness Consensus Committee) guidelines for stimulation implant.
4. Patients are called at 5-day pre-op, to reiterate steps 1–3.
5. At 48 h:
   (a) Patient is called at 48 h to again confirm steps 1–3.
   (b) Confirm appropriate imaging will be available to the surgeon on the day of surgery.
   (c) Document patient has educated themselves on the associated risks so that formal consenting process goes smoothly.
   (d) Ensure facility has preoperative antibiotics consistent with allergy profile of patient and all other equipment and medicines are available (catheters, needles, syringes, local anesthetic contrast appropriate to patient).
   (e) Ensure facility has surgical equipment readied and sterilized.
   (f) Confirm patient has transportation and observer at home for postsurgical neurological surveillance.

Perioperative Risk Reduction Strategies

1. Confirm all steps of preoperative RR above.
2. Full consenting process with family present.
3. Educate observer on the sentinel signs of worsening neural compression as can be seen in evolving epidural hematoma such as leg weakness, numbness or bowel or

J.E. Pope, T.R. Deer (eds.), *Treatment of Chronic Pain Conditions*, DOI 10.1007/978-1-4939-6976-0_71

bladder incontinence, and how to recognize and regularly assess signs.
4. Confirm and then carry out anesthesia plan of minimal sedation to no sedation, with excellent local anesthesia to the lamina so as to allow the patient the ability to give intraoperative feedback regarding neural compromise.
5. Preoperative IV antibiotics given in a timely manner.
6. Wide and adequate surgical prep.

Intraoperative RR Strategies

1. As noted above arousable level of sedation for surgical steps near the canal.
2. Maintain good imaging and refresh contrast as necessary or use an epidural catheter such as Epimed Brevi-XL to delineate the posterior confines of the epidural space.
3. Good anesthesia to the periosteum of the superior and inferior lamina and block of the medial branches and along the intended surgical tract will not only allow for arousable patient, but will also reduce movement from procedural discomfort.
4. Copious irrigation to clear upon conclusion of the case diminishes infection risk as does use of intra-wound antibiotics.
5. Multilayer closure with excellent skin approximation diminishes dead space formation, risk of dehiscence, and infection risk.

Discharge RR Approaches

1. Document any changes in neurologic status.
2. Document and again educate caregivers on the sentinel signs of worsening neural compression as can be seen in evolving epidural hematoma such as leg weakness, numbness or bowel or bladder incontinence, and how to recognize and regularly asses signs and have plan of return to ER for surgical decompression ASAP. Provide written instruction.
3. Document and then have discussion and provide written instructions regarding the prevention of, surveillance for, and action plan for infection control.
4. Document and have wound care discussion and provide written instructions.
5. Document and have discussion regarding re-initiation of anticoagulants and provide written instruction.
6. Provide for postoperative oral pain management.
7. Consider a short course of oral postsurgical antibiotic.
8. Schedule surgical follow-up in timely manner.

Conclusion

PILD is a neurosurgical procedure and demands the same attention to surgical risk reduction, as does any open surgery. Properly training staff, discussing each step with staff, and then using checklists to mitigate risk minimize the burden of remembering each step. PILD enjoys as a primary attribute its low surgical hazard; however, complacency is the ally of risk regardless of the innate nature of PILD's surgical safety.

Suggested Reading

1. Deer, et al. The appropriate use of neurostimulation: avoidance and treatment of complications of neurostimulation therapies for the treatment of chronic pain. Neuromodulation. 2014;17:571–98.

Part XII

Selected Chronic Pain Disease XII

Complex Regional Pain Syndrome (CRPS): Type I and Type II

72

Reda Tolba

Key Concepts

- Complex regional pain syndrome (CRPS) is a disorder characterized by pain as well as myriad of sensory, motor, and autonomic dysfunction.
- Diagnosis of CRPS is mostly clinical, based on the findings in history and physical examination.
- Interdisciplinary approach is required for treatment of CRPS with the primary goal of functional restoration of the affected extremity.

Introduction and Terminology

Complex regional pain syndrome (CRPS) is a disorder characterized by pain as well as myriad of sensory, motor, and autonomic dysfunction. CRPS usually follows a noxious event such as trauma or surgery. CRPS can be subdivided into two categories, CRPS I and CRP II. *CRPS I*, formerly known as reflex sympathetic dystrophy (RSD), does not involve definable major nerve injury. The symptoms are not limited to a territory of a single peripheral nerve. On the other hand, *CRPS II*, formerly known as causalgia, involves definable major nerve injury. CRPS is characterized by spontaneous pain, which is associated with *sensory changes* such as allodynia and hyperalgesia. Allodynia is defined as pain perception to a stimulus that is not noxious. Hyperalgesia is defined as exaggerated pain response to a painful stimulus. *Autonomic changes* can happen such as color changes, increase or decrease sweating, temperature changes (cold or hot), and edema of the affected extremities. The affected extremity usually has trophic and dystrophic changes of the skin (thin or thickened), nails (thickened), and hair (increased or decreased hair growth). Motor changes such as weakness, dystonia, and tremors can eventually happen. Patients can eventually suffer from significant depression and anxiety.

R. Tolba, MD (✉)
200 west Esplanade Avenue, Kenner, LA 70005, USA
e-mail: redatolba@hotmail.com

Diagnosis

The diagnosis of CRPS is clinical, based on the findings in history and physical examination. According to the Budapest Diagnostic Criteria for CRPS, to make a clinical diagnosis of CRPS, the following criteria must be met:

1. Continuing pain, which is disproportionate to any inciting event.
2. Must report at least one symptom in *three of the four* following categories:
   - *Sensory*: reports of hyperesthesia and/or allodynia
   - *Vasomotor*: temperature asymmetry and/or skin color changes and/or asymmetry
   - *Sudomotor/Edema*: edema and/or sweating changes and/or sweating asymmetry
   - *Motor/Trophic*: decrease range of motion and/or motor dysfunction (weakness, tremors, dystonia) and/or trophic changes (hair, nail, skin)
3. Must display at least one sign at time of evaluation *in two or more* of the following categories:
   - *Sensory*: evidence of hyperalgesia or allodynia
   - *Vasomotor*: evidence of temperature asymmetry and/or skin color changes and/or asymmetry
   - *Sudomotor/Edema*: evidence of edema and/or sweating changes and/or asymmetry
   - *Motor/trophic*: evidence of decrease range of motion and/or motor dysfunction (weakness, tremor, dystonia) and/or trophic changes (hair, nail, skin)
4. There is no other diagnosis that better explains the signs and symptoms.

Radiological studies, such as bone scan and MRI, are important to rule out underlying orthopedic anomalies that

J.E. Pope, T.R. Deer (eds.), *Treatment of Chronic Pain Conditions*, DOI 10.1007/978-1-4939-6976-0_72

may explain symptomatology and, if present, would exclude the diagnosis of CRPS. There are no laboratory tests used to confirm the diagnosis of CRPS. CRPS is primarily a clinical diagnosis; however, functional imaging, visual analog scales, and devices to quantify temperature and mechanical allodynia are available to corroborate physical exam findings.

Treatment

The goal of the treatment is to functionally restore the affected extremity and prevents motor weakness. Aggressive physical therapy is the mainstay of treatment. However, to achieve the goal, pain control is essential to be able to effectively participate in physical therapy. An interdisciplinary approach is used. That involves the following:

Physical and occupational therapy: including desensitization, isometric and isotonic strengthening, and postural normalization.

Pharmacological treatment: including membrane-stabilizing medications such as gabapentin, pregabalin; tricyclic antidepressants such as amitriptyline and nortriptyline; and selective norepinephrine-serotonin reuptake inhibitors (SNRIs) such as duloxetine – all used for the treatment of neuropathic component of the pain. Opioid medications can also be used in conjunction. NSAIDs and steroids can be used if there is an inflammatory component. N-methyl-D-aspartate (NMDA) receptors antagonists such as ketamine infusion can also be considered. If the pain is believed to be sympathetically mediated, alpha receptor blockers such as terazosin (Hytrin) can be considered.

Interventional therapies: interventional pain procedures can be considered in refractory cases to help with progression of physical therapy. Sympathetic blocks such as lumbar sympathetic blocks for lower extremities and stellate ganglion block for upper extremities can be considered if pain is suspected to be sympathetically mediated. Upper and lower extremity blocks and local anesthetic catheter continuous infusion can be considered as well (such as supraclavicular and axillary for upper extremities, sciatic for lower extremities). Tunneled epidural catheter with local anesthetic/opioid infusion has been described. In chronic refractory CRPS, spinal cord stimulation can be considered.

Psychological therapy: patients with chronic CRPS could suffer from depression and anxiety. Individual psychotherapy, cognitive behavioral therapy, and medications such as anxiolytics and antidepressants should be considered.

Suggested Reading

1. Benzon H, Raja SN, Fishman SM, Liu S, Cohen SP. Essentials of pain medicine. 3rd ed. 2011. Paperback ISBN: 9781437722420; eBook ISBN: 9781437735932.
2. Freedman M, Greis AC, Marino L. Complex regional pain syndrome. Phys Med Rehabil Clin N Am. 2014;25:291–303. http://dx.doi.org/10.1016/j.pmr.2014.01.003
3. Goldsmith DP, Vivino FB, Eichenfield AH, et al. Nuclear imaging and clinical features of childhood reflex neurovascular dystrophy: comparison with adults. Arthritis Rheum. 1989;32:480–5. http://dx.doi.org/10.1002/anr.1780320419
4. Laxer RM, Allen RC, Malleson PN, et al. Technetium 99m-methylene diphosphonate bone scans in children with reflex neurovascular dystrophy. J Pediatr. 1985;106:437–40. http://dx.doi.org/10.1016/S0022-3476
5. Scott M, Ballantyne JC, Rathmell JP. Bonica's management of pain. 4th ed. Fishman, Bonica's pain management; LWW; 2009. Language: English; ISBN-10: 0781768276; ISBN-13: 978-0781768276.
6. Sherry DD, Wallace CA, Kelley C, et al. Short- and long-term outcomes of children with complex regional pain syndrome type I treated with exercise therapy. Clin J Pain. 1999;15:218–23. http://dx.doi.org/10.1097/00002508-199909000-00009
7. Stanton RP, Malcolm JR, Wesdock KA, et al. Reflex sympathetic dystrophy in children: an orthopedic perspective. Orthopedics. 1993;16:773–9.

Failed Surgery Syndrome

73

Mehul J. Desai

Key Concepts

- Failed surgery syndrome likely represents a spectrum disorder rather than a truly distinct clinical entity.
- A thorough timely work-up to elucidate the etiology of continued pain following spine surgery may provide an opportunity for successful intervention.

Introduction

Failed back surgery syndrome represents a constellation of symptoms encapsulating a failure of expected outcomes following spine surgery. This may affect spinal segments ranging from the cervical through lumbar regions. A wide range of incidence rates is reported in the literature. The diagnostic category remains challenging to treat due to its heterogeneity.

Background

In order to truly address persistent issues following spine surgery, one must take a moment to appreciate the nomenclature surrounding this disease state. Often labeled as failed back or neck surgery syndrome or post-laminectomy syndrome, these terms are anachronisms as they do not adequately describe the disease state in an era when most cervical spine surgery is performed from an anterior approach without laminectomy. Further, the preponderance of emerging lumbar techniques including anterior interbody fusion and extreme lateral approaches that do not include laminectomy renders PLS a relic from a bygone era. FBSS denotes blame of a technical nature when in fact a myriad of reasons may result in unanticipated or adverse outcomes following surgery. Predominant among these baseline factors is the behavioral and psychological state of the patient. For these reasons, we would suggest that the current terminology is inadequate, and a redefinition of this disease state should undergone consideration.

The comprehensive evaluation of FBSS, in an effort to truly identify the etiology of persistent or recurrent pain, requires a comprehensive interdisciplinary history and examination consisting of medical, behavioral, functional, and radiographic components. It is vital to identify acute surgical factors that may remit upon correction (i.e., misplaced pedicle screw). Particular care must be focused on assessing psychosocial comorbidities including depression, anxiety, sleep disorders, and personality disorders. It may be useful to categorize FBSS into more manageable categories (Table 73.1). These categories may be further subdivided into likely etiological factors (Tables 73.2, 73.3, 73.4 and 73.5).

A thorough radiographic assessment may include magnetic resonance imaging (MRI) with gadolinium enhancement, computed tomography (CT) with digital reconstruction, and dynamic standing radiographs in anterior-posterior, lateral, flexion, and extension. These modalities are useful in identifying pathologies including recurrent disc herniation, pseudarthrosis, recurrent or new spondylolisthesis, hematoma, and infection.

In fact one may ascertain that a systematic attempt to identify a root cause (when possible) may be the single most important aspect of achieving successful future treatment.

Treatment

Despite the myriad of reports detailing various treatments for FBSS, very little robust data exist regarding successful treatment in randomized trials. Certainly the very nature of the disorder precludes elements of study design. A recent

M.J. Desai, MD, MPH (✉)
MAPS Minnesota Advanced Pain Specialists,
9550 Upland Lane North, Maple Grove, MN 55369, USA
e-mail: mehuljdesaimd@gmail.com

J.E. Pope, T.R. Deer (eds.), *Treatment of Chronic Pain Conditions*, DOI 10.1007/978-1-4939-6976-0_73

Table 73.1 PSSS categorization

Time course	Early	Late	
Etiology	Nociceptive	Neuropathic	
Impairment	Pain	Function	Behavioral
Region	Axial	Extremity	

Table 73.2 Early (<6 months) versus late complications

Early	Late
Hardware malpositioning	Psychosocial
Hematoma	Degenerative spondylolisthesis
Recurrent herniation	Zygapophyseal disease
Spondylolisthesis	Sacroiliac dysfunction
Infection	Pseudarthrosis
Nerve root traction	Adjacent level degeneration
Abscess	Neuropathic back pain
Adjustment disorder	Radiculopathy
	Epidural adhesion/scar
	Arachnoiditis
	Discogenic pain

Table 73.3 Nociceptive and neuropathic etiologies

Nociceptive	Neuropathic
Hardware	Nerve root traction
Abscess	Recurrent disc herniation
Hematoma	Radiculopathy
Recurrent disc herniation	Arachnoiditis
Infection	Epidural scar/adhesions
Spondylolisthesis	Neuropathic low back pain
Zygapophyseal	Discogenic pain
Pseudarthrosis	Recurrent disc herniation
Sacroiliac joint dysfunction	Spondylolisthesis
Discogenic pain	
Adjacent level degeneration	
Epidural scar/adhesions	

review of the literature surrounding pharmacological, behavioral, and therapeutic treatments noted support for cognitive-behavioral therapy, intensive residential therapy, and some forms of structured rehabilitation.[2] Interestingly there were no significant trials in support of opioids or any other monotherapy, be it tricyclic antidepressants, muscle relaxants, or antiepileptics. As a result, the pharmaceutical approach to these patients often takes an empiric approach with multimodal options including the above categories of medications used in concert.

Table 73.4 Psychosocial issues

Psychosocial
Somatization
Anxiety
Family support issues
Depression
Personality disorder
Medication related
Hypochondriasis
Poor coping
Litigation
Adjustment disorder

Table 73.5 Functional impairment

Function
Gait abnormality
Impairment in activities of daily living
Use of assistive device
Neurogenic edema

From an interventional standpoint, there is more compelling evidence particularly with regard to the use of neuromodulatory techniques such as spinal cord stimulation. Here, it is once again important to note that accurate identification of etiological factors is more likely to portend success. Specifically, understanding the biomechanics of the operated spine allows for more successful isolation of causative factors such as cervical zygapophyseal dysfunction in axial neck pain or sacroiliac dysfunction in patients with prior lumbar fusion suffering with persistent low back or buttock pain. Grasping these nuances allows the pain practitioner to utilize appropriate therapies such as radiofrequency ablation in these patients.

Suggested Reading

1. Chan CW, Peng P. Failed back surgery syndrome. Pain Med. 2001;12(4):577–606.
2. Desai MJ, Nava A, Rigoard P, Shah B, Taylor RS. Optimal medical, rehabilitation and behavioral management in the setting of failed back surgery syndrome. Neurochirurgie. 2015;61(Suppl 1): S66–76.
3. Kumar K, Taylor RS, Jacques L, et al. Spinal cord stimulation versus conventional medical management for neuropathic pain: a multicentre randomised controlled trial in patients with failed back surgery syndrome. Pain. 2007;132(1-2):179–88.
4. North RB, Kidd DH, Farrokhi F, Piantadosi SA. Spinal cord stimulation versus repeated lumbosacral spine surgery for chronic pain: a randomized, controlled trial. Neurosurgery. 2005;56(1):98–106.

Radiculopathy

74

Reda Tolba

Key Concepts

- Radicular pain and radiculopathy are characterized by pain, usually electric or shooting in nature that radiates to one or more dermatomes whether it is cervical, thoracic, lumbar, or sacral.
- Diagnosis of radiculopathy and radicular pain is mostly clinical, based on the findings in history and physical examination. Imaging studies might be needed to confirm the diagnosis.
- Treatment of radiculopathy and radicular pain includes conservative treatment such as physical therapy, neuro-modulating medications, NSAIDs, and opioids. Interventional treatment such as epidural steroid injections can be helpful in resistant cases. Surgery might be indicated in case of presence of any neurological deficits.

Introduction and Terminology

Radicular pain and radiculopathy are characterized by pain, usually electric or shooting in nature that radiates to one or more dermatomes whether it is cervical, thoracic, lumbar, or sacral (see Fig. 74.1). Radicular pain and radiculopathy are two interchangeable terms, but not synonyms. While radicular pain is usually characterized by pain across a certain dermatomal distribution, radiculopathy includes neurological manifestations such as sensory and/or motor changes. It can be caused by variety of conditions that lead to nerve root irritation and inflammation. Most common causes include disc herniation causing chemical irritation of the nerve roots and degenerative changes in the spine causing neural foraminal stenosis such as lumbar spondylosis, spondylolisthesis that can cause mechanical compression of the nerve roots.

R. Tolba, MD (✉)
200 west Esplanade Avenue, Kenner, LA 70005, USA
e-mail: redatolba@hotmail.com

Diagnosis

Diagnosis of radiculopathy is mostly clinical based on findings in history and physical examination. Imaging studies such as X-ray, MRI, and CT scan can be helpful to confirm the diagnosis and correlate the symptoms to the underlying pathology.

History

Patient usually complains of radiating electric and shooting pain across a certain dermatomal distribution. Other descriptions such as dull, burning, throbbing, or piercing have been described. The pain can be accompanied by paresthesia across the affected dermatomes. However, there are variations among the distribution of pain across the affected area, and sometimes the pain does not follow a specific dermatomal distribution. The patient is asked about duration of symptoms, pain location, intensity and character, aggravating and relieving factors, and previous treatments. Red flags should be ruled out such as motor deficits, loss of sensations, urine or bowel incontinence and unintentional weight loss, fever or evidence of infection, history of cancer, and drug use. In the presence of red flags, immediate imaging and possible urgent decompressive surgeries might be needed.

Physical Examination

A focused neurological and muscular skeletal examination should be performed. Specific test such as straight leg test can be helpful to diagnose lumbosacral radiculopathy. The patient is asked to raise his leg straight. If the pain is elicited below 60°C, there is a large possibility there is a lumbar disc herniation. Spurling test can be used to help diagnosis of cervical radiculopathy. In the test, the neck is extended with the head rotated to affected shoulder while axially loaded.

J.E. Pope, T.R. Deer (eds.), *Treatment of Chronic Pain Conditions*, DOI 10.1007/978-1-4939-6976-0_74

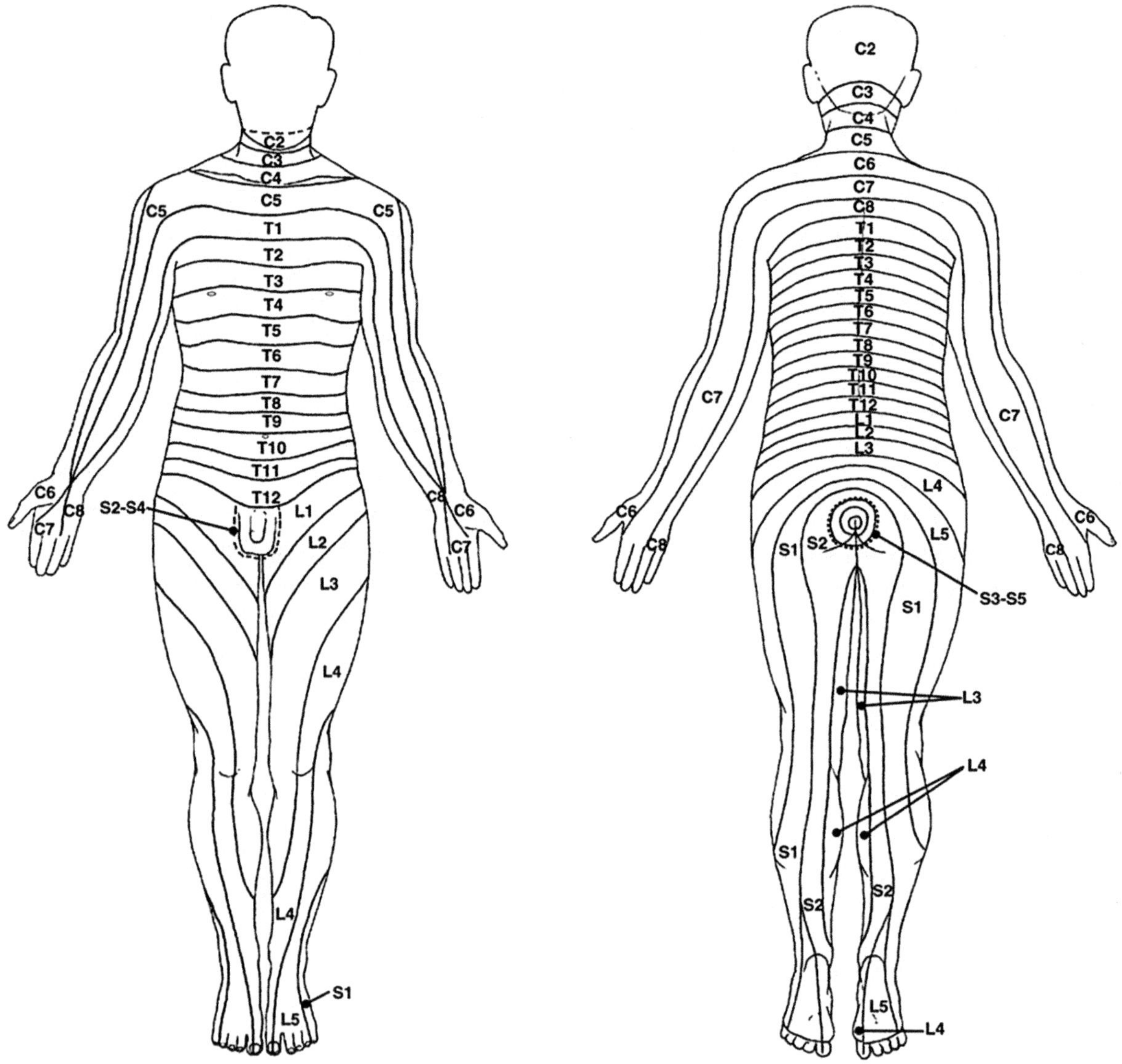

Fig. 74.1 Dermatome chart (With permission © Springer)

Clinicians should correlate the patient's symptoms with physical examination. Motor weakness or decrease/loss of sensations in the affected nerve root can be observed. For instance, drop foot suggests L5 nerve root paresis (weakness in dorsiflexion of the ankle). Absent patellar reflex suggests affection of L4 nerve root. Another example is absent biceps reflex, which is suggestive of C6 nerve root affection.

Imaging Studies

X-ray can be used as an initial low-cost test. MRI is the preferred method for visualization of soft tissue structures. However, correlation with the history and physical examination is essential to reach a clinic diagnosis and establish an adequate treatment plan. While MRI and CT can be helpful in confirming the diagnosis, it is important to know that sometimes the pathology found in the imaging studies could be asymptomatic. Clinicians should be aware of that, and correlation with the symptoms and signs should be done to avoid unnecessary procedures.

Treatment

Conservative Treatment

Conservative care includes physical and aquatic therapy as well as medications. Medications include over-the-counter medications such as NSAIDs and Tylenol. Neuromodulating medications such as gabapentin and pregabalin can help neuropathic pain. Other medications such as tricyclic antidepressants

(TCAs) (e.g., amitriptyline, nortriptyline) and serotonin-norepinephrine reuptake inhibitors (SNRIs) (e.g., duloxetine) could be helpful for chronic radiculopathy. Opioids can be used as a temporary tool for acute radicular pain, but long-term use is not advised. Medrol dosepak can be used to relief severe acute radicular symptoms especially if there is an inflammatory component to the pain.

Interventional Treatment

Epidural steroid injections using transforaminal, interlaminar, or caudal approaches can be useful to treat acute and chronic radicular pain. Pain relief achieved by those interventions could help the patients to progress into a physical therapy program and potentially improve functional level. Imaging studies should be reviewed, and correlation with symptoms and signs should be done before planning any intervention.

Surgery

Surgery is indicated in the presence of any neurological loss of function or in the presence of any red flags suggesting cauda equina syndrome, or evidence of progressive myelopathy symptoms. Surgery could also be considered in case of persistence of symptoms despite conservative and interventional treatment.

Spinal Cord Stimulation

Neuromodulation of targeted neural structures such as dorsal column, dorsal root ganglion, and peripheral nerves can be considered in refractory pain despite conservative treatment. Dorsal column stimulation has been used for years for treatment of post-laminectomy syndrome refractory to conservative treatment. It could be an option for patients with chronic radicular symptoms who are not candidates for surgery, or patient who have persistent symptoms despite having surgery.

Suggested Reading

1. Benzon H, Raja SN, Fishman SM, Liu S, Cohen S. Essentials of pain medicine. 3rd ed.
2. Fishman SM, Ballantyne JC, Rathmell JP. Bonica's management of pain. 4th ed.
3. Van Boxem K, Cheng J, Patjin J, et al. Lumbosacral radicular pain: evidence-based medicine: evidence-based interventional pain medicine according to clinical diagnoses. © 2010 World Institute of Pain, 1530–7085/10/$15.00 Pain Practice. 2010;10(4):339–358.
4. Van Zundert J, Huntoon M, Patjin J, et al. Cervical radicular pain: evidence-based medicine: evidence-based interventional pain medicine according to clinical diagnoses. © 2009 World Institute of Pain, 1530–7085/10/$15.00 Pain Practice. 2010;10(1):1–17.

Facet Arthropathy

75

Eduardo Jusino and Maged Guirguis

Key Concepts

- The most commonly affected facet joints are L3-4, L4-5, and L5-S1 for the lumbar region and C2-3, C4-5, and C5-6 for cervical region.
- Radiographic studies are neither sensitive nor specific for diagnosis of facet syndrome. The most reliable diagnostic method is with image-guided medial branch block (MBB) or intraarticular facet joint blocks.
- Treatment options include corticosteroid injection into the joint or neuroablation of the corresponding medial branch nerves.

Introduction

The zygapophysial (facet) joint is a potential source of primary and referred pain in the head, neck, shoulder, mid back, low back, and legs. Facet joint interventions are the second most common pain procedures performed in the United States after epidural steroid injections. The function of the facet joint is to provide support, stability, and mobility to the vertebrae.

Etiology

Degeneration/arthritis, trauma, and repetitive strain are the most common associated factors. This concurs with the disease being more common in the elderly. The facet joints and intervertebral discs work together such that degeneration of one produces strain on the other and vice versa. The facet joints normally fit together smoothly without pressure. If pressure develops where the joint meets, the cartilage on the joint erodes. The body responds by developing bone spurs. These bone spurs enlarge the joints causing hypertrophy. The joint surfaces become arthritic with associated inflammation, swelling, and pain. The three most common types of joint arthritis are osteoarthritis, rheumatoid arthritis, and traumatic arthritis. Arthropathy occurs when arthritis affects the facet joints.

Cervical

The most common causes of cervical facet pain include acceleration-deceleration injuries and cervical compression trauma. The most affected cervical spine facet joint is the C2-3 joint followed by the C5-6 joint. Generalized posterior neck pain, suboccipital pain, and localized tenderness over the posterolateral aspect of the neck are the most common complaints. These joints may refer pain from the midthoracic spine to the cranium. Neurologic symptoms are not expected in patients with primary cervical facet pain. Nerve root or spinal cord injury is more likely if patients present with sensory complaints and/or muscle weakness.

Thoracic

Trauma and degenerative changes are the most common causes of thoracic facet pain. Most major pain is associated with disc lesions in the lower thoracic spine.

Lumbar

Degenerative lumbar disc, fracture, and ligamentous injury are the most common causes of lumbar facet arthropathy. The most affected lumbar spine facet joints are the L4-5 and L5-S1 joints (Fig. 75.1).

E. Jusino, MD
Cleveland Clinic Foundation, Cleveland, OH, USA

M. Guirguis, MD (✉)
Ochsner Health System, Pain Management, Department of Anesthesiology & Critical Care Medicine, New Orleans, LA, USA
e-mail: magedaziz@gmail.com

J.E. Pope, T.R. Deer (eds.), *Treatment of Chronic Pain Conditions*, DOI 10.1007/978-1-4939-6976-0_75

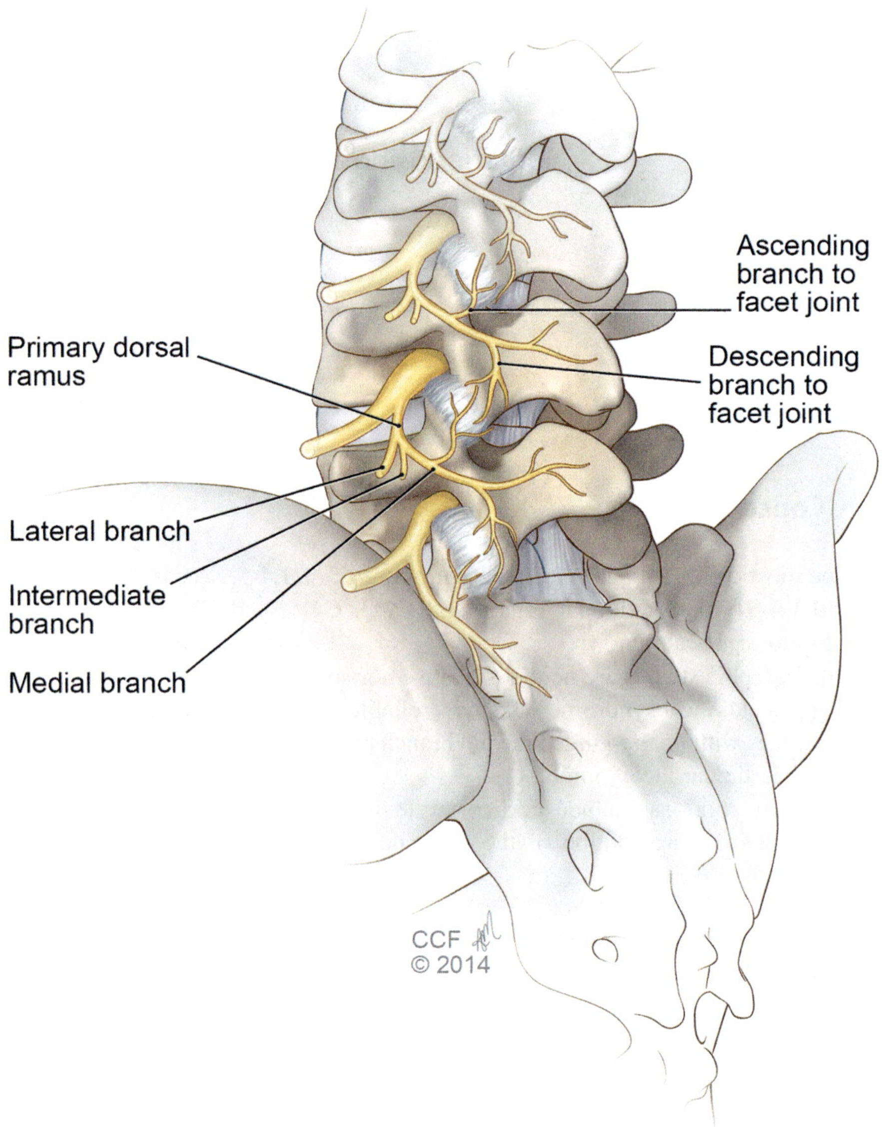

Fig. 75.1 Lumbar and pelvis posterolateral (Reprinted with permission, Cleveland, Clinic Center for Medical Art & Photography © 2014. All Rights Reserved)

Anatomy

The spine is composed of 7 cervical, 12 thoracic, and 5 lumbar vertebrae. Facet joints are true synovial joints formed from the superior articular process of one vertebra and the inferior articular process of the vertebra above. On the ventral aspect, the capsule is deficient, and the joint is in contact with the ligamentum flavum. These joints support, stabilize, and prevent injury to the spine by limiting range of motion in all planes. The dorsal ramus of the spinal nerve is divided into the medial, intermediate, and lateral branches. The medial branch provides sensory innervation to the facet joint, multifidus muscle, interspinal muscle, and periosteum of the neural arch. The intermediate branch innervates the longissimus muscle. The lateral branch innervates the paraspinous muscles, skin, and sacroiliac joint (lumbar spine). For all cervical, thoracic, and lumbar facet joints, there are two medial branches that innervate each facet joint: the medial branch at the same level and the level above. The two exceptions to this dual nerve supply are single nerve supply to the atlanto-occipital joint, atlanto-axial joint, and C2/3 facet joint, which are innervated by C1, C2, and C3 nerves, respectively.

Cervical

The cervical facets change significantly in position and shape in order to facilitate the complex motions of the neck; they are oriented in an oblique coronal plane, angled superior to inferior in a posterior direction. The first seven cranial nerves exit the intervertebral foramen above the vertebral body of the same number. The medial branch nerves at the cervical spine curve around the waist of the articular pillars and then branch out to supply two joints. The volume capacity of the cervical facet joints is 0.5–1.0 mL.

Thoracic

The thoracic facets are the most vertical and coronal in orientation, rotating toward the sagittal plane near the thoracolumbar junction. In the low thoracic spine, the angle transitions from a frontal orientation to the sagittal orientation of the lumbar facets. The transition generally occurs between T11 and L1. The anatomy of the thoracic spine facet joints and nerves varies significantly. The superolateral corner of the transverse process is the most accurate target point for diagnostic blockade and denervation of the thoracic facet joints.

Lumbar

The lumbar facet's inferior articular process faces anterolateral, and the superior articular process faces posteromedial. The volume capacity of the joints is 1–1.5 mL in the lumbar area.

Diagnosis

Facet arthropathy can be diagnosed with a detailed history, physical examination, radiographic studies, and diagnostic local anesthetic blocks. The symptoms of facet syndrome are nonspecific and overlap with other diagnosis. Physical examination findings include pain aggravated by palpation of the paraspinal muscles, standing, spinal extension, and facet joint loading with rotation. Sitting and flexing the spine usually ameliorate pain. Facet arthropathy and myofascial pain are usually associated with pain on extension, while disc pain is worsened with flexion. Radiographic or scintigraphic studies are neither sensitive nor specific for diagnosis of facet syndrome. The most reliable method to determine facet joint pain is with image-guided medial branch block (MBB) or intraarticular facet joint blocks (Figs. 75.2 and 75.3).

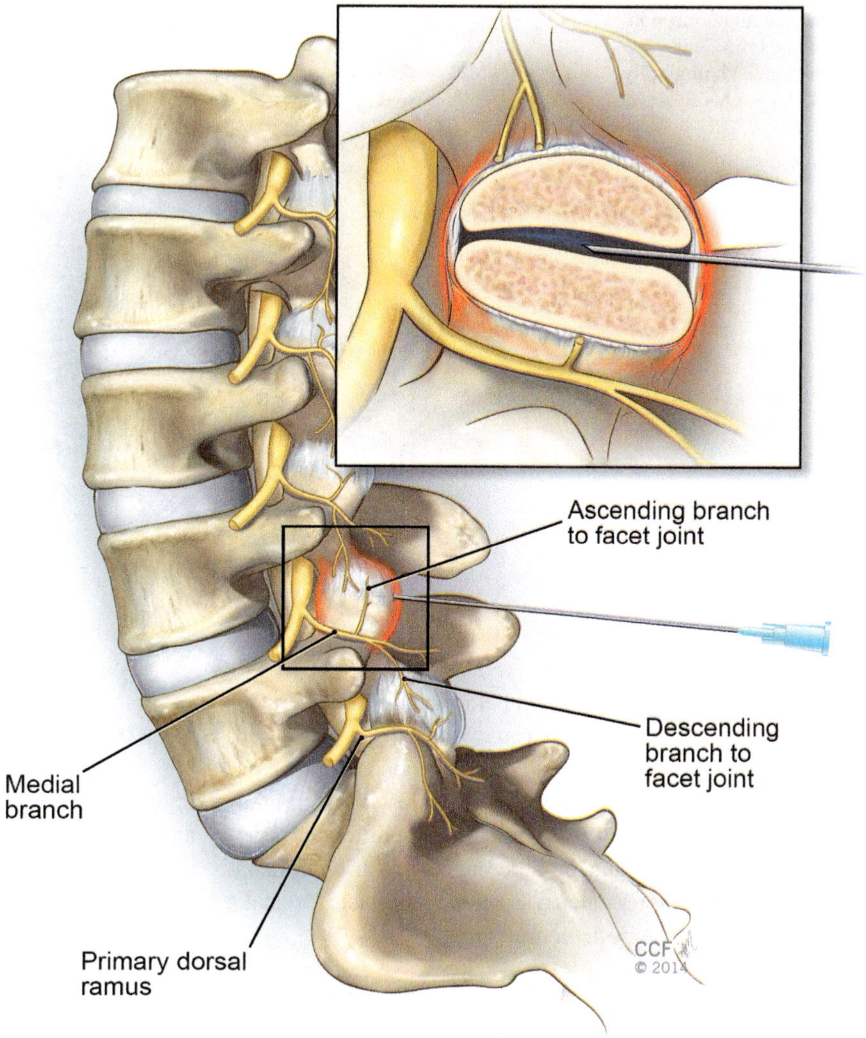

Fig. 75.2 Lumbar facet injection (Reprinted with permission, Cleveland Clinic Center for Medical Art & Photography © 2014. All Rights Reserved)

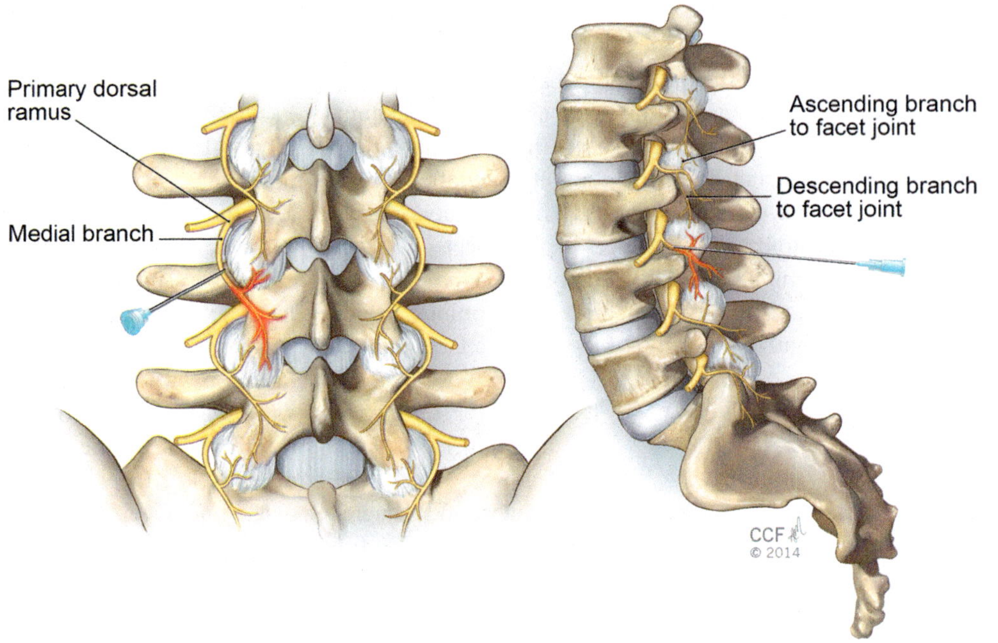

Fig. 75.3 Medial branch block (Reprinted with permission, Cleveland Clinic Center for Medical Art & Photography © 2014. All Rights Reserved)

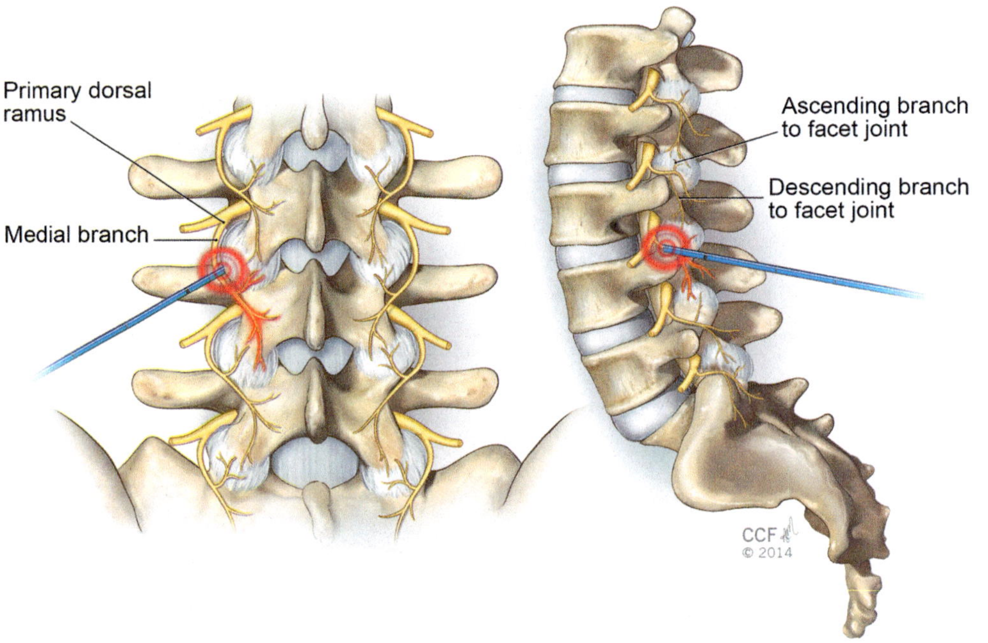

Fig. 75.4 Lumbar RFA (Reprinted with permission, Cleveland Clinic Center for Medical Art & Photography © 2014. All Rights Reserved)

Differential diagnosis of spinal pain includes degenerative disc disease, myofascial pain syndrome, internal disc disruption, disc herniation, spinal stenosis, nerve root compression, spondylolysis, spondylolisthesis, spondylosis, tumor, infection, and facet arthropathy. Other medical conditions producing undistinguishable pain include cancer, gastric/duodenal ulcer, pancreatitis, aortic aneurysm, nephrolithiasis, prostatitis/cystitis, and postherpetic neuralgia.

Treatment

Pharmacotherapy (NSAIDs, acetaminophen, antidepressants, and muscle relaxants) has been shown to have a small effect on spinal pain. Noninterventional modalities (physical activity, weight loss, exercise, yoga, acupuncture, and psychotherapy) were shown to be essential to optimize outcomes.

Intraarticular steroid injections are utilized for therapeutic purposes. Radiofrequency ablation of the medial branch is the most favorable and long-term treatment for facet joint pain (Fig. 75.4). Surgery is not recommended.

Conclusion

Facet pain is usually due to degeneration. The diagnosis requires detailed clinical assessment to rule out different sources of pain and to select the correct candidates for intervention. Intraarticular and medial branch blocks remain the "gold standard" for facet joint pain diagnosis.

Suggested Reading

1. Brummett CM, Cohen SP. Facet syndrome: facet joint injections, medial branch blocks, and radiofrequency denervation. In: Essentials of pain medicine. 3rd ed. Philadelphia: Saunders; 2011. p. 322–9.
2. Grabow TS, Block BM. Facet joint injection. In: Image-guided interventions. 2nd ed. Philadelphia: Saunders; 2014. p. 1234–40.
3. Greher M. Ultrasound-guided lumbar spine injections. In: Spinal injections and peripheral nerve blocks. Vol. 4. Philadelphia: Saunders; 2012. p. 200–9. A Volume in the Interventional and Neuromodulatory Techniques for pain management series.
4. King W, Borowczyk JM. Zygapophysial joint pain: procedures for diagnosis and treatment. In: Pain procedures in clinical practice. 3rd ed. Philadelphia: Elsevier; 2011. p. 357–89.
5. Pope JE. Complications of facet joint injections and medial branch blocks. In: Interventional and neuromodulatory techniques for pain management: reducing risks and complications of interventional pain procedures. 1st ed. Philadelphia: Elsevier; 2012a. p. 117–25.
6. Pope JE. Complications of radiofrequency rhizotomy for facet syndrome. In: Interventional and neuromodulatory techniques for pain management: reducing risks and complications of interventional pain procedures. 1st ed. Philadelphia: Elsevier; 2012b. p. 126–31.
7. Steiner AS, Gray DP. Facet syndrome. In: Principles & practice of pain medicine. 3rd ed. McGraw-Hill Education/Medical; 2004. Access Anesthesiology. Web. 10 Jul. 2014. ISBN-10: 0071766839; ISBN-13: 978- 0071766838.

Discogenic Pain

76

Sherief Zaky

Key Concepts

- Discogenic pain accounts for about 40% of all causes of persistent low back pain.
- The intervertebral disc consists of an outer fibrous ring called annulus fibrosis that surrounds a central gelatinous core known as nucleus pulposus.
- The intervertebral disc is supplied by two interconnected nerve plexuses: the anterior and the posterior nerve plexuses.
- Disc degeneration is associated with dehydration and desiccation of the nucleus causing morphological changes that can lead to annular tears.
- Pain associated with degenerative discs is caused by proliferation of the nerve endings deep into the inner layers of the annulus.
- Radiologic findings that are commonly associated with discogenic pain are high-intensity zone lesions and modic changes.

Introduction

Discogenic pain or pain originating from the intervertebral discs has been a debatable condition for many decades. In the 1940s, investigators found that pressing on the intervertebral discs in patients undergoing spine surgery under local anesthesia causes pain. The presence of nerve supply to the intervertebral discs was later demonstrated in 1980 and 1981.

Internal disc disruption is recognized to be the most common cause of axial pain and represents about 40% of chronic low back pain conditions. Chronic low back pain is ranked as the number one cause of disability in individuals between the ages of 45 and 65.

Anatomy of the Intervertebral Disc

The intervertebral disc consists of an outer fibrous layer called the annulus fibrosis, an inner gelatinous core known as nucleus pulposus, and vertebral end plates. The annulus is made up of type I collagen that is arranged in a series of 15–25 concentric layers or lamellae. The inner nucleus pulposus contains randomly organized collagen and radially organized elastin fibers. These fibers are embedded in a proteoglycan-containing gel called aggregan.

The vertebral end plate is composed of a thin layer of hyaline cartilage close to the vertebral body and fibrocartilage near the nucleus pulposus. The end plates completely envelop the nucleus pulposus centrally and taper off peripherally where they attach to the vertebral bodies. The intervertebral discs are basically avascular with nutrition being supplied through vertebral end plates and annulus fibrosis via passive diffusion.

Innervation of the Intervertebral Discs

Intervertebral discs are innervated by two interconnected plexuses: the anterior and posterior nerve plexuses. The anterior plexus supplies the anterior part of the disc and is formed of branches of the two sympathetic plexuses, the proximal ends of the gray rami communicans and the perivascular nerve plexuses of the segmental arteries. The posterior plexus supplies the posterior part of the disc and is formed primarily by the sinuvertebral nerves. The two plexuses supply only the layer of the annulus fibrosis in normal discs.

S. Zaky, MD, MSC, PhD (✉)
Pain Management Service, Firelands Regional Medical Center, Case Western Reserve University, 703 Tyler St Ste 352, Sandusky, OH 44870, USA
e-mail: zakys1@gmail.com

J.E. Pope, T.R. Deer (eds.), *Treatment of Chronic Pain Conditions*, DOI 10.1007/978-1-4939-6976-0_76

Pathogenesis of Discogenic Pain

Disc Degeneration

Reduced blood flow to the end plates leads to diminished nutrition through the end plates to the matrix. This leads to fragmentation of the matrix proteoglycans followed by decrease in proteoglycan and water concentration. This process is typically asymptomatic and eventually leads to dehydration and desiccation of the nucleus. These changes in the disc morphology lead to weakening of the annulus predisposing it to tears.

The sensory nerve endings extend only to the outer third of the annulus fibrosis in normal human discs. In degenerated or herniated discs, the sensory innervation extends deeply and more extensively to the inner layers of the annulus fibrosis and even to the nucleus pulposus.

The intervertebral discs contain numerous inflammatory mediators such as calcitonin gene-related peptide (CGRP), substance P, vasoactive intestinal peptide (VIP), and phospholipase A2. As the annulus starts to break and tear, the nucleus material leaks outside and comes in contact with the nerve roots causing inflammation and pain.

Internal Disc Disruption Syndrome (IDDS)

IDDS has been described since the 1970s as a condition that is associated with severe back pain secondary to occult discogenic pathology. The morphology of the disrupted disc was described in later studies as degenerated nucleus pulposus with radial tears or fissures extending to the periphery of the annulus.

Pain in patients with IDDS is typically described as dull axial pain that is difficult to localize.

Radiologic Findings Associated with Discogenic Pain

Two features on MRI correlate strongly with the affected disc being painful upon disc stimulation:

High-Intensity Zone (HIZ) Lesions

HIZs are defined as spots of intensely high signal within the posterior annulus of a disc viewed in T2-weighted MR images. They represent the appearance, in sagittal images, of large radial or circumferential fissures.

Modic Changes

Type 1 changes appear hypointense of T1-weighted MR images and hyperintense on T2-weighted images. Type 1 changes represent inflammatory edema surrounding the disc.

Type 2 changes appear hyperintense on both T1-weighted and T2-weighted images. Type 2 changes represent fatty infiltration.

Type 3 changes appear hypointense on both T1-weighted and T2-weighted images. Type 3 changes represent sclerosis of the vertebral body.

Suggested Reading

1. Bogduk N, Aprill C, Derby R. Lumbar discogenic pain: state of the art review. Pain Med. 2013;14:813–36.
2. Cohen SP, Larkin TM. Lumbar discography. In: Raj's practical management of pain. 4th ed. Elsevier Press. Philadelphia; 2008.
3. Walker III J, El Abd O, Isaac Z, Muzin S. Discography in practice: a clinical and historical review. Curr Rev Musculoskelet Med. 2008;1:69–83.

Sacroiliitis and Sacroiliac Joint Dysfunction

77

George C. Chang Chien, Radhika P. Grandhe, and Joseph D. Fortin

Key Concepts

- The sacroiliac joint (SIJ) joins the sacrum to the pelvis, transmitting the forces from the axial skeleton above to the lower extremities. SIJ dysfunction is a common cause of low back pain.
- History will reveal pain with maneuvers that stress the pelvic ring.
- Look for contributing factors such as a history of pelvic girdle trauma, repetitive asymmetric axial loading, pregnancy, or spondyloarthropathy (ankylosing spondylitis).
- No single physical exam maneuver is indicative of sacroiliac joint dysfunction, but a composite of exam maneuvers has been positively correlated to confirmatory diagnostic joint injection.
- The diagnostic gold standard remains image-guided intra-articular joint injection.
- There are myriad treatment options including corticosteroid injection and radiofrequency ablation.

Introduction

Sacroiliac joint (SIJ) arthropathy is a common cause of acute and chronic low back pain. It is estimated to be the cause of up to 30% of low back pain. In a recent multicentric study, Cher and colleagues found that the overall health burden endured by chronic SIJ pain sufferers was greater than cohorts with COPD, coronary artery disease, and asthma.

The SIJ is a mechanical relay station – transmitting loads to and fro the trunk and lower extremities while simultaneously providing logic functions as position sense and loading behavior. As such, it provides a unique role in human locomotion and serves as the driving impulse of truncal counterrotation.

SIJ pathology is commonly associated with other conditions including trauma to the pelvis, ankylosing spondylitis, psoriatic arthritis, Reiter's syndrome, inflammatory bowel disease, and pregnancy.

Anatomy

The sacroiliac joints are a pair of diarthrodial L-shaped joints that join the sacrum to the ilium bones. The articular surface of the ilium is made up of fibrocartilage, while the sacral surface is made up of much thicker hyaline cartilage. There are interosseous sacroiliac ligaments that maintain tight adherence between the sacrum and ilium. In addition to the primary SI ligaments, the sacrotuberous and sacrospinous ligaments further stabilize the sacrum to the pelvic girdle. These ligaments have also been implicated as potential pain generators. The orientation of the SIJs within the pelvis renders them particularly vulnerable to axial loading to failure. In fact, Miller found the SIJ to be 20 times more susceptible to axial overloading than the lumbar motion segments. Commensurate with Miller's report, Fortin and Roberts observed a high incidence of SIJ pain in competitive figure skaters – who repetitively land their jumps on the same lower extremity. Normal motion within the paired joints includes a small amount of movement (2–18°) in the transverse plane called nutation (forward rotation of the sacrum between the ilium) and counternutation (backward rotation of the sacrum between the ilium). In addition to the

G.C. Chang Chien, DO (✉)
Cleveland Clinic, Anesthesia Institute Pain Management, 9500 Euclid Ave, Dept C-25, Cleveland, OH 44195, USA
e-mail: gchangchien@gmail.com

R.P. Grandhe, MBBS, MD
Cleveland Clinic, Department of Pain Management, Cleveland, OH, USA

J.D. Fortin, DO
Spine Technology and Rehabilitation, Indiana School of Medicine, Fort Wayne, IN, USA

J.E. Pope, T.R. Deer (eds.), *Treatment of Chronic Pain Conditions*, DOI 10.1007/978-1-4939-6976-0_77

amount of nutation/counternutation, the existence of an oblique axis (implicated in normal reciprocal gait mechanics) has been the subject of debate.

Innervation

The common pathways of innervation revealed by recent investigations include the lateral branches of the sacral dorsal rami, the medial branch of the L5 dorsal rami, and variable innervation from the superior gluteal nerve (see Fig. 49.1). Several investigators have also reported on the branches from the lumbosacral plexus and obturator nerve. Innervation of ventral rami origin has been questioned by the absence of ventral receptors in fetal SIJ capsules. This complex innervation pattern has implications for the treatment of SIJ arthropathy.

Physical Examination

Patients with symptomatic sacroiliac joints often present to their physicians pointing at the SIJ (immediately medial and inferior to the PSIS) as the source of their pain (i.e., a positive Fortin finger test or FFT). Upon experimental stimulation of the SIJ capsules of asymptomatic volunteers, Fortin and coworkers observed that all volunteers referred evoked symptoms below their PSIS with some extending toward the ipsilateral greater trochanter. These observations are congruent with the aforementioned cadaveric reports demonstrating dense innervation in the same area below the PSIS. While primary buttock pain is the most common presentation, it is not unusual for patients with symptomatic SIJs to report symptoms radiating as far distal as the foot. Accordingly, Fortin and colleagues employed arthrography, post arthrography CT, and capsular immunohistochemical techniques to link the SIJ to sciatica.

There are a number of physical examination provocative maneuvers for identifying symptomatic sacroiliac joints including Gillet's test, Patrick's maneuver (FABER), Gaenslen's test, anterior-posterior compression, thigh thrust, and sacral compression (Table 77.1). While no single exam maneuver is diagnostic for SIJ pathology, Laslett and others have demonstrated that combining multiple stress tests greatly enhances the diagnostic yield. As the pelvic girdle is a ring (consider Pascal's principle), examine patients with putative SIJ pain for tenderness of the surrounding ligaments, as well as the pubic symphysis.

Diagnostic Modalities

Plain films (X-rays) are a common screening method for suspected sacroiliac joint pathology but are often nondiagnostic for early stages of degenerative or inflammatory pathology. They do play an important role in the setting of trauma, when evaluating a patient for gross fracture, dislocation, or dynamic instability. CT can show evidence of degenerative, erosive, or destructive joint changes earlier than radiographs. While MRI is more sensitive than CT or scintigraphy for evaluating the evolution of marrow space pathology (associated with stress fracture or inflammatory sacroiliitis), CT outperforms MRI when assessing osseous

Table 77.1 Provocative physical exam maneuvers

Exam maneuver	Description	Patient position	Action	Findings
Distraction or anterior-posterior compression	This test applies anterior-posterior shear stress on the bilateral sacroiliac joints	Supine, legs in neutral position	Apply gradual, sustained downward pressure on the bilateral anterior-superior iliac spine	Reproduction of pain localized to the sacral sulcus or sacroiliac joint
Thigh thrust	This test applies anterior-posterior shear stress on unilateral the sacroiliac joint	Supine, hip flexed to 90° with the knee relaxed	Apply gradual, sustained, vertically directed force through the femur	Reproduction of pain localized to the sacral sulcus or sacroiliac joint
Sacral thrust	This test applies forces to the bilateral sacroiliac joint	Prone, legs in neutral position	Apply gradual, sustained downward pressure on the superior sacrum	Reproduction of pain localized to the sacral sulcus or sacroiliac joint
Patrick's maneuver (FABER)	This test applies tensile forces to the anterior sacroiliac joint ligaments	Supine, the hip flexed, abducted, and externally rotated and the foot resting on the opposite knee	The examiner then applies gradual, sustained downward pressure on the flexed knee	Reproduction of pain localized to the sacral sulcus or sacroiliac joint, *not* the anterior groin which would suggest femoral-acetabular dysfunction
Fortin finger test	The patient is asked to point to the area of maximum pain	Standing	The patient points with one finger	Patient points immediately posteromedial to PSIS

contour abnormalities. Structural findings on imaging studies are not prima facie evidence of pain. In fact, degenerative changes in asymptomatic SIJs are common, after the age of 30.

While image-guided anesthetic blockade of a putatively painful joint is the standard for diagnosis (as no single physical exam maneuver is indicative of sacroiliac joint dysfunction), the intervention should be considered an extension of a careful history and physical examination.

Treatment Options

Conservative treatment should include cold application, anti-inflammatory medication or anti-inflammatory nutritional supplements, and relative rest (in the acute stage). Once pain has subsided, further efforts should be employed to restore normal mechanics, including manual medicine techniques, pelvic stabilization exercises to allow dynamic postural control, and muscle balancing of the trunk and lower extremities. SIJ belts or pelvic stabilization orthoses will provide confidence and proprioceptive awareness for sacroiliac joint dysfunction sufferers. A properly positioned cinch-type pelvic stabilization orthotic (worn directly superior to the greater trochanters) can significantly limit sacroiliac motion and thereby decrease pain.

If conservative treatment fails, SIJ intra-articular injections should be considered, not only as a therapeutic intervention but also to confirm the diagnosis (see Fig. 49.2). Mitigation of symptoms by analgesic block is the most reliable and reproducible means by which a painful SIJ can be identified.

Once the diagnosis is confirmed by profound relief of symptoms (lasting at least as long as the duration of the local anesthesia) following a diagnostic block, long-standing relief can often be obtained by radiofrequency ablation treatment of the sacral lateral branches and dorsal ramus of the L5 nerve (Fig. 77.1).

Dorman and coworkers observed in vitro that injecting chemical irritants into ligamentous tissue incites collagen proliferation. Theoretically, scarring and tightening of the ligaments results in stabilization of the joint. Hence, proliferant therapies may have a role in addressing an unstable SIJ.

Autologous mesenchymal stem cells (which morph in to the bone, cartilage, and connective tissue) combined with platelet-derived growth factors have also been the subject of considerable research focus for joint conditions, including the SIJ. These biologic media are generally administered by image-controlled injections. While more research and development of this technology is warranted, regenerative approaches to SIJ pathology hold great promise.

Arthrodesis of the sacroiliac joint for chronic, nontraumatic, painful dysfunction is controversial but may be considered if all nonsurgical treatments have failed. Moore found a 75% success rate employing an open, modified Smith-Pederson fusion technique with AO hardware. Since Moore's study there have been at least ten reports in the peer review literature suggesting that minimally invasive ("closed") fusion with instrumentation approaches is also effective for a subset of patients. Clinical judgment should be used if lumbar spine pathology coexists with sacroiliac joint dysfunction, as this information should factor in the treatment algorithm.

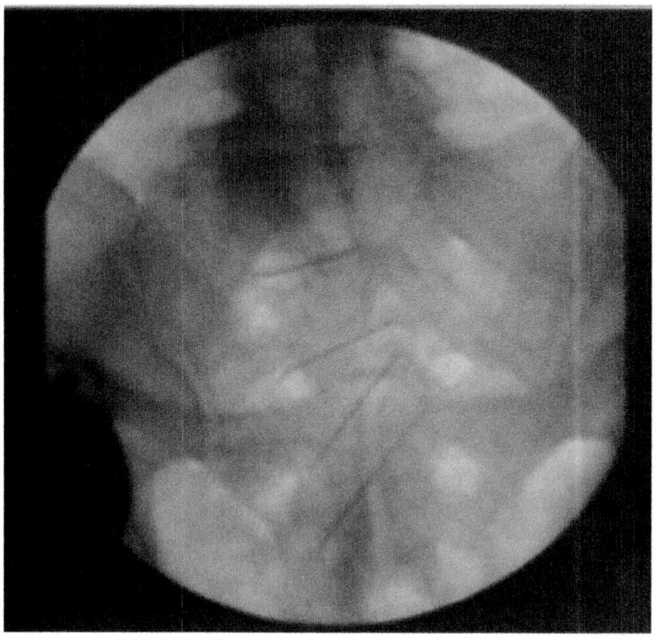

Fig. 77.1 AP plain film projection. Radiofrequency probes (with 10 mm tips) are oriented across the S1–S4 dorsal foramina (medial to lateral)

Summary

On balance, look for a history of trauma to the pelvic ring or repetitive asymmetric axial loading. Many patients with SIJ dysfunction present with primary buttock pain, as well as those who point directly at the joint as the source of their symptoms (i.e., positive FFT). Some patients will report symptoms suggestive of instability – the so-called "slipping clutch" syndrome. Palpatory examination reveals sacral sulcus, joint line, and surrounding ligamentous tenderness. Pubic symphysis tenderness further implicates pelvic girdle versus primary lumbar pathology. Several PE stress maneuvers also substantiate the diagnosis of SIJ dysfunction.

The history and physical findings should be confirmed by an image-guided direct intra-articular diagnostic block. Treatment options range from anti-inflammatory medications and physical therapy to radiofrequency ablation, stem cell therapy, and surgical fusion.

Suggested Reading

1. Cher D, Polly D, Berven S. Sacroiliac joint pain: burden of disease. Med Devices (Auckl). 2014;7:73–81.
2. Cox RC, Fortin JD. The anatomy of the lateral branches of the sacral dorsal rami: implications for radiofrequency ablation. Pain Physician. 2014;17:459–64.
3. Dorman T. Pelvic mechanics and prolotherapy. In: Vleeming A, Mooney V, Dorman T, Snijders C, Stoeckart R, editors. Movement, stability, and low back pain: the essential role of the pelvis. New York: Churchill Livingstone; 1997. p. 501–22.
4. Elgafy H, Semaan HB, Ebraheim NA, Coombs RJ. Computed tomography findings in patients with sacroiliac pain. Clin Orthop Relat Res. 2001;382:112–8.
5. Fortin JD. An algorithm for understanding spine imaging. Pain Physician. 2002;5(1):102–9.
6. Fortin JD, Falco FJE. The Fortin finger test: an indicator of sacroiliac joint pain. Am J Orthop. 1997;26(7):477–80.
7. Fortin JD, Roberts D. Competitive figure skating injuries. Pain Physician. 2003;6(3):313–8.
8. Fortin JD, Dwyer A, West S, Pier J. Sacroiliac joint pain referral patterns upon application of a new injection/arthrography technique – part I, asymptomatic volunteers. Spine. 1994;19(13):1475–82.
9. Fortin J, Falco F, Washington W. Three pathways between the sacroiliac joint and neural structures exist. Am J Neuroradiol. 1999;20(8):1429–34.
10. Fortin JD, Vilensky JA, Merkel GJ. Can the sacroiliac joint cause sciatica? Pain Physician. 2003;6(3):269–71.
11. Fortin JD, Wahezi SE, Mintz D, Chang A. Diagnostic imaging of painful sacroiliac joints. In: DePalma MJ, editor. iSpine evidence-based interventional spine care. New York: Demos Medical; 2013.
12. Laslett M, Young SB, Aprill CN, McDonald B. Diagnosing painful sacroiliac joints: a validity study of a McKenzie evaluation and sacroiliac provocation tests. Aust J Physiother. 2003;49:89–97.
13. Miller JAA, Schultz AM, Anderson GBJ. Load-displacement behavior or sacroiliac joints. J Orthrop Res. 1987;5:92–101.
14. Moore MR. Surgical treatment of chronic painful sacroiliac joint dysfunction. In: Vleeming A, Mooney V, Dorman T, Snijders C, Stoeckart R, editors. Movement, stability, and low back pain: the essential role of the pelvis. New York: Churchill Livingstone; 1997. p. 563–72.
15. Nakagawa T. A study on the distribution of nerve filaments of the iliosacral joint and its adjacent region in the Japanese. J Jap Orthop Assoc. 1966;40:419–30.

Piriformis Muscle Syndrome

78

Navdeep Singh Jassal

Key Concepts

- Pain caused by piriformis syndrome is located in the buttock with/without radiation to the ipsilateral leg.
- Physical examination signs can be used to help in confirmation, including Pace, Lasegue, and Freiberg Sign, and may occur in a setting of trauma.
- Perisciatic and piriformis muscle injections with steroid and local anesthetic may provide several months of pain relief and improved function. If transient, botulinum toxin may be used.

Introduction

The incidence rate of piriformis syndrome has typically ranged from 5% to 8% but has been cited as high as 36% among patient with low back pain. Although uncommon, piriformis syndrome is often misdiagnosed as a cause of buttock and leg pain.

Anatomy of the Piriformis Muscle

Origin

Anterior surface of the S2–S4 sacral vertebrae, the sacroiliac joint capsule, and the gluteal surface of the ilium.

N.S. Jassal, MD (✉)
Florida Pain Medicine, University of South Florida, Department of Neurology, James A. Haley VA Medical Center, Number 127, Tampa, FL 33612, USA
e-mail: navdeepjassal@gmail.com

Insertion

Runs through the greater sciatic foramen and inserts into the piriformis fossa at the medial aspect of the greater trochanter of the femur.

Innervation

Branches of the ventral rami of the L5, S1, and S2 spinal nerves.

Actions on the Femur

Lateral (external) rotator of the femur in the hip joint.

It is important to understand that there can be six possible anatomic relationships that can occur between the sciatic nerve and piriformis muscle. These anomalies can cause the patient's hip and buttock pain and sciatica.

1. Undivided sciatic nerve that passes above the piriformis muscle
2. Undivided sciatic nerve that passes below the piriformis muscle (most common)
3. Undivided sciatic nerve passing through the piriformis
4. A divided sciatic nerve passing through and above the muscle
5. A divided sciatic nerve passing through and below the muscle
6. A divided sciatic nerve passing above and below the muscle

Etiologies

Etiology can include trauma to the pelvis or buttock, hypertrophy/spasm of the piriformis muscle, female gender, pregnancy, and anatomic abnormalities that exist between piriformis muscle and sciatic nerve, as described above.

J.E. Pope, T.R. Deer (eds.), *Treatment of Chronic Pain Conditions*, DOI 10.1007/978-1-4939-6976-0_78

Also, greater than half an inch leg length discrepancies, cerebral palsy with hypertonicity, obesity, and lumbar hyperlordosis can also predispose factors of this syndrome. There is often a history of microtrauma to the piriformis muscle in up to 50% of the cases that can occur months prior to the start of symptoms. It can be seen after total hip replacement or laminectomy, in which scar tissue can impinge on nerve roots of the sciatic nerve.

Differential Diagnosis

May include causes of low back pain with sciatic including lumbar facet syndrome, sacroiliac joint dysfunction, trochanteric/ischial bursitis, endometriosis, pelvic neoplasm, or myofascial pain syndrome. Diagnosis is often achieved after exclusion of the above differential.

Signs and Symptoms

On history taking, patients typically complain of buttock pain (sacrum to the greater trochanter) with/without radiation down the ipsilateral leg or paralumbar pain. Patient's pain is generally aggravated by activities such as biking or driving, as it includes prolonged sitting posture. Aggravation can also occur from sitting to standing positions, bowel movements, and sitting hard surfaces. On physical examination there may be a pelvic tilt on inspection and tenderness in the buttock (greater sciatic foramen to the greater trochanter) upon palpation. Neurologic weakness is usually absent; however, there may be numbness of distal lower extremity from sciatic nerve compression from the piriformis muscle. There may be normal or limited straight leg raise.

There are also three notable signs that can be characteristic for piriformis syndrome, including Pace, Lasegue, and Freiberg sign.

- Pace sign: pace and weakness upon resisted abduction of the hip, while the hip is in flexed position (or seated).
- Lasegue sign: pain on voluntary flexion, adduction, and internal rotation (FAIR position) of the hip.
- Freiberg sign: pain on forced internal rotation of the extended thigh.

Diagnosis is made mainly clinically, although electromyography (myopathic or neuropathic changes including delayed H-reflex in FAIR position), computed tomography, magnetic resonance imaging (enlargement of piriformis muscle), and bone scan (increased radioactive uptake) may reveal abnormalities.

Treatment

The mainstay of treatment of piriformis syndrome includes physical therapy in combination with the use of anti-inflammatory drugs, analgesics, and muscle relaxants for reduction of inflammation, pain, and muscle spasms. Physical therapy modalities, such as moist heat (superficial heat) and/or ultrasound (deep heat), are often beneficial forms of treatment when used in conjunction with stretching and manual therapy. Stretching of the piriformis muscle involves flexion, adduction, and internal rotation of the hip adductors and the knee while the patient lies supine. This may be followed by the physical therapist performing a muscle energy technique. Abnormal biomechanics including poor posture, leg length discrepancies, and pelvic obliquities should be corrected.

If unresponsive to conservative treatment, patients often benefit from injections into the piriformis muscle with or without per sciatic nerve injections. This can be done with an injectate containing 40 mg of Depo-Medrol and 3–5 ml of local anesthetic (lidocaine or bupivacaine). Initially performed blindly, newer techniques are performed with fluoroscopic (X-ray), with or without EMG, or ultrasound needle guidance in order to confirm proper placement of the needle. The piriformis muscle lies deep to the buttock adipose tissue and gluteus maximus muscle.

Technique (Under Fluoroscopic Guidance)

- A 22-gauge 3.5″ or 5″ (depending on patient body habitus) Quincke needle is used to advance down and contact the very tip of the inferior sacroiliac joint. Make note of the approximate needle depth.
- The needle is then withdrawn and redirected to a final target site 1 cm inferior, 1 cm lateral, and 1 cm deeper than the SI joint.
- AP view should demonstrate contrast flow in a diagonal pattern from cephalad to caudad as it goes toward the femoral attachment site of the piriformis muscle.

Botulinum toxin may also be injected into the piriformis muscle if the response to steroid/anesthetic is transient. Botulinum toxin specifically cleaves SNARE protein, preventing neurosecretory vesicles from docking/fusing with the nerve synapse plasma membrane, preventing acetylcholine release, and causing prolonged relaxation (~3 months). BTX-A (Botox) or botulinum toxin type B (Myobloc) may be utilized.

Surgery may be considered in recalcitrant cases and includes the muscle excision, division, or thinning.

Suggested Reading

1. Barton PM. Piriformis syndrome a rational approach to management. Pain. 1991;47:345–52.
2. Beason LE, Anson BJ. The relation of the sciatic nerve and its subdivisions to the piriformis muscle. Anat Rec. 1937;70:1–5.
3. Benzon HT, et al. Essentials of pain medicine. Philadelphia: Elsevier Saunders; 2011.
4. Papadopoulos EC, Kahn SN. Piriformis syndrome and low back pain a new classification and review of the literature. Orthop Clin North Am. 2004;35:65–71.
5. Parziale JR, Hudgins TH, Fishman LM. The piriformis syndrome. Am J Orthop. 1996;25:819–23.

Migraine/Headache

79

Navdeep Singh Jassal

Key Concepts

- Headaches are divided into primary and secondary headaches, and classification is according to the International Headache Society's (IHS) classification (ICHD –II).
- Pharmacologic treatment of migraine can involve both acute and preventive interventions.

Classification

Headaches can be divided into two groups:

1. *Primary headaches* – including a group of remarkable disorders in which headache and associated features are seen in the absence of any exogenous cause
2. *Secondary headaches* – including group of disorders in which headache is secondary to an organic or physiologic process, either intracranially or extracranially

According to the ICHD–II, primary headache entities include:

1. Migraine (*emphasis will be made on migraine in this chapter)
   1.1 Migraine without Aura
   1.2 Migraine with Aura
   1.3 Childhood Periodic Syndromes
   1.4 Retinal Migraine
   1.5 Complications of Migraine (Including Chronic Migraine and Status Migrainosus)
   1.6 Probable Migraine
2. Tension-Type Headache (TTH)
3. Cluster Headache *and* Other Trigeminal Autonomic Cephalalgias
4. Other Primary Headaches

Secondary headache entities include headaches attributed to head and/or neck trauma (whiplash injury, traumatic intracranial hematoma, postcraniotomy), cranial or cervical vascular disorder (CVA, TIA, cerebral venous thrombosis), nonvascular intracranial disorder (intracranial neoplasm, epileptic seizure), substance or its withdrawal (medication overuse headache), infection (HIV/AIDS, intracranial infection), homeostasis, and psychiatric disorders.

Migraine

Migraine headaches are prevalent in 12–17.6% among females and 4–6% among males in North America. Prevalence increases among females until the age of 40. More than 80% of severe migraine patients experience headache-related disability and totals greater than 20 billion dollars in cost in productivity in the USA.

Migraine without aura occurs without clear prior headache symptomatology, unlike migraine with aura. The more common auras can include visual symptoms such as bright spots, dark spots, zigzag lines, or tunnel vision. Others can include numbness/paresthesias in an upper extremity or side of the body. Diagnosis is made by a suggestive clinical history (see Table 79.1).

Treatment modalities include nonpharmacologic such as regular sleep, exercise, meals, stress management, biofeedback, and cognitive behavioral therapy. Avoidance of aggravating factors including psychosocial stress; frequent intake of alcohol and food high in tyramine (including chocolate and aged cheese), high in nitrates (hot dogs, salami, and bacon), and high in additives including aspartame; and wearing optical quality glasses are examples self-help strategies.

Pharmacologic treatment (see Tables 79.2 and 79.3) of migraine can involve both acute and preventive

N.S. Jassal, MD (✉)
Florida Pain Medicine, University of South Florida, Department of Neurology, James A. Haley VA Medical Center, Number 127, Tampa, FL 33612, USA
e-mail: navdeepjassal@gmail.com

J.E. Pope, T.R. Deer (eds.), *Treatment of Chronic Pain Conditions*, DOI 10.1007/978-1-4939-6976-0_79

Table 79.1 Diagnostic criteria for migraine – according to the HIS (2nd edition)

A. At least five attacks[1] fulfilling criteria B–D
B. Headache attacks lasting 4–72 h (untreated or unsuccessfully treated)
C. Headache has at least two of the following characteristics: Unilateral location Pulsating quality· moderate or severe pain intensity Aggravation by or causing avoidance of routine physical activity (e.g., walking or climbing stairs)
D. During headache at least one of the following: Nausea and/or vomiting Photophobia and phonophobia
E. Not attributed to another disorder

Table 79.2 Migraine pharmacologic treatment

Abortive/acute	Prophylactic
Triptans (5HT 1D/1B receptor agonists) – sumatriptan, rizatriptan, zolmitriptan, frovatriptan, eletriptan, naratriptan	*Beta-blockers* – propranolol, metoprolol, atenolol, timolol, nadolol
Ergot derivatives (5HT agonist) – ergotamine	*Anticonvulsants* – valproic acid, carbamazepine, topiramate
Isometheptene	*Antidepressants* – TCAs (amitriptyline, nortriptyline, imipramine, desipramine), SNRIs
Narcotics – *should be used as a last resort secondary to short- and long-term complications associated with frequent use	*Calcium channel blockers* – verapamil
Butalbital – *major concerns for overuse and withdrawal. Use should be limited	*Lithium carbonate*
Antinauseants – (D2 dopamine receptor antagonists) – prochlorperazine, chlorpromazine, metoclopramide	*Botulinum toxin A* (inhibits acetylcholine release from nerve endings) – *first/only preventive treatment approved by the FDA for adults with chronic migraine (15 or more headache days a month, each lasting 4 h or more)
Dihydroergotamine (DHE)	
NSAIDs – ibuprofen, indomethacin, diclofenac potassium, ketorolac	
Corticosteroids	

Table 79.3 Botox dosing for chronic migraine by muscle

Head/neck region	Recommended dose
Frontalis	20 units divided in 4 sites b/l
Corrugator	10 units divided in 2 sites b/l
Procerus	5 units in 1 site
Occipitalis	30 units divided in 6 sites b/l
Temporalis	40 units divided in 8 sites b/l
Trapezius	30 units divided in 6 sites b/l
Cervical paraspinals	20 units divided in 4 sites b/l
Total dose:	155 units over 31 sites

Each IM site =0.1 ml = 5 units of Botox; b/l = bilaterally

interventions. Patients with frequent headache may require both approaches. Acute treatment is aimed at aborting the headache, whereas preventive treatment is geared toward reducing the frequency and severity of anticipated attacks. In evaluating therapy, it is important to give sufficient trial to the initial acute medication agent. Treat at least two or three attacks before judging the effectiveness of the therapeutic choice. Note that the chronic use (>10×/month) of any triptan, acetaminophen, NSAIDs, butalbital, narcotics, or ergotamine can lead to medication overuse headache. Lastly, there are hospital/rehabilitation programs.

Suggested Reading

1. Benzon HT, et al. Essentials of pain medicine. Philadelphia: Elsevier Saunders; 2011.
2. Ferrari MD, Roon KI, Lipton RB, Goadsby PJ. Oral triptans (serotonin 5-HT(1B/1D) agonists) in acute migraine treatment: a meta-analysis of 53 trials. Lancet. 2001;358(9294):1668–75.
3. Fishman SM, et al. Bonica's management of pain. Baltimore: Lippincott Williams & Wilkins; 2010.
4. Silberstein SD, Saper JR, Freitag FG. Migraine diagnosis and treatment. In: Silberstein SD, Lipton RB, Dalessio DE, editors. Wolff's headache and other head pain. 7th ed. Oxford: Oxford University Press; 2001. p. 121–237.

Occipital Neuralgia

80

Alexander Feoktistov and Sherif Zaky

Key Concepts

- Occipital neuralgia is a secondary headache that lends itself to direct treatment.
- Treatment strategies include systemic neuropathic pain medications to peripheral nerve block, to ablative therapies, to stimulation therapies.

Introduction

Occipital neuralgia is a form of neuropathic pain characterized by paroxysmal, sharp, severe, short-lasting electric shock like painful attacks located in the distribution of greater, lesser, or third occipital nerves. It is one of the most over diagnosed pain conditions and is frequently confused with tension-type headache, migraines, and cervicogenic headaches. Treatment of occipital neuralgia is quite specific and may differ significantly from treatment of other pain conditions that involve occipital region; thus, good understanding and accurate diagnosis are essential.

Anatomy

Occipital neuralgia most commonly involves greater occipital nerve, lesser occipital nerve, and, in some cases, third occipital nerve.

Greater occipital nerve is one of the main sensory nerves of the occipital region, and it supplies sensory innervation to the proximal part of the neck/suboccipital area and posterior and medial portion of the scalp from the occipital region all the way up to the vertex.

Greater occipital nerve mainly originates from dorsal ramus of C2 and to a lesser degree from C3 cervical spinal nerve root. Once leaving C2 dorsal ramus, it proceeds more superficially and proximally traversing semispinalis capitis and trapezius muscles and emerging to the surface shortly after piercing the fascia just below superior nuchal ridge along with occipital artery.

Lesser occipital nerve supplies sensory information to the scalp located laterally to the area innervated by the greater occipital nerve and to the area behind and superior to the ear. Lesser occipital nerve arises from the second and third cervical nerve roots, and it travels up the neck along the posterior margin of the sternocleidomastoid muscle. Just like greater occipital nerve, it penetrates the fascia just below superior nuchal ridge few inches laterally from the greater occipital nerve.

Third occipital nerve innervates posterior portion of the neck and suboccipital region. It originates from the medial branch of the dorsal ramus of the third cervical spinal nerve root. It penetrates the trapezius muscle as it ascends toward the head.

Etiology

Occipital neuralgia most commonly results from blunt trauma to the described nerves. Interestingly, the trauma does not need to be severe, and, frequently, chronic repetitive microinjury to the greater or lesser occipital nerves as seen with chronic hyperextension of the neck may be sufficient to cause occipital neuralgia. Whiplash injury is another common cause of occipital neuralgia.

Occipital neuralgia may also be caused by compression by occipital artery that frequently passes next to greater occipital nerve. Occasionally occipital neuralgia may occur spontaneously as well.

A. Feoktistov, MD
Staff Physician and Director of Clinical Research, Diamond Headache Clinic, Chicago, IL, USA

S. Zaky, MD, MSC, PhD (✉)
Pain Management Service, Firelands Regional Medical Center, Case Western Reserve University, Sandusky, OH, USA
e-mail: zakys1@gmail.com

J.E. Pope, T.R. Deer (eds.), *Treatment of Chronic Pain Conditions*, DOI 10.1007/978-1-4939-6976-0_80

Despite the fact that entrapment theory remains most commonly utilized explaining occipital neuralgia symptoms, multiple surgical studies performed in the past failed to provide supporting evidence to this "convenient" theory.

Clinical Presentation and Diagnosis

Occipital neuralgia present as severe, sharp, lancinating, short-lasting, paroxysmal pain in the occipital region. The pain may radiate to the top of the head and behind one of the ears. It is usually unilateral (although bilateral cases have been described). The pain appears to be sudden, and patients frequently describe it as electric shocklike pain that lasts from several seconds to 1 to 2 min. Usually occipital neuralgia presents as a series of sudden brief attacks that may occur multiple times per day. Occasionally patients may experience dull, low-grade constant pain in the occipital regions between severe exacerbations.

On physical examination there is usually increased tenderness in the distribution of the greater and lesser occipital nerve. Occasionally patients may report presence of scalp hypersensitivity (allodynia or dysesthesia) in the affected area. Frequently, applying pressure at the point of greater occipital nerve may trigger an actual neuralgia attack or produce paresthesia in the distribution of greater or lesser occipital nerves (Table 80.1).

Differential diagnoses for occipital neuralgia include cervical facet arthropathy (especially when affecting proximal zygapophyseal joints) and myofascial pain syndromes affecting proximal paracervical spinal muscles and trapezius muscles. Certain lesions in the cervical spinal cord and posterior cranial fossa such as meningiomas and cerebral artery aneurysms may also produce occipital pain. Occasionally migraine headaches may present as predominantly occipital pain and should be distinguished from occipital neuralgia. Thus history and physical examination are important in making diagnosis of occipital neuralgia. Some patients with abnormal neurological examination may require neuroimaging (MRI) of the brain and possibly cervical spine.

Finally patients with suspected occipital neuralgia may undergo occipital nerve block and if the diagnosis is correct should experience prompt pain resolution.

Table 80.1 The international classification of headache disorders, 3rd edition (beta version)

13.4 Occipital neuralgia
A. Unilateral or bilateral pain fulfilling criteria B–E
B. Pain is located in the distribution of the greater, lesser, and/or third occipital nerves
C. Pain has two of the following three characteristics:
1. Recurring in paroxysmal attacks lasting from a few seconds to minutes
2. Severe intensity
3. Shooting, staging, or sharp in quality
D. Pain is associated with both of the following
1. Dysesthesia and/or allodynia apparent during innocuous stimulation of the scalp and/or hair
2. Either or both of the following
(a) Tenderness over the affected nerve branches
(b) Trigger points at the emergence of the greater occipital nerve or in the areas of distribution of C2
E. Pain is eased temporarily by local anesthetic block of the affected area
F. Not better accounted for by another ICDH-3 diagnosis

https://www.ichd-3.org/1-migraine/

Treatment

When dealing with acute, recent onset of occipital neuralgia, the patient may respond to local heat or cold applications. Short courses of muscle relaxants and nonsteroidal anti-inflammatory drugs may also be beneficial. Finally occipital nerve block should also be considered. In fact, in patents with occipital neuralgia, occipital nerve block may serve not only diagnostic purposes but also provide rapid therapeutic response.

In some cases, the abovementioned treatment modalities provide only temporary or limited relief (as frequently seen among patients with intractable or chronic occipital neuralgia), and in these cases, use of prophylactic daily medications may be warranted.

When starting long-term prophylactic therapy, multiple factors such as coexisting depression and anxiety, compliance with treatment, sleep pattern, and other comorbidities should be considered.

One of the most well-studied and effective medications for occipital neuralgia is carbamazepine. Treatment usually starts at a dose of 100 mg per day and the dose may be gradually increased by 100 mg per day every 2–3 days up to a maximum dose of 1200 mg per day. Common side effects include drowsiness and dizziness. Rare, yet significant, side effects include aplastic anemia; thus, serum carbamazepine levels as well complete blood count and comprehensive metabolic panel should be routinely monitored.

Other treatment options include tricyclic antidepressants such as amitriptyline or nortriptyline. Patients with coexisting depression and insomnia may especially benefit from this medication. Treatment may start at 10–25 mg nightly and gradually increased up to 100–150 mg/day.

Other alternative therapy options may include gabapentin, topiramate, topical applications of lidocaine, and capsaicin.

Finally for more intractable and resistant cases not responding to traditional therapy, occipital nerve stimulation may be considered.

Suggested Reading

1. Ashkenazi A, Levin M. Three common neuralgias. How to manage trigeminal, occipital, and postherpetic pain. Postgrad Med. 2004; 116(3):16–8.
2. Bogduk N. The neck and headaches. Neurol Clin. 2004;22(1):151.
3. Handel TE, Kaplan RJ. Occipital neuralgia. In: Essentials of physical medicine and rehabilitation. Philadelphia: Lippincott Williams and Wilkins; 2002.
4. Headache Classification Committee of the International Headache Society (IHS). The international classification of headache disorders, 3rd edition (beta version). Cephalalgia. 2013;33(9): 629–80.
5. Reed KL. Peripheral neuromodulation and headaches: history, clinical approach, and considerations on underlying mechanisms. Curr Pain Headache Rep. 2013;17(1):305.

Cancer Pain

81

Gassan Chaiban and Maged Guirguis

Key Concepts

- Majority of patients with cancer will experience pain secondary to either the pathology or the treatment.
- Pain needs to be continually reassessed because worsening or changing pain can signify cancer recurrence or metastasis
- Through a team-based multimodal approach including interventions, majority of cancer pain can be adequately controlled.

Background

Approximately 90% of patients with advanced stage cancer will experience pain, 70% of patients will have pain associated with the primary tumor, and 20% will have pain associated with cancer treatments including chemotherapy, radiation therapy, and surgery. The remaining 10% will have coincident pain from other chronic pain syndromes such as chronic back pain or migraines. The pain can be experienced as nociceptive, neuropathic, or a combination of the two. Cancer-related pain can originate from spread of the tumor into viscera, nerves, or bone either directly or through metastasis. Patients with advanced stage cancers can have multiple sites causing concurrent pain problems, which may need to be treated separately. Additionally, pain associated with treatment may be severe enough for an oncologist or patient to limit treatment that could potentially improve survival rates. Currently, adequate pain control can be achieved in 90–95% of patients with opioids and adjuvants. The remaining 5–10% may benefit from advanced techniques including interventions. Treatment of pain has been linked to improved survival and improved quality of life. Despite this, pain tends to be undertreated in the cancer patient population.

G. Chaiban, MD
Interventional Pain Management, Ochsner Medical Center, Department of Anesthesiology, New Orleans, LA, USA

M. Guirguis, MD (✉)
Ochsner Health System, Pain Management, Department of Anesthesiology & Critical Care Medicine, New Orleans, LA, USA
e-mail: magedaziz@gmail.com

Assessment of Pain

A thorough history and physical examination needs to be performed on every patient with cancer pain. In addition to a detailed history of the current pain problem, the patient's oncologic history needs to be addressed. The type of cancer, staging, and current sites of disease need to be included in the assessment. Additionally, treatments that have been performed (past and ongoing) can affect the patient's pain through direct effects of the treatment (chemotherapy, radiation therapy, or surgery) or side effects associated with the treatments (see Table 81.1). Detailed discussion with the patient's treating oncologist regarding current prognosis and future treatment plans may also affect pain management decisions. Most importantly the patient's pain needs to be continually reassessed throughout treatment. Worsening or changing pain may indicate reoccurrence or spread of disease, causing patients to be reluctant in discussing their pain. Appropriate laboratory and radiologic studies may need to be performed in order to address changes in the disease course.

Treatment

The goals of pain management in cancer pain should be to relieve suffering while preserving function. A multidisciplinary team consisting of oncologists, psychologists, and pain specialists can collaborate to create a comprehensive plan that helps the patient effectively deal with all of the psychosocial aspects of a cancer diagnosis and its associated treatments. Whenever possible, the most effective treatment of cancer-related pain is treatment of the cancer itself through chemo- and radiation therapy.

J.E. Pope, T.R. Deer (eds.), *Treatment of Chronic Pain Conditions*, DOI 10.1007/978-1-4939-6976-0_81

Table 81.1 Side effects of interventions for cancer pain

Intervention	Side effects	Causes
Surgery	Postmastectomy syndrome	
	Post-thoracotomy syndrome	
	Radical neck dissection	
	Limb amputation	
Chemotherapy	Oral mucositis	Methotrexate, doxorubicin, daunorubicin, bleomycin, etoposide, 5-fluorouracil, dactinomycin
	Painful polyneuropathy	Vinca alkaloids (vincristine,vinblastine) Taxanes (paclitaxel, docetaxel) Platinum-based compounds (cisplatin, oxaliplatin) Proteosome inhibitors (bortezomib, disulfiram)
	Phlebitis	
	Hemorrhagic cystitis	Cyclophosphamide, ifosfamide
Radiation therapy	Mucositis	
	Cutaneous burns	
	Myelopathy	
	Plexopathy	
	Soft tissue fibrosis	
	Radiation-induced peripheral nerve tumors	
Medications	Sedation	
	Constipation	
	Nausea/vomiting	
	Itching	
	Delirium/confusion	

Medical Management

Majority of cancer pain can be treated with simple oral analgesics. In order to help standardize cancer pain treatment, the WHO outlined a three-step analgesic ladder which is tailored to pain intensity. The first step for mild pain includes non-opioid-based analgesics (NSAIDs, acetaminophen, and adjuvant agents). The second step introduces weak opioids (codeine, tramadol) plus adjuvants for moderate pain. Major opioids (morphine, methadone, hydromorphone) plus adjuvants are used in combination with interventions as the third step. Different routes of administration such as transdermal, transmucosal, or neuraxial administration can be considered based on patient's needs (i.e., inability to swallow). Long-acting or sustained-release opioids should be used in combination with immediate-release opioids for breakthrough pain with the majority of total daily opioid requirement being administered in long-acting preparations allowing for around-the-clock pain control. Interventions have traditionally been reserved for patients who remain in pain despite treatment with oral opioids, but arguments have been made to introduce interventions earlier to the treatment algorithm to help minimize medication doses and their associated side effects.

Typical adjuvants used for neuropathic pain include tricyclic antidepressants (TCAs), serotonin-norepinephrine reuptake inhibitors, and anticonvulsants. Corticosteroids (clodronate, pamidronate, zoledronic acid) can also be used. Bisphosphonates (which inhibit osteoclast activity and reduce bone resorption) can be used for bone pain. They are recommended for early use with identification of bone metastasis to help prevent fractures and reduce bone pain. Radionuclides (strontium-89, samarium-153, phosphorus-32) are absorbed into areas of high bone turnover such as metastatic lesions and may help relieve pain over 1–6 months.

Side effects of medications should be aggressively treated including treatment of sedation with amphetamines such as methylphenidate so that the patient can remain alert while receiving adequate analgesia.

Interventional Management

Appropriate interventional therapies can be added to the treatment plan to help decrease overall pain and limit medication use.

Neurolytic Blocks

Sympathetically maintained pain can be treated with diagnostic blocks to be followed by chemical neurolysis with absolute alcohol or phenol (Table 81.2).

Peripheral neuralgias such as intercostal neuralgia in the setting of post-thoracotomy syndrome can be treated with radiofrequency ablation following successful diagnostic blocks.

Neuraxial Analgesia

Neuraxial analgesia can be used to introduce multiple agents to target neuropathic, somatic, and visceral components of pain. Medications such as opioids can be used in combination with bupivacaine, clonidine, ziconotide, or baclofen. One of the advantages of neuraxial analgesia is that the amount of drug administered is decreased, reducing side effects. Implanted intrathecal pumps are generally used in

Table 81.2 Neurolytic blocks

Block	Areas innervated
Stellate ganglion	Brain, meninges, eyes, ears, tongue, skin of the head and neck, and upper extremities
Thoracic ganglion	Trachea, bronchi, esophagus, pericardium, heart, thoracic aorta, pleura, lungs
Celiac plexus	Distal esophagus to transverse colon, liver, pancreas, adrenals, ureters, abdominal vessels
Lumbar plexus	Skin and vessels of lower extremities, kidneys, ureters, transverse colon, testes
Hypogastric plexus	Descending and sigmoid colon, rectum, vaginal fundus, bladder, prostate, prostatic urethra, testes, seminal vesicles, uterus and ovaries
Ganglion impar	Perineum, distal rectum and anus, distal urethra, vulva and distal third of vagina

patients who have a prognosis of greater than 3 months, whereas a tunneled epidural catheter can be used in a patient who has a shorter life expectancy.

Spinal Cord Stimulation

Spinal cord stimulation is effective in the treatment of neuropathic or sympathetically maintained pain. Concerns related to the further need of imaging need to be taken into consideration prior to implanting a spinal cord stimulator because MRI compatibility may be an issue.

Vertebroplasty and Kyphoplasty

Vertebroplasty and kyphoplasty can be used to treat movement-associated pain from compression fractures caused by metastatic bone lesions.

Surgical Procedures

Less favorable secondary to many reversible alternatives and typically used as a last resort surgical cordotomy, pituitary ablation, and punctate midline myelotomy are examples of pain-relieving procedures that can be performed in carefully selected patients.

Suggested Reading

1. Adult Cancer Pain (version 1.2014). NCCN clinical practice guidelines in oncology. National Comprehensive Cancer Network. Retrieved from http://www.nccn.org.
2. Parris W, Eriator I. Chapter 14 cancer pain management. In: Smith HS, editor. Current therapy in pain. Elsevier Health Sciences/Saunders; 2008. p. 97–106. eBook ISBN: 9781437710090; eBook ISBN: 9781455757640.
3. Sharma V, Casasola O. Chapter 23 cancer pain. In: Benzon H, Rathmell JP, Wu CL, Turk DC, Argoff CE, Hurley RW, editors. Practical management of pain. 5th ed. Elsevier Health Sciences/Mosby; 2013. p. 335–45. Language: English, ISBN-10: 0323083404, ISBN-13: 978-0323083409.
4. Waldman SD. Chapter 208 cancer pain. Pain review (346–349). Elsevier Health Sciences; 2009.

Phantom Limb Pain

82

George C. Chang Chien and Robert Bolash

Key Concepts

- There are three principle neuroanatomical theories describing pain generators in phantom limb pain: peripheral neuromas at the site of the residual limb, hyperexcitability of pain afferents in the dorsal horn, and somatosensory cortical reorganization.
- Somatosensory cortical reorganization accounts primarily for the generation of phantom pain, with afferent signals from dysfunctional peripheral nerves and dorsal horn neurons provoking further maladaptive reorganization at the cortical level.
- Mind–body therapies including biofeedback, mirror therapy, mental imagery, hypnosis, and meditation have proven clinical efficacy in the treatment of phantom pain.
- Neuromodulation with spinal cord, motor cortex, or deep brain stimulation are established options for the treatment of refractory phantom pain in subjects who have failed more conservative therapies.

Introduction

Phantom sensations are characterized by cortical sensory perception of an amputated body part. These phenomena can be painful, such as seen in phantom limb pain (PLP), or non-painful, such as seen in patients with phantom sensation alone. Non-painful sensations are more prevalent and can be kinetic (perceived as movement), static (limb is held in a particular posture), or exteroceptive (possessing sensations of touch, temperature, itch, pressure, and vibration). Post-amputation pain can manifest as either pain in the residual limb pain known as residual limb pain (RLP) or stump pain, which occurs at the most distal aspect of the residual extremity.

Descriptors of phantom pain can be diverse but commonly include burning, gnawing, stabbing, pressure, and aching sensations. Sufferers also describe sharp muscle spasms or the sensation of a painfully clenched fist in an absent upper extremity. Phantom pain has been described after the loss of limbs or organs such as the tongue, eye, breast, or tooth. Phantom limb pain has also been described in brachial plexus avulsion and in people with congenitally absent limbs.

Currently there are over 1.6 million people in the United States that live with limb loss, and that number is expected to double by the year 2050. The primary causes of limb amputation include peripheral vascular disease, trauma, and malignancy, with the lower limbs five times more likely to be affected than the upper extremities. As many as 80% of patients experience either phantom sensation or phantom pain following an amputation.

Pathophysiology of Phantom Pain

The mechanism of phantom limb pain has yet to be fully elucidated, though it is widely believed that pain is largely neuropathic in origin. Models describing at least three possible pain generators have been proposed: peripheral neuromas at the site of the residual limb, hyperexcitability of pain afferents in the dorsal horn, and somatosensory cortical reorganization.

Peripheral Neuroma Theory

The neuroma theory posits that aberrant clusters of nerve endings formed as a result of transection of the peripheral nerves in the residual limb tissue generate afferent impulses

G.C. Chang Chien, DO (✉)
Cleveland Clinic, Anesthesia Institute Pain Management, 9500 Euclid Ave, Dept C-25, Cleveland, OH 44195, USA
e-mail: gchangchien@gmail.com

R. Bolash, MD
Cleveland Clinic, Anesthesia Institute Pain Management, 9500 Euclid Ave, Dept C-25, Cleveland, OH 44195, USA

J.E. Pope, T.R. Deer (eds.), *Treatment of Chronic Pain Conditions*, DOI 10.1007/978-1-4939-6976-0_82

perceived as pain. The theory is partially supported by the observation that there is some diminution of the pain following peripheral nerve blocks, application of local anesthetic to the neuromas, or destruction of the neuroma resulting in improvement in pain in select individuals. The peripheral neuroma theory likely represents an oversimplification of the complexity of phantom pain generation, especially in the setting of advanced disease, which typically demonstrates a centralized component.

Dorsal Horn Theory

The dorsal horn theory hypothesizes that sensitization occurs in the dorsal horn of the spinal cord. A loss of afferent signaling from peripheral nerves causes neuroma formation in lamina II of the dorsal horn, an area responsible for nociceptive input from afferent neurons. An increase in NMDA receptor activity has also been described at the dorsal horn after loss of sensory afferent input. These changes in the dorsal horn result in increased neural excitability and decreased response to cortical inhibition, leading to unregulated afferent pain signaling to the brain. The observation that patients with complete spinal cord transection are still able to experience phantom limb pain indicates a central pain generator and disputes both the peripheral neuroma theory and the dorsal horn theory.

Somatosensory Cortex Theory

Indeed phantom limb pain is likely to have some influence from the somatosensory cortex. In 1915, a case report indicated that a patient's phantom leg pain completely disappeared following a cortical lesion that included the territory of the somatosensory cortex.

Cortical reorganization leads to the development of abnormal circuitry and firing patterns that encode pain signals and, notably, are associated with phantom pain, but not non-painful phantom limb sensations. The changes of cortical reorganization are seen more extensively following amputation in patients with chronic pain preceding their amputation. This observation is consistent with the fact that patients with chronic limb pain prior to their amputation typically suffer proportionately more severe phantom limb pain post-amputation. Imaging studies have correlated a greater extent of cortical reorganization with more intense phantom limb pain.

It is likely that somatosensory cortical reorganization primarily accounts for the generation of phantom pain, with afferent signals from dysfunctional peripheral nerve and dorsal horn neurons provoking further maladaptive reorganization at the cortical level.

Evidence-Based Management

A recent systematic review identifies the highest level of evidence for phantom limb pain (level 2) exists for the use of IV ketamine and IV morphine in the perioperative treatment of PLP and oral morphine for intermediate- to long-term treatment (8 weeks to 1 year). Level 2 evidence is mixed for the efficacy of perioperative epidural anesthesia with morphine and bupivacaine for short- to long-term pain relief (perioperatively up to 1 year) as well as for the use of gabapentin for pain relief of intermediate duration (6 weeks). An adapted evidence-based medication summary can be found in Table 82.1. Table 82.2 describes phantom limb pain pharmacotherapy.

Table 82.1 Evidence-based medication summary

Hormonal	Calcitonin Intravenous	Level 2: mixed Evidence for efficacy acutely
NMDA Receptor Antagonists	Ketamine Intravenous Epidural	Level 2: effective Acute but not long-term relief of PLP
	Memantine Oral	Level 2: short term to subacute Persistence of relief of PLP Level 2: no efficacy for the treatment of chronic PLP
	Dextromethorphan Oral	Level 3: long-term treatment of PLP

Table 82.2 Phantom limb pain pharmacotherapy

Peripheral-acting agents		
Sodium channel blockers	Amitriptyline – oral	Level 3 evidence: no effect on long-term relief of PLP
	Ropivacaine – perineural catheter	Level 3 evidence: effective for acute PLP, but mixed for long-term treatment
Neuromuscular junction inhibition	Botulinum toxin – IM	Level 2 evidence: no reduction in the severity of PLP
Centrally acting agents	Gabapentin	Level 2: mixed evidence for reduction in PLP
	Topiramate	Level 3 evidence: significant reduction in PLP compared to placebo
	Opioids Morphine	Intravenous: level 2 evidence, effective for acute treatment of PLP, in the short term Oral: level 2 evidence, effective long-term treatment of PLP, compared to placebo
NMDA receptor antagonists	Ketamine	Level 2 evidence: effective for acute but not long-term relief of PLP
	Memantine	Level 2 evidence: short-term to subacute relief of PLP

Rehabilitation

Mind–body therapies represent both cost-effective and well-tolerated treatments for phantom limb pain. These modalities include biofeedback, mirror therapy, mental imagery, hypnosis, and meditation. Techniques such as mental imagery and mirror therapy are easy to implement, while biofeedback requires specialized equipment such as an electromyography device or virtual reality simulator. These therapies have many distinct advantages over more invasive interventions; they have little to no side effects and can be taught to patients for self-delivery.

The Role of Preemptive Analgesia

The observation that pre-amputation pain was a risk factor for developing PLP prompted the idea that peri-surgical pain control may represent a method for decreasing the incidence of developing PLP. Many authors have hypothesized that a pain-free interval may prevent peripheral sensitization of injured nerves and that the reduction in afferent nerve impulses may decrease the cortical reorganization seen after amputation. The evidence currently supports the utility of perioperative analgesia in treating acute post-amputation pain. Disappointingly, the evidence for pre-amputation pain control is not proven to prevent phantom limb pain.

Interventional Management

Invasive Techniques

Increasingly invasive therapies have been trialed to treat phantom and stump pain refractory to medications and conservative modalities. Surgical techniques such as spinothalamic tractotomy, stump neuroma excision, dorsal root entry zone lesion, ganglionectomy, and anterior cingulotomy are meant to interrupt the sensory pathways to the brain, or within the brain itself. These are reserved for patients with a short life span, due to the observation that the transient interval of decreased pain was often followed by high rates of recurrence at pain levels greater than pre-procedure.

Sympathectomy is an attempt to interrupt the sympathetic nervous system and is based upon the belief that select neuropathic pain syndromes are, in part, sympathetically mediated. Sympathectomy can be accomplished with radiofrequency ablation, chemical denervation, or open dissection of the sympathetic chain. If successful, pain relief may last for weeks to months. Partial pain relief may be a sign of incomplete neurolysis, and the procedure can be repeated. The most common cause of an unsuccessful sympathectomy is failure to successfully or adequately target the sympathetic chain.

Neuromodulation

Spinal cord stimulation can be considered in patients who have not obtained adequate relief from medical management and therapies. Though the mechanism underlying neuromodulation has not been fully understood, clinical application of neurostimulation has been adapted for the treatment of phantom limb pain. Using implantable electrodes, an electrical stimulus is delivered to either the brain, spinal cord, or peripheral nerves. Patients retain control of the device and are able to match the intensity of neurostimulation to their pain complaint.

Deep brain stimulation is performed through surgically implanted electrodes using stereotactic guidance and may be more effective for nociceptive pain than for deafferentation pain. Motor cortex stimulation has been shown to be effective for treating central neuropathic pain. In patients with phantom limb pain, reduction in pain scores can decrease by up to 70% through the use of these technologies.

Conclusion

Despite a growing body of evidence, phantom limb pain remains a challenging condition to treat. Current best evidence supports the use of a multimodal approach to treatment including medication management, aggressive physical and occupational therapy, and interventional techniques such as spinal cord or deep brain stimulation after the exhaustion of more conservative modalities. Despite the utility of these techniques, in a large number of patients with phantom limb pain, satisfactory analgesia is never achieved. There remains a large potential for innovation in improving the treatment strategies for these patients.

Cross-References to Articles Within the Work

Neuropathic Pain
Spinal Cord Stimulation
Physical Therapy
Chronic Pain Rehabilitation

Suggested Reading

1. Flor H, Elbert T, Muhlnickel W, et al. Cortical reorganization and phantom phenomena in congenital and traumatic upper-extremity amputees. Exp Brain Res. 1998;119:205–12.
2. Hunter JP, Katz J, Davis KD. Stability of phantom limb phenomena after upper limb amputation: a longitudinal study. Neuroscience. 2008;156(4):939–49.
3. Jensen TS, Krebs B, Nielsen J, Rasmussen P. Nonpainful phantom limb phenomena in amputees: incidence, clinical characteristics and temporal course. Acta Neurol Scand. 1984;70(6):407–14.

4. McCormick Z, Chang-Chien G, Marshall B, Huang M, Harden RN. Phantom limb pain: a systematic neuroanatomical-based review of pharmacologic treatment. Pain Med. 2014;15(2):292–305.
5. Ramachandran V, Sltschuler E. The use of visual feedback, in particular mirror visual feedback, in restoring brain function. Brain. 2009;132:1693–710.
6. Ramachandran VS, Stewart M, Rogers-Ramachandran DC. Perceptual correlates of massive cortical reorganization. Neuroreport. 1992;3:583–6.
7. Woolf CJ, Mannion RJ. Neuropathic pain: aetiology, symptoms, mechanisms, and management. Lancet. 1999;353:1959–64.

Ultrasound Guidance in Interventional Pain Medicine

83

Alexander Bautista, Enrique Galang, and George C. Chang Chien

Key Concepts

- Ultrasound has experienced explosive growth in popularity for advanced imaging in interventional pain management.
- Real-time needle visualization may improve success rate of interventions and avoid trespassing vital structures.
- Ultrasound is a reliable alternative to fluoroscopy in terms of reproducibility, accuracy, and safety for optimal image-guided pain procedures.
- Lack of ionizing radiation exposure makes the use of ultrasound appealing in both diagnostic and therapeutic image-guided injections.
- Knowledge of basic anatomy, ultrasound machine, and having a systematic approach are essential in the success of ultrasound imaging.

Introduction

Ultrasound is a growing technology in the field of interventional pain management and the treatment of musculoskeletal injuries. It has been adopted for both diagnostic and image-guided blocks. Table 83.1 summarizes the advantages and disadvantages of ultrasound.

A. Bautista, MD
Cleveland Clinic, Anesthesia Institute Pain Management, Cleveland, OH, USA

E. Galang, MD
Orthopaedic and Rheumatologic Institute, Cleveland Clinic, 9500 Euclid Ave, Cleveland, OH, 44195, USA

G.C. Chang Chien, DO (✉)
Cleveland Clinic, Anesthesia Institute Pain Management, 9500 Euclid Ave, Dept C-25, Cleveland, OH 44195, USA
e-mail: gchangchien@gmail.com

Basic Concepts of Ultrasound Imaging

- The brightness-mode (B-mode) display with a pulse-echo approach involves transmission of small pulses of ultrasound echo from a transducer into the body.
- The image is generated by the returned echo signals from many sequential coplanar processed pulses.
- The ultrasound transducer contains piezoelectric crystals that vibrate after application of electrical current. The machine in turn decodes the reflected waves to make the picture.
- Medical ultrasound utilizes sound waves and can be described in terms of frequency, wavelength, and amplitude.
- The frequency and wavelength are inversely related and help determine resolution and tissue penetration.
  - High frequency/high resolution/low penetration
    - Better for superficial structures
  - Low frequency/low resolution/more penetration
    - Better for deeper structures
- Image artifact as seen with ultrasound occurs most frequently in the fat-soft tissue interface and is caused by refraction. This is due to the difference in the speed of sound transmission as it travels through the interface of two tissues. The speed of sound is low in fat and high in soft tissues.
- The intensity of ultrasound pulses is reduced and attenuated as it traverses through tissue as a result of scattering and reflection of waves.

Knobology: Understanding Your Machine

- Understanding the operative functions of the ultrasound machine will help optimize imaging. Although ultrasound machines look different, basic functions are the same.

J.E. Pope, T.R. Deer (eds.), *Treatment of Chronic Pain Conditions*, DOI 10.1007/978-1-4939-6976-0_83

Table 83.1 Pros and cons of ultrasound

Pros	Cons
More accurate than landmark techniques	2D representation of 3D structure (1 mm wide slice)
Precise needle placement leads to less risk of inadvertent trauma	Poor penetration for visualization of deep structures
Affordable	Prone to artifacts
Portable	User-dependent, advanced skills needed
No radiation	Contrast-guided injection not appreciated
Dynamic – scanning while moving the relevant anatomy	Anatomical variation (e.g., obesity) may cause technical difficulty
Sonoauscultation – place ultrasound probe directly onto the point of pain	

- Selection and adjustment of the appropriate frequency helps optimize image and albeit most crucial in ultrasound technique.
  - Usual frequency used is in the range of 8–12 MHz and 10–15 MHz.
  - Higher-frequency waves are *attenuated*, have a gradual loss in intensity, are more in comparison to lower frequency waves as they penetrate through the tissue.
- Probe selection
  - Ultrasound probes come in a variety of shapes and sizes. The primary distinction between ultrasound probes is based on classifications on frequency, shape, and size.
  - Lower-frequency probes (2–5 MHz) are used to visualize deeper structures.
  - Higher-frequency probes (>5 MHz up to 18 MHz) are most often used for superficial structures.
- *Depth* adjustment is necessary to enable the structure of interest to fall within the field of view.
  - Set the depth of the survey a little deep to begin. Be mindful that excessive depth will degrade the picture unnecessarily.
  - Minimizing the depth will lead to better temporal resolution.
  - The trick is "get target in view and then adjust image."
  - Machines will try to improve lag by reducing the width of image.
- *Gain* dictates the brightness and darkness as the image appears on the screen. The image that is bright is termed *hyperechoic* and dark is *hypoechoico*
  - Increasing the gain amplifies electrical signal that thereby increases the brightness of the image, which also includes the background noise and vice versa.
  - Louder is *not* always better as this may distort the subtle differences between adjacent tissues.
- *Time gain compensation* (TGC) allows the operator to control brightness at specific depth independently. This property basically allows the machine to create a uniform image to compensate for attenuation.
- The *focus* dial helps to optimize lateral resolution. This may not be always present in all ultrasound machines.
  - Lateral resolution is the ability of the ultrasound machine to discern two objects lying next to each other at the same depth.
  - Always adjust focus to the depth of target.
- *Color Doppler* technology allows identification and quantification (velocity, direction) of blood flow.
- *Power Doppler* is a newer ultrasound technology that is more sensitive, almost angle-independent, and detects blood flow that is harder to detect with standard color Doppler. However, it does not demonstrate direction of flow and is highly vulnerable to motion artifact.
- The *freeze* button allows the machine to display the current image on the screen.

Needle Visualization and Managing Ultrasound

- The use of echogenic needle technology helps in the direct visualization of the needle as it traverses the tissues to hit the target.
- The image quality in itself is also dependent on the appropriate-sized probe and properties of the ultrasound machine to obtain an optimal image resolution.
  - Sonographic artifacts impede visualization of targeted structure and real-time needle visualization, caused by acoustic beam misalignment, termed as *anisotropy*.
  - The ultrasound beam that is emitted from the probe is very narrow, about 1 mm, and misalignment during the procedure may cause difficulty in needle visualization.
    - *Anisotropy* – "directionally dependent" produces focal areas of hypo-echogenicity when the probe is not at 90 to the linear structure being imaged.
- There are two ways by which optimal needle visualization can be achieved:
  - "In-plane" approach: The needle is inserted midline, parallel, and under the long axis of the probe. Visualization of the entire needle and the tip can be achieved.
  - "Out-of-plane" approach: The needle is inserted under, midline, and perpendicular to the probe in the short axis view. The needle tip/shaft appears as a hyperechoic dot.

Ultrasound Guidance for Musculoskeletal and Interventional Pain

- Ultrasound has been used to perform nerve blocks involving the brachial and lumbar plexus, including their distal branches.
- It has been a useful tool in blockade of sensory and mixed nerves that include ilioinguinal, lateral femoral cutaneous, pudendal, and intercostal nerves.
- Intraarticular injections of medications (e.g., corticosteroids) may increase the rate of responders and even decrease discomfort in patients compared to surface landmark techniques. However, benefits in long-term outcomes are controversial with mixed results.
- The use of ultrasound may decrease complication rate associated with trigger point injections and deep muscular injections (e.g., pneumothorax).
- Blockade of medial branch blocks and zygapophyseal joints has been done using ultrasound. The third occipital nerve block is one of the few that has been studied and demonstrated accurate localization in comparison to fluoroscopy. However, its superiority over the standard fluoroscopy on this particular block remains to be elucidated.
- Epidural blocks have been performed under ultrasound guidance but only caudal has been the most promising to date. The inherent issue with ultrasound like lack of contrast dye and failure to visualize the needle as it traverses bony structures limit its use.
- Direct visualization of neurovascular structures with ultrasound such as stellate ganglion block makes this modality particularly appealing.

Conclusion

The use of ultrasound in today's practice of pain management has many benefits including lack of radiation and improved visualization of soft tissue structures. However, clinicians should be mindful of the inherent risk, requiring proper training, and disadvantages associated with its use. Knowledge of basic anatomy, ultrasound machine, and having a systematic approach are essential in the success of ultrasound imaging.

Suggested Reading

1. Narouze SN. Atlas of ultrasound guided procedures in interventional pain management. New York: Springer; 2010.

Central Poststroke Pain Syndrome

84

Prin X. Amorapanth and George C. Chang Chien

Key Concepts

- Central pain is a form of neuropathic pain caused by damage or dysfunction within the central nervous system.
- Central poststroke pain (CPSP) syndrome is characterized by pain occurring after stroke that is due to disordered sensory processing in areas of the brain affected by the stroke.
- CPSP is an underrecognized entity. Diagnosis requires clinical suspicion and an awareness of disease course.
- Treatment is centered around antidepressant medications leveraging noradrenergic and dopaminergic pathways, as well as anticonvulsants. Newer modalities include electrical stimulation of the brain and spinal cord.

History and Epidemiology

Pain is a common complication in the poststroke population and may manifest musculoskeletally (shoulder subluxation, muscle spasticity, support limb osteoarthritis) or neurologically [headaches, central poststroke pain (CPSP)]. CPSP is a type of central neuropathic pain characterized by dysesthesia and allodynia on the side contralateral to the stroke. One of the first descriptions of CPSP was by Adolf Wallenberg in his description of his eponymous syndrome, where he noted pain and hyperesthesia located in areas of the body contralateral to the lateral medullary stroke. This was followed by Dejerine and Roussy's description of intractable pain secondary to thalamic stroke, which was part of a syndrome including hemianesthesia, hemi-ataxia, and chorioathetoid movements on the hemiplegic side. Work by further investigators has determined that damage anywhere along the thalamocortical or spinothalamic tracts may result in pain.

CPSP has an incidence of 8% after stroke, making it less common than many other peripheral causes of poststroke pain. CPSP rarely presents within the acute period, but will commonly declare itself within a month of stroke onset, with the majority of cases presenting within a year.

Pathophysiology

Theories on the root causes of CPSP comprise several main concepts. One is that disruption of neural function anywhere along the spino-thalamocortical pathway that conveys afferent pain information to the brain may result in CPSP. Another is that maladaptive neuroplasticity may contribute to the development of CPSP, with strong parallels between the plasticity involved in learning and memory processes in cortex and hippocampus and the plasticity in areas that may underlie chronic pain development and maintenance, such as anterior cingulate cortex and areas carrying afferent sensory information. These latter regions also provide a pathway by which the emotional state of the patient may augment the perception of pain. At a pharmacologic level, the involvement of various neuromodulators has been advanced based on the various medications that have been used to treat CPSP, ranging from decreased aminergic (adrenergic, serotonergic) modulation to alteration of glutamatergic function, particularly changes in N-methyl D-aspartate (NMDA) receptor activity. Finally, there is research suggesting that interfering with the reconsolidation of painful memories with agents such as ζ-pseudosubstrate inhibitory peptide may be an effective way of decreasing the strength of painful memories.

P.X. Amorapanth, MD
Brain Injury Medicine, Rusk Rehabilitation, NYU Langone Medical Center, Department of Physical Medicine and Rehabilitation, New York, NY, USA

G.C. Chang Chien, DO (✉)
Cleveland Clinic, Anesthesia Institute Pain Management, 9500 Euclid Ave, Dept C-25, Cleveland, OH 44195, USA
e-mail: gchangchien@gmail.com

J.E. Pope, T.R. Deer (eds.), *Treatment of Chronic Pain Conditions*, DOI 10.1007/978-1-4939-6976-0_84

Diagnosis

CPSP typically presents with severe neuropathic pain contralateral to the side of cerebral pathology. The quality is most commonly burning or aching, though it may also be described as lacerating or pricking. The time course is variable and can be episodic or continuous. This pain may be associated with sensory changes, both of normal and painful stimuli; allodynia and hyperpathia are common, with up to 59% of patients displaying the latter. Nonphysical stimuli, such as negatively valenced emotions, may elicit or exacerbate pain as well. An association with ataxia is more common (62%) and is more common than hemiplegia (48% with moderate to severe hemiplegia). In order to accurately diagnose CPSP, the physician must eliminate other peripheral causes of pain, ranging from musculoskeletal to rheumatologic to peripheral neuropathic (diabetes especially), and must make sure that the site of cerebral lesion is consistent with the distribution of suspected CPSP (Table 84.1).

Table 84.1 Proposed criteria for central poststroke pain syndrome

A history suggestive of stroke
Pain with a distinct neuroanatomically plausible distribution
Indication of distinct neuroanatomically plausible distribution by clinical examination
Indication of the relevant vascular lesion by imaging
Exclusion of other likely causes of pain

Treatment

Oral Medications

Pharmacologics for CPSP fall broadly into several categories: aminergic agents, calcium channel blockers, GABA-ergics, glutamate antagonists, and membrane stabilizers (Table 84.2). Amitriptyline is considered to be the first-line treatment for CPSP; however, anticholinergic side effects may limit use.

Nonpharmacologic Approaches to CPSP

When patients have severe CPSP that is refractory to pharmacotherapy, they may benefit from surgical or neuromodulation techniques to manage their pain (Table 84.3). Motor cortex stimulation (MCS), deep brain stimulation (DBS), and noninvasive brain stimulation (NIBS), encompassing both transcranial magnetic stimulation (TMS) and transcranial direct current stimulation (tDCS), are all experimental modalities that have been demonstrated to provide some benefit in CPSP in research studies.

Conclusion

CPSP is a rare complication of stroke, but it is one of the most common causes of central pain. Pharmacological treatment of CPSP includes amitriptyline, lamotrigine, gabapen-

Table 84.2 Medications to treat central poststroke pain syndrome

Class	Aminergics	Calcium channel blockers	GABA-ergics	Glutamate antagonists	Membrane stabilizers
	Amitriptyline	Gabapentin	Thiopental	Ketamine	Carbamazepine
	Fluvoxamine	Pregabalin	Propofol	Dextromethorphan	Lidocaine
			Baclofen	Lamotrigine	Mexiletine
			Midazolam		

Table 84.3 Non-pharmacotherapy treatment of CPSP

Treatment	Description
Deep brain stimulation (DBS)	DBS is a neurosurgical procedure involving insertion of deep stimulating electrodes through burr holes into target brain regions. In patients with chronic pain, target structures include the periaqueductal gray matter or sensory thalamus
Motor cortex stimulation (MCS)	Motor cortex stimulation was initially introduced for the treatment of central poststroke and thalamic pain. Most surgeons prefer a small craniotomy for electrode implantation. The motor cortex of the corresponding pain topography is exposed and identified. Electrodes are positioned over the area of the motor cortex where stimulation will elicit contraction of the affected muscles
Transcranial magnetic stimulation (rTMS)	tDCS is a type of NIBS that alters neuronal excitability by using a handheld electromagnetic induction coil firing at regular pulses to induce changes in electrical current in the underlying cortex. When these pulses are administered in rapid succession, this is call "repetitive TMS" or "rTMS," which can have longer lasting changes in brain excitability. Advantages over tDCS include improved spatial selectivity and strength of effect
Transcranial direct current stimulation (tDCS)	tDCS is a type of noninvasive brain stimulation(NIBS) that alters neuronal excitability through application of direct current electricity via surface electrodes, with a nodal (+) stimulation increasing and cathodal (−) stimulation decreasing neuronal excitability. Central pain syndromes associated with functional reorganization and cortical hyperexcitability may benefit from cathodal stimulation over somatosensory or motor cortex. Advantages over TMS include ease of use, increased subject tolerability, and decreased risk of seizure

tin, or pregabalin. Emerging technologies in the treatment of CPSP include both invasive (motor cortex stimulation, deep brain stimulation) and noninvasive brain stimulation (transcranial magnetic stimulation, transcranial direct current stimulation).

Suggested Reading

1. Klit H, Finnerup NB, Jensen TS. Central post-stroke pain: clinical characteristics, pathophysiology, and management. Lancet Neurol. 2009 Sep;8(9):857–68.
2. Kumar S, Selim MH, Caplan LR. Medical complication after stroke. Lancet Neurol. 2010;9:105–18.
3. Li XY, Ko HG, Chen T, Collingridge GL, Kaang BK, Zhuo M. Erasing injury-related cortical synaptic potentiation as a new treatment for chronic pain. J Mol Med (Berl). 2011;89(9):847–55.
4. O'Connell NE, Wand BM, Marston L, Spencer S, Desouza LH. Non-invasive brain stimulation techniques for chronic pain. Cochrane Database Syst Rev. 2010;9:CD008208.
5. Owen SLF, et al. Deep brain stimulation for the alleviation of post-stroke neuropathic pain. Pain. 2006;120:202–6.

History and Physical Evaluation of Headache

85

George C. Chang Chien and Zachary McCormick

Key Concepts

- A thorough history is the most revealing tool in the evaluation of headaches.
- Screening for health or life-threatening causes of headache must be performed.
- The most common primary headaches disorders include tension-type, migraine, and cluster headache.
- Secondary headaches commonly referred to pain medicine specialists are often related to medication overuse or cervical spine disease/dysfunction.
- Patients often have more than one type of headache. It is helpful to differentiate the most common or primary headache type.
- A headache diary is a useful tool to characterize patterns and triggers.
- The physical examination may provide no positive findings in most patients with primary headaches but can provide vital information in diagnosing health or life-threatening secondary headaches.
- Imaging is indicated when a health or life-threatening secondary headache is suspected. The decision to image may be informed by guidelines developed by the American Association of Neurology.

Introduction

According to some sources, headache is the most common complaint that leads people to seek medical care. Thus, the pain medicine specialist must be comfortable with a thorough yet efficient evaluation of headache. The evaluation of headache begins with a targeted history and physical examination. A health or life-threatening cause of headache must first be ruled out. If reason for concern is identified, the workup must progress rapidly. If suspicion for a health- or life-threatening headache is alleviated, a reasonable approach involves determining whether symptoms are related to a benign secondary headache disorder versus a primary headache disorder. Headaches may resolve without further need for treatment if a secondary cause of headache can be identified and eliminated. Alternatively, if symptoms appear to be related to a primary headache disorder, establishing a correct diagnosis is vital to subsequently developing a treatment plan.

History

A thorough interview that includes key elements of history (Table 85.1) is necessary to distinguish primary versus secondary causes of headache. Attention to potential "red flags" is important in order to determine the urgency of imaging or other intervention. Elements of history that should provoke concern include a new headache of unusual severity or a sudden change in typical headache pattern; a rapid progression to peak symptoms, associated with traumatic onset, exertion, or Valsalva maneuver; and nocturnal symptoms, associated with recumbent positions, projectile vomiting, neurologic dysfunction, or evidence of other associated systemic illness.

If potential "red flag" symptoms are not present, the focus of interview can shift to distinguishing whether the headache is related to primary or secondary cause. While there are numerous primary causes of headache (Table 85.2), pain medicine specialists tend to encounter tension-type head-

G.C. Chang Chien, DO (✉)
Cleveland Clinic, Anesthesia Institute Pain Management, 9500 Euclid Ave, Dept C-25, Cleveland, OH 44195, USA
e-mail: gchangchien@gmail.com

Z. McCormick, MD
Northwestern University, The Rehabilitation Institute of Chicago, Department of Physical Medicine and Rehabilitation, Chicago, IL, USA

J.E. Pope, T.R. Deer (eds.), *Treatment of Chronic Pain Conditions*, DOI 10.1007/978-1-4939-6976-0_85

Table 85.1 Key elements of a headache history

Onset
Progression
Temporal pattern (frequency, duration, time of day, menstruation, etc.)
Location
Quality
Severity
Premonitory symptoms
Triggers
Exacerbating and relieving factors
Associated symptoms
Family headache history
Past medical history
Social history – occupation, habits, diet
Medication reconciliation

Table 85.2 Primary headache disorders

Most common	Common
	Paroxysmal hemicrania
Migraine with or without aura	Paroxysmal short-lasting unilateral neuralgiform attacks (SUNCT)
Tension-type headache	Hemicrania continua
Cluster headache	Cold-stimulus headache
	Benign cough headache
	Benign exertional headache

ache, migraine, and cluster headaches most commonly. Typical features of these headache types are shown in Table 85.3. Likewise, of the numerous types of secondary headaches (Table 85.4), pain specialists are most likely to see patients with cervicogenic or medication overuse as the underlying etiology of secondary headache. Typical features of these headache types are shown in Table 85.5.

It is important to recognize that patients may experience more than one type of headache, which may be related. For example, cervicogenic headache may provoke tension-type headache due to reactionary guarding or head, neck, and shoulder girdle postural changes. Any headache type may be associated with independent analgesic-rebound headache due to frequent nonsteroidal anti-inflammatory drug (NSAID) use. In cases where headache type is not easily categorize due to symptom overlap or in adequate history, instructing the patient to keep a headache diary may be useful. A sample template for a headache diary useful for clinical practice is shown in Table 85.6.

Physical Examination

In general, physical examination in the headache patient will provide less diagnostic information than the history. However, the physical exam can provide vital clues that indicate a health or life-threatening type of headache. Thus, a thorough but targeted physical exam in the evaluation of headache is necessary and, with repetition, can be performed in approximately 3 min.

A systematic approach to the physical exam will ensure thorough screening and efficiency. Key elements of the targeted headache physical exam are shown in Table 85.7. "Red flag" features on physical exam include Horner's syndrome (arterial dissection, malignancy), oculomotor deficits particularly with pupil asymmetry (aneurysm), and combined

Table 85.3 Typical features of common primary headache

Tension-type headache
Mild/moderate intensity paroxysmal, bilateral "band-like" lasting 30 min to 7 days
Migraine headache
Moderate/severe unilateral paroxysmal "throbbing" headache lasting 4–72 h associated with nausea, vomiting, photo-/phonophobia with or without aura, with predictable environmental or dietary triggers, possible relation to menstrual cycle, aggravated by routine physical activity, improved with sleep, often with a family history of similar headaches
Cluster headache
Severe unilateral orbital/temporal "stabbing/piercing" headache with possible tearing, rhinorrhea, miosis, ptosis, eyelid edema, or facial diaphoresis, lasting 15–180 min occurring more than 5x per day, often predictable times during the day, in cycles of 2 weeks to 3 months

Table 85.4 Secondary headache disorders

Benign	Health or life-threatening
Medication overuse headache	Cerebrovascular dissection, thrombosis, or vasculitis
Cervicogenic headache	Intracranial hemorrhage
Sinusitis	Subdural hemorrhage
Dental	Hydrocephalus
	CSF leak
	Idiopathic intracranial hypertension
	Neoplasm
	Meningitis
	Abscess
	Open-angle glaucoma

Table 85.5 Common, benign secondary headaches most often encountered by pain medicine specialists

Cervicogenic headache
Occipitofrontal unilateral headache with predominant neck pain, worsened by movement of the cervical spine, potentially in the setting of recent trauma/whiplash-type injury or osteoarthritis: cervicogenic headache
Medication overuse headache
Insidious, progressive onset of frequency and intensity, associated with regular analgesic use, temporally related to the last dose or just prior to the next scheduled dose of an analgesic medication (most often ergotamines, triptans, opioids, or NSAIDs), with possible development of drug dependence behavior

Table 85.6 Sample headache diary template

Date:
Time started/ended:
Warning signs:
Quality of pain ("stabbing," "throbbing," etc.):
Pain intensity (0–10):
Location:
Other symptoms (nausea, photophobia, etc.):
Treatment or medication tried and effect:
Hours of sleep:
Food eaten today:
Events prior to headache (activity, stress, etc.):
Other comments:

Table 85.7 Key elements of a targeted headache physical exam

Vital signs
Mental status
Speech
Cranial nerves: particular attention to pupil symmetry, ocular movement, facial symmetry, and strength
Sympathetics: Horner's syndrome (ipsilateral ptosis, miosis, facial anhidrosis)
Funduscopic exam for papilledema if increased intracranial pressure is suspected
Muscle stretch reflexes, Hoffman's sign, and Babinski sign
Motor function
Sensation
Balance
Gait
Musculoskeletal assessment of the cervical spine and shoulder girdle: posture, cervical range of motion, palpation for tender, and trigger points
Temporomandibular joint assessment: range of motion, and palpation
Palpation of the sinuses and teeth

facial weakness and numbness (head and neck malignancy). In general, any cranial nerve palsy or neurologic deficit should raise concern for a potentially life-threatening cause of headache.

Aside from screening for potentially sinister causes of headache, a careful examination of the cervical spine and shoulder girdle is often illuminating given that pain medicine specialists often see patients with cervicogenic symptoms. Complete assessment includes postural assessment with attention to cervical spine and scapular position, cervical range of motion in all planes, palpation for tender and trigger points, as well as zygapophysial joint and occipital nerve regional tenderness.

Imaging

No particular imaging is indicated for a primary headache disorder. However, if there is clinical suspicion for a secondary headache disorder, imaging must be considered. While consensus does not exist, an imaging guideline to inform clinical management of non-acute headache was developed by the American Academy of Neurology (Table 85.8). Imaging may also be considered when cervicogenic headache is suspected, as zygapophysial arthropathy, cervical foraminal stenosis, or other structural findings may provoke such symptoms. Corroborating clinical and imaging findings in such cases may inform the diagnosis as well as identify potential targets for therapeutic intervention.

Table 85.8 American Academy of Neurology imaging guideline for non-acute headache

1. Non-contrast computed tomography
(a) Recommended when urgent neuroimaging is necessary in cases of:
(i) Suspected intracranial hemorrhage
(ii) Suspected elevated intracranial pressure or focal neurologic deficit prior to lumbar puncture
(iii) Headache associated with neurologic changes
(iv) Headache presenting with a substantial change in previously experienced headache characteristics
2. Contrast-enhanced computed tomography
(a) Recommended if abnormality is found on noncontrast CT or a vascular abnormality or tumor is suspected and an urgent evaluation is necessary
3. Magnetic resonance imaging
(a) Recommended as an initial or urgent diagnostic examination if there is suspicion of venous sinus thrombosis or vasculitis
(b) Recommended when an abnormality is suspected in the posterior cranial fossa or at the craniocervical junction
(c) Recommended when an aneurysm or vascular malformation is suspected, evaluated with magnetic resonance angiography (MRA)
(d) If an abnormality is detected on CT, MRI may further define the abnormality

Conclusion

A thorough, targeted history and physical exam is vital in the evaluation of headache. Pain medicine specialists should be familiar with the commonly encountered types of headache but should also systematically screen for potentially health- or life-threatening causes of headache.

Suggested Reading

1. Donohoe CD. The role of the physical examination in the evaluation of headache. Med Clin North Am. 2013;97(2):197–216.
2. Frishberg B, Rosenberg JH, Matchar DB, et al. Evidence-based guidelines in the primary care setting: neuroimaging in patients with nonacute headache. www.aan.com/go/practice/guidelines.
3. Waldman SD. Targeted headache history. Med Clin North Am. 2013;97(2):185–95.

Part XIII

Business of Pain Medication: XIII. Practice Types

Office-Based Pain Management Practices

86

Denis G. Patterson

Key Concepts

- Physician owners must be aware of the financial outcomes of their practices.
- Physician owners must manage and plan daily business transactions of the practice.
- Having a good business plan while providing good quality care is extremely important.

Introduction

Office-based physician practices are generally owned by some or all of the physicians working in the practice. As a result, the physician owners are at risk for the financial outcomes of the practice. Any profit generated by the practice, and therefore made available to the owners, is dependent upon the financial and operational performance of the practice. In order to ensure a favorable outcome, physician owners and their business managers must be diligent and thoughtful when it comes to managing and planning the daily business aspects of an office-based practice. Key areas that require constant planning and attention include customer service, business development, clinical operations, revenue cycle operations, and finance.

Customer Service

In an office-based pain management practice, customer service is a critical element of daily work, and it can be a challenge. Many of our patients suffer from serious illnesses, and whether or not they are the kind of illnesses that our providers have been trained to treat, they deserve our compassion and respect. This genuine level of personal care should not just come from the physicians, but it should be expected of all of the office staff as well. A physician who has excellent "bedside manner," but whose staff are not as welcoming, will see his reputation suffer.

Two important aspects of customer service delivery are a demeanor that is positive, pleasant, and personable as well as a simultaneous focus on teamwork and communication. A very effective way to achieve excellent customer service is to clearly and consistently communicate those expectations and the reasons for them, throughout the hiring and onboarding processes for all staff. People who want to work in that type of environment will gravitate to it. Another effective method is to design processes in such a way that they are customer-oriented and promote teamwork among staff. For example, if your new patient scheduling process wasn't designed with great customer service in mind, you will lose many of the patients referred to your office before you have a chance to see them.

Business Development

Business development is the next key area of office-based practices. "If you build it, they will come" is a famous line from the movie "Field of Dreams." Fortunately or not, Hollywood endings rarely happen in business. When it comes to running a business, you can build anything you want, but if you don't tell anyone about it, they won't come. A business owner simply must budget and plan for marketing and business development activities.

In most office-based pain management practices, marketing efforts should be made toward referring physician offices, such as primary care providers, orthopedic surgeons, and neurosurgeons. Of course, each physician practice should have at least a website, with business cards for each provider, and ready-to-share information about the practice, its providers, and their services. In addition to those marketing

D.G. Patterson, DO (✉)
Nevada Advanced Pain Specialists, Department of Pain Medicine, 10715 Double R Blvd, Ste 101, Reno, NV 89521, USA
e-mail: patterson@nvadvancedpain.com

J.E. Pope, T.R. Deer (eds.), *Treatment of Chronic Pain Conditions*, DOI 10.1007/978-1-4939-6976-0_86

basics, there are endless opportunities to network with your referral sources, such as lunches at their offices, conferences, local medical society gatherings, one-on-one dinners, golf course meetings, etc. A physician who puts energy into networking himself will gain much more business than one who neglects these activities, regardless of clinical skill. A financially successful practice is a building full of patients, not an empty one.

Clinical Operations

Clinical operations is another key area of office-based pain management practices. Designing and implementing processes that allow your patients to flow through the office in a smooth, efficient, and timely manner will make a big difference for your patients, your staff, and your providers' quality of life. There are countless physician practices that run hours behind schedule every day. This leads to staff that are stressed out, providers in a rush, providers who see fewer patients per day, and patients who feel that their time has been disrespected. In other words, nothing good comes out of it. It is wise to invest time to set up the right processes, train the staff properly, and then continue to be open to tweaking it as needed.

In order to prevent a decline in the provider's work-life balance, it is also advisable to hire competent business leaders into the practice so that they can focus on running daily operations which in turn allows providers to focus on treating patients. A leader hired specifically to run the office-based clinic should be responsible for controlling expenses such as staffing and supplies. That same leader should also be able to improve provider productivity (which is measured using a simple calculation of patients seen per workday) by tweaking staffing and processes. It is also very important to have an EMR system that works effectively and efficiently throughout the clinic.

Revenue Cycle Operations

In all types of healthcare providers, not just office-based practices, revenue cycle operations occur alongside the clinical operations. The "revenue cycle" is the set of processes that ensure providers get paid appropriately and timely for the work they do. The scope of revenue cycle operations includes many of the business activities that occur between new patient registration and when the patient's bill gets paid in full.

A simplified summary of those steps includes:

- Starting with new patient registration; information such a demographic data and insurance data is entered into the EMR.
- Insurance verification, patient-specific benefits information, and authorization for services are obtained from insurance companies and entered into the EMR.
- Next, the provider sees the patient, which generates charges for services provided (in the form of CPT codes) as well as clinical documentation that is entered into the EMR system.
- The EMR system organizes all of the above information and sends electronic bills to most insurance companies or prints bills to send to patients and some workers' compensation companies.
- The billing office oversees the collection of all accounts and manages the unpaid accounts.

All of the above processes must happen accurately and timely, on every patient every time, in order to get paid appropriately for the services provided in the clinic. There must be close operational ties between the billing office and the clinic in order for this process to work more effectively. Many insurance companies will send denials instead of payments, and those typically are the result of some error or oversight that was made in the clinic. If the billing office and clinic aren't communicating effectively, then the opportunities to correct those problems at their source in the clinic will be missed, and as a result the denials will keep coming instead of payments.

Finance

Finally, the role of finance in an office-based physician practice can vary depending on the size and complexity of the practice. For a single practitioner with a small practice, the finance role can be simplified to simply processing invoices and payroll, while making daily deposits to the bank, and doing the bookkeeping. However, as the practice grows in size and complexity, the role of finance expands because there will be opportunities to perform better and avoid mistakes, and good finance support can help a physician on both ends of that spectrum.

As a practice takes on physician partners, a seasoned finance person can help the managing physician with communication about individual physician performance as well as overall entity performance, which takes some heat off of the managing physician. It goes without saying that the same person would be the one preparing that information so that the managing physician doesn't have to.

Other duties of finance can include developing and implementing strategies for the practice; creating detailed projections of business ideas; understanding and managing the strengths, weaknesses, opportunities, and threats of the practice; being the practice's liaison between accountants, attorneys, and other business professionals; overseeing the revenue cycle operations; and effectively managing daily cash flows. A practice that fails to recognize the value of good finance support will fail to meet its full financial and operational potential.

The Business of Pain Medicine

87

Diedra Dias and Maged Guirguis

Key Concepts

- Appreciating the concepts of coding a billing is critical to understand when considering remuneration for services surrounding the clinical encounter.
- Engagement models for clinical encounters are vast and vary from employee to various partnership models.
- Everything is negotiable.

Introduction

An array of practice types and compensation models are available to physicians in the healthcare industry today. Physicians may practice independently or seek employment or alignment with a hospital or major health system. The American Medical Association's (AMA) recent report shows that "as of 2012, 60% of physicians worked in physician-owned practices. Only 23% were in practices that are wholly or partially owned by a hospital, and 5.6% were direct hospital employees." Although several options are available, healthcare reform has initiated a model shift from volume-based to value-based reimbursement, and this transition will drive increased alignment of independent physicians. Merritt Hawkins' most recent Review of Physician and Advanced Practitioner Recruiting Incentives revealed that 64% of their current searches were for hospital-employed physicians. Compensation models can range from salary only to production based, value based, or a hybrid based on components of these. As physician employment rises in conjunction with the emergence of healthcare reform, the pay for performance will follow, and pure salary or production only models will be replaced with value-based compensation.

D. Dias, MD
Ochsner Health System, Department of Anesthesia and Interventional Pain Medicine, Jefferson, LA, USA

M. Guirguis, MD (✉)
Ochsner Health System, Pain Management, Department of Anesthesiology & Critical Care Medicine, New Orleans, LA, USA
e-mail: magedaziz@gmail.com

Physician Practice Types

Independent Contractor

Physicians in a solo or group practice who operate independently and are not formally employed but rather are contracted by a hospital or healthcare system. The formal definition of an independent contractor is "a worker or business entity that provides a good and/or service to another individual or business entity under the terms of a specified contract. The independent contractor is not subject to the employer's control or guidance except for what is designated in a mutually binding agreement."[9] The contract typically prescribes the desired outcome or results of the arrangement but not the process or means by which the service is completed. Physicians who are entrepreneurial in nature, have an interest in small business ownership, and highly value autonomy tend to prefer private practice as independent contractors.

Employed Physician

Physicians directly employed by a hospital or group practice of a large health system. This model typically represents physicians who favor financial predictability and better work-life balance in lieu of greater financial risk or reward. They also prefer to focus predominantly on clinical care without added administrative responsibilities.

Aligned Physician

Physicians that remain independent but more formally align with a health system or hospital via an accountable care organization, clinical integration network, or co-management

J.E. Pope, T.R. Deer (eds.), *Treatment of Chronic Pain Conditions*, DOI 10.1007/978-1-4939-6976-0_87

agreement. Alignment serves as a middle ground or a bridge during the shift from volume to value-based reimbursement whereby the physician still maintains their independence but also partners to create value by improving quality and/or reducing cost. In this scenario, they receive a portion of the shared benefit created.

Physician Compensation Models

Salary

In a salary model, physician compensation is based on a fixed annual rate. "The salary-only model once common in academic centers, government practice settings, and some health maintenance organizations remains prevalent in some settings but is gradually giving way to structures that combine a base salary with a bonus based on the physician's productivity, performance on quality metrics, or increasingly both."

Relative Value Unit (RVU)-Based Model

In an RVU-based model, physician compensation is determined by RVU production. "An RVU is a productivity measure that reflects the relative level of time, skill, training and intensity required of a physician to provide a given service. RVUs, therefore are a method for calculating the volume of work or effort expended by a physician in treating patients." There are three components that make up the RVU value assigned to a medical service:

- "Work RVUs (reflect the relative time and intensity associated with providing a service and equal approximately 50 percent of the total payment)
- Practice Expense (PE) RVUs (reflect costs such as renting office space, buying supplies and equipment, and staff)
- Malpractice (MP) RVUs (reflect the relative costs of purchasing malpractice insurance)"

Value-Based Model

Value-based models encourage alignment of physicians and physician behavior with organizational goals, strategy, and reimbursement. These models aim to create value for patients by improving quality while decreasing cost. Although hospitals and healthcare systems have historically relied on RVU-based models for compensation, value-based models will become increasingly prominent with the emergence of accountable care.

Suggested Reading

1. Darves B. Retrieved from www.nejmcareercenter.org. 2011, Oct 30.
2. Duffy JH, Green T. Monogram series: hospital-physician clinical integration. Chicago: The American Hospital Association's Center for Healthcare Governance; 2007.
3. Halim L. The future of physician practice: Employed, independent, or something unexpected? Retrieved from www.advisory.com. 2013, Sept 30.
4. How to use the searchable Medicare Physician Fee Schedule (MPFS). Retrieved from cms.gov. 2014, April.
5. Independent Contractor vs. Employee: no simple definition. Retrieved from HRM-Partners.com. 2011.
6. Merritt Hawkins 2014 Review of physician and advanced practitioner recruiting incentives An overview of salaries, bonuses, and other incentives customarily used to recruit physicians, physician assistants and nurse practitioners. 21. Ivring; 2014. p. 1–30.
7. Rosenthal E. Apprehensive, many doctors shift to jobs with salaries. 2014, Feb 13. The New York Times. https://www.nytimes.com/2014/02/14/us/salaried-doctors-may-not-lead-to-cheaper-health- care.html.
8. RVU Based physician compensation and productivity: ten recommendations for determining physician compensation/productivity. 2011. Retrieved Aug 8, 2014.
9. Deane J. How physicians can achieve success in the arriving population health model. September 26, 2013. https://www.medicalcenter.virginia.edu/clinicalstaff/doc/UVA%20Pop%20Health%20-%20Sep%2026%20Final.pdf.

Office Based and Surgery Center

88

Denis G. Patterson

Key Concepts

- When a physician performs a procedure in his office, he/she gets a global fee (which consists of a professional fee and a facility fee) from the insurance company.
- If a physician performs a procedure in a hospital or at an ambulatory surgery center, he/she only receives the professional fee.
- Pain management physicians can own ambulatory surgery centers and generate significant profits from them.

Introduction

An office-based pain management practice with a surgery center can be an effective business structure for optimizing revenue for pain management physicians. Most interventional pain management services can be provided in an office-based setting because they do not require significant clinical resources. However, some of the services must be performed at an ambulatory surgery center (ASC) or hospital. Most insurance companies pay for services in two ways: a professional fee for the physician and a facility fee for the location. If a physician performs a service in their office, he gets both of these payments in one lump sum that is referred to as a global fee. If he performs the service at an ASC or hospital, he receives only the professional component of the fee, and the ASC or hospital receives the facility component of the fee. So the physician receives less money for a service he does not perform in his own office, and the facility payment to an ASC or hospital is usually much higher than the facility fee paid to the physician office. This is because the ASCs and hospitals are required to have significantly more fixed costs in order to be licensed as such entities.

Opportunities exist for pain management physicians to be owners of ASCs. Depending on state regulations, which vary widely for treatment of ASCs, a physician or group of physicians can join together to build or purchase an ASC. If the ASC's fixed costs can be effectively minimized, and the physicians involved in the ASC can effectively bring and build surgery and procedure volume in a consistent manner, the ASC can generate significant profits from the facility fees it earns. Depending on the exact legal structure and compensation arrangements, a physician who is a partner in an ASC can improve his revenue by performing appropriate cases in the ASC as opposed to a hospital. The physician and his office scheduling staff must be trained to know which procedures should be performed at which locations in order to optimize this opportunity.

Emerging Concepts

Practice development and management of the complexities of the clinical encounter is critical when deciding where to perform or the "site of service." Trends can be forecasted based on remuneration changes, both for the clinical provider payment and the facility payment. Hospitals traditionally are paid more than the ASC for facility fees, which vary based on the procedure.

Suggested Reading

1. ASIPP Fee Schedule. https://www.asipp.org/feeschedules.html.
2. Falowski SM, Pope JE, editors. Integrating pain treatment into your spine practice. New York: Springer; 2016.

D.G. Patterson, MD (✉)
Nevada Advanced Pain Specialists, Department of Pain Medicine, 10715 Double R Blvd, Ste 101, Reno, NV 89521, USA
e-mail: patterson@nvadvancedpain.com

J.E. Pope, T.R. Deer (eds.), *Treatment of Chronic Pain Conditions*, DOI 10.1007/978-1-4939-6976-0_88

Contract Considerations

89

Denis G. Patterson

Key Concepts

- Contracting with insurance companies is beneficial to the practice.
- The contract may be negotiable.
- When a practice is not contracted with an insurance company, they have access to fewer patients, more difficulty getting interventional services authorized, and inconsistent payment amounts.
- Contracts between physicians and their employers are very important.
- Contracts can help both parties avoid potential legal problems.
- Incentives for the physicians are typically written into the contracts.
- Based on the physician's performance, there may be an opportunity for partnership.

Introduction

Contracting is a key component of office-based pain management practices. The term "contracting" can simply be defined as managing all of the contracts that may exist between the practice and other companies. There are two general types of contracts: insurance contracts for revenues and vendor contracts for expenses.

D.G. Patterson, MD (✉)
Nevada Advanced Pain Specialists, Department of Pain Medicine, 10715 Double R Blvd, Ste 101, Reno, NV 89521, USA
e-mail: patterson@nvadvancedpain.com

Insurance Contracting

The process of insurance contracting can be simple or challenging depending on the approach of the practice. Insurance companies will typically offer low reimbursement rates, and other terms favorable to the insurance company, to a practice requesting a contract. At that point, the practice has three basic options: it can simply accept those terms in order to become a provider for that insurance company's patients, it can try to negotiate for improvements in reimbursement rates and other terms (which can be a long and arduous process in order to get to a successful ending), or the practice can choose to not sign the contract.

The benefits of being contracted with an insurance company include having access to more patients, achieving consistent payment amounts for services provided by the practice, and being able to get interventional services authorized. If a practice is not contracted with an insurance company, it will be tougher to access those patients, it may be paid significantly more or less for services (and the patients will have to pay significantly more out of their own pockets), and interventional services will generally not be authorized or paid.

Vendor Contracting

Vendor contracts are advisable as a way to control expenses so that the practice is not subject to the whim of a vendor's desire to change key terms such as products, prices, and delivery. Typically the negotiations for vendor contracts are a much easier process than the insurance company negotiations. In all contract negotiations, having a good personal relationship with the other party can be a very effective way to get the best possible terms.

J.E. Pope, T.R. Deer (eds.), *Treatment of Chronic Pain Conditions*, DOI 10.1007/978-1-4939-6976-0_89

Physician Employment Contracts

Contracts between physicians and their employers, and the details within the contracts, are very important to both the physician and the employer. Whether the employer is a physician practice or a hospital, a contract is generally offered to a physician by the employer, and then it is carefully refined through negotiations between the two parties over the course of one or several months before signatures occur. Because of the importance of the contract, as well as the potential legal nuances that must be taken into account when developing medical service contracts, it is always advisable to have an attorney involved with the development and ratification of physician employment contracts, for the benefit and protection of all parties involved.

Typically, physicians are incentivized in their contracts to produce income into the business. These incentives can be structured a number of different ways, from very complicated formulas involving combinations of productivity, cost, and quality of care to very simple arrangements, wherein the physician simply gets paid a percentage of the revenue he generates. Based on the physician's performance and the employer's organizational structure, there may be an opportunity for partnership if the physician performs well over a period of time. If a partnership opportunity exists for the physician, some of the basic parameters of the partnership topic should be included in the contract. Examples of these parameters include the performance level required to earn a partnership offer and the basic components of the partnering process.

Any verbal promises made or "handshake" terms should be included in the written contract. There should not be a contract that only includes some of the terms and also a side verbal understanding of other terms. It is in the best interest of all parties to have clear and complete terms in a written contract. After all, a contract will determine each party's actions not only when things are going well but also if things don't go well. Issues such as a noncompete, termination processes, and other "divorce" terms should also be spelled out in the contract. A noncompete clause can potentially force a physician to move to a different city or state and restart his practice there, so it is a crucial component of the employment contract. Again, it is advisable to get an attorney involved early and often in a contracting process. It is wise to choose an attorney based on trust and to keep in mind that his fees are a small price to pay for the legal protection that he provides.

Suggested Reading

1. American College of Physicians. Physican employment contract guide. Copyright 2017. Washington, DC; 2017.

Part XIV

Business of Pain Medication: XIV. Risk Mitigation

Drug Divergence and Vigilance

90

Kasra Amirdelfan

Key Points

- Opioids and opiates for acute and chronic pain
- Risk of noncompliance, abuse, and diversion with opioids
- Risk mitigation
- Utilization of opioid agreement for patient compliance guidelines
- Appropriate documentation for reasonable pain management
- Prescription Drug Monitoring Program (PDMP) as a risk management tool
- Urine toxicology examination as an objective measure of compliance

Introduction

Opioid and opiate medications are also among the most abused substances for recreational purposes due to their euphoric effect. These substances have been shown to have direct activity on the ventral tegmental area and the nucleus accumbens in the central nervous system (CNS). It is certainly not surprising that opioid prescriptions are also the subject of diversion and abuse in the United States and around the world. However, these medications continue to be an integral tool for the treatment of acute and chronic pain, largely due to the lack of equivalent efficacy in other analgesic medication groups available.

As such, the prescribing clinician not only has a professional obligation to treat the pain patients with the most efficacious medications but he/she also has the task of doing so in a safe and responsible manner in order to mitigate any risk of diversion or abuse. The management of such a risk is possible by the utilization of some proven tools in the daily practice of pain management by any provider.

Background

Opioid analgesics have been shown to have the highest rate of diversion and recreational abuse, among other medications with such a potential. Benzodiazepines are the second most abused family of prescription medications. Although there is no absolute indication to utilize benzodiazepines in pain management, many pain physicians in the United States and around the world continue to use these medications as adjuvant therapy for pain control.

As pain management continues to gain popularity as a specialty, the rate of prescriptions for such medications is on the rise. The treatment of chronic pain with scheduled medications is also increasing in the primary care clinics. A responsible and educated treatment plan is the only method to provide the patient with appropriate pain control. Such a plan will also safeguard both the provider and the patient from aberrant drug behavior including untoward severe side effects.

Implementation

Opioids and opiates are some of the most effective molecules in the control of nociceptive pain. As such, their utilization for pain management will continue to grow. However, with overdoses, diversion, and drug abuse on the rise all around the world, the spotlight is on responsible prescribing in order to mitigate all risks, as much as possible. The governing agencies have a particular goal in accomplishing this task. Although, there is never a substitute for sufficient provider education and a responsible approach to any treatment, there are three key methods, which will assist the prescribing provider in the reduction of diversion and risk mitigation. The authors would

K. Amirdelfan, MD (✉)
IPM Medical Group, Inc, Department of Interventional Pain Management, 450 N. Wiget Lane, Walnut Creek, CA 94598, USA
e-mail: delfan@yahoo.com

J.E. Pope, T.R. Deer (eds.), *Treatment of Chronic Pain Conditions*, DOI 10.1007/978-1-4939-6976-0_90

like to emphasize that the described methods below are not the only ways to reduce risk. But these methods have indeed gained increasing popularity due to their effective implementation as the standard of care for responsible controlled substance prescribing in the United States and the developed world.

Opioid Agreement

The opioid agreement (See Appendix 4), otherwise known as the "opioid contract," is currently the standard of care for all providers who prescribe controlled substances to treat chronic pain. Despite its prevalence, there is a lack of unified approach to this document. However, it maintains its roles as an effective tool in risk mitigation. The primary purpose of this document is to establish mutual understanding of the level of discipline required for the prescription and consumption of opioids and other controlled substances between the doctor and the patient. It is important to note that the agreement is not a binding "contract" which would hold anyone legally liable; however, it is a written documentation outlining the guidelines required by the physician and the clinic. The guideline will likely contribute to improved patient compliance and understanding of the prescribing process at any given healthcare center. Such a document will prevent misunderstandings and potential conflicts between the prescriber and the patient. For example, the document may outline the clinic's policy on after hours refill requests, frequent emergency room visits, or overconsumption of medications. Although there are always exceptional circumstances to any guideline, the opioid agreement sets forth an initial theme for the patient's treatment at any pain physician's office.

Moreover, the opioid agreement may also provide additional information regarding the nature of opioids and the reason they are typically prescribed for pain as an informative to alleviate the patient's concerns regarding such medications. This portion of the agreement, also known as the "opioid monograph" (Appendix 5), may also provide further information regarding abuse, addiction, and overdose in order to educate the patient about the nature of these medications and their potential risks.

The opioid agreement is typically given to the patients as part of their initial intake packet. The patient and the physician both sign this document in order to acknowledge its content as part of the patient's permanent clinical record. If the patient chooses not to sign the opioid agreement, a discussion between the doctor and the patient, regarding the reason why, may be warranted. The most common reason for this inaction is a lack of understanding of what this document entails. Despite a discussion, should the patient refuse to acknowledge the agreement, the physician may choose to refrain from prescribing any controlled substances for the patient as a mutual protective measure. As an additional informative effort, the physician and the clinic may ask the patient to revalidate their opioid agreement on a periodic basis, for example, annually. Although there is no guarantee, such an informed consent can potentially mitigate risk through education and encourage compliance with the treatment regimen. Retrospective studies have demonstrated high rates of compliance with opioid agreements among the pain patient population. As such, opioid agreements, including opioid monographs, are universally used at facilities providing care for pain patients with controlled substances. A sample of an opioid agreement is provided at the end of this chapter.

Documentation and Prescription Drug Monitoring Program

The importance of documentation has been instilled in every provider's skill set from the beginning of his or her training. The significance of good documentation takes a new level of importance in the treatment of pain patients. Thorough documentation will chronicle the appropriate and necessary care provided for the pain patient from their first evaluation. Moreover, it will provide historical data on the discipline of the provider in responsible prescribing, as well as the patient's level of compliance. The records will of course also reflect the treatment outcomes throughout the patient's care.

Organized documentation will also provide a clear level of communication among providers who may care for the same patient at the same or various treatment centers. Some of the key points which should be documented throughout the patient's pain treatment are the informed consent via opioid agreement, precautions and education regarding all prescribed treatment, potential hazards and drug interactions, and any history of aberrant drug behavior.

The Prescription Drug Monitoring Program (PDMP) has quickly become an invaluable tool for the pain practitioner in the ongoing risk mitigation process. The program, initially designed by the Department of Justice, is a statewide electronic database containing controlled substances dispensed for each individual within that state. Providers are then authorized to utilize the database in order to mitigate aberrant behavior such as obtaining pain medications from multiple prescribers. The pain practitioner is able to check a patient's prescription history by signing on to the PDMP portal within his or her state in order to evaluate each patient's prescription medication behavior. If the patient has obtained similar medications from other physicians while under the care of one provider, the risk of abuse and diversion is likely to be much higher. This is especially true if there is a signed opioid agreement in place with the patient and the physician.

The provider may choose to taper and discontinue controlled substance prescriptions for that patient to reduce risk to the patient and potential diversion.

Although there are no clear recommendations on the frequency of PDMP checks, quarterly evaluations on at-risk individuals may be warranted. Despite the fact that the program was conceived through the Department of Justice, it is important to note that each state has complete jurisdiction on their respective PDMP programs. As such, there are variations in its implementation and the reported medications based on the legislative regulations of that particular state. Currently 49 states and the District of Columbia have operational PDMP programs). Of course, the prescriber's participation and utilization of the program is absolutely necessary to mitigate the risk of prescription drug abuse and diversion.

Urine Toxicology Examination

The physician may, in good faith, prescribe the appropriate medications for the patient for optimal pain relief due to a diagnosed condition. The patient may not only be obtaining the prescription from the physician but he or she may also be reporting to be fully complaint with the regimen. However, the only objective manner in which the physician may at least ensure some compliance with the medication consumption is a toxicology examination. The urine toxicology examination or the urine drug test (UDT) is the most common method to obtain this information; however toxicology examination can be done through other methods, such as blood or saliva samples. The physician may request a sample from the patient at the initial evaluation, and at random, thereafter. Lack of the prescribed medication or the presence of other medications or street drugs in the UDT may demonstrate the risk of abuse and/or diversion for that patient. The physician will need to have a clear understanding of the metabolism of each controlled substance in order to be able to appropriately interpret the UDT results. For example, hydromorphone is a metabolite of hydrocodone. Therefore a patient who has been prescribed a hydrocodone prescription will likely test positive for both hydrocodone and hydromorphone. Moreover, it is important to understand that the UDT will not provide a quantified measure of how much medicine the patient may have consumed. The provider will need to be aware that despite the fact that the patient may test positive for a prescribed medication, it is possible that some of the medication may have been diverted elsewhere.

It is important to note that UDT should not be reserved for patients at higher-risk levels since inherent risk may not be readily apparent in patients with a history of compliance and lower-risk profiles. Although the physician may choose to test such patients at a lower frequency, some UDT testing for all pain patients on controlled substances is recommended. Current guidelines suggest testing patients at high risk in a range of 4 times per year (quarterly) up to monthly, depending on the physician and clinic preferences. The low-risk individuals would be tested at a much lower frequency, but at least annually. All UDTs should be administered at random for obvious reasons.

Conclusion

The notion of substance abuse has long been present as an aberrant human behavior within our very nature. The advent of modern pharmaceutical-grade medications, with abuse potential, has created a new epidemic of substance abuse in the United States and around the world. The epicenter of prescription medication abuse is the continuation prescription of such medications to individuals at risk and their subsequent diversion of these medications to the "street user." The provider has a professional obligation to treat pain in the best of his or her ability. However, the provider also has the professional and moral obligation to monitor at-risk behavior to prevent abuse and diversion. Although there are no absolute safety measures, which can ensure the prevention high-risk behavior, certain actions by the provider can help reduce such a risk to a reasonable degree.

The opioid agreement and monograph have become the standard of care as a first-line measure to outline the patient's, as well as the provider's, obligations to ensure compliance with the prescribed regimen. Diligent documentation of the treatment plan will assist in providing consistent care and mutual protection. It will also help the provider against any potential conflicts or discrepancies regarding the care of the patient. The utilization of the PDMP program in each state in the United States will ascertain the prescriber is the only individual prescribing the controlled substances for any particular patient. Finally the UDT will be an objective measure of the patient's consumption of the prescribed medication, as well as the consumption of other controlled substances, prescribed or illegal, which have not necessarily been reported to the healthcare provider. The employment of these efforts in any healthcare practice caring for pain patients will ensure that all patients may obtain the care they need and reduce the risk to the patient, provider as well as the society by a reasonable degree.

Suggested Reading

1. Administration DE. U.S. Department of Justice. [Online]. [cited 2015 May 8]. Available from: deadiversion.usdoj.gov.
2. Fishman SM, Kreis PG. The opioid contract. Clin J Pain. 2002;18(4):70–5.
3. Gouraly D, Heit H, Almahrezi A. Univeral precuations in pain medicine: a rational approach to the treatment of chronic pain. Pain Med. 2005;6(2):107–12.

4. Gourlay D, Heit H, Almaherzi A. Universal precautions in pain management: a rational approach to the treatment of chronic pain. Pain Med. 2005;6(2):107–12.
5. Hariharan J, Lamb G, Neuner J. Long-term opioid contract use for chronic pain management in primary care practice: a five year experience. J Gen Intern Med. 2007;22(4):485–90.
6. Heit H, Gourlay D. Urine drug testing in pain medicine. J Pain Symptom Manag. 2004;27(3):260–7.
7. Heit, H, Gourlay, D. Philosophy of urine drig testing in pain management. [Online]. [cited 2015 May 8]. Available from: prescriberesponsibly.com.
8. Manubay J, Muchow C, Sullivan M. Prescription drug abuse: epidemiology, regulartory issues, chronic pain management with narcotic analgesics. Priamry Care. 2011;38(1):71–5.
9. McCabe SE, Boyd C, Teter C. Medical use, illicit use, and diversion of abusable prescription drugs. J Am Coll Health. 2006;54(5):269–78.
10. Micha E, Jamison RN. Urine toxicology screening among chronic pain patients on opioid therapy: frequency and Predictiblity of abnormal findings. Clin J Pain. 2007;23(2):173–9.
11. Owen G, Burton A, Schade C, Passik S. Urine drug testing: current recommendations and best practices. Pain Physician. 2012a;15:119–33.
12. Owen G, Burton A, Schade C, Passik S. Urine drug testing: current recommendations and best practices. Pain Physician. 2012b;15: 119–33.
13. PDMP Information.: www.DEAdiversion.USdoj.gov
14. Portenoy RK, Payne R, Passik S, Lowinson JH, Ruz P, Millman RB, et al. Substance abuse: a comprehensive textbook. 4th ed. Philadelphia: Lippincott, Wlillams & Wilkins; 2004.
15. Reddy S, Patt RB. The benzodiazepines as adjuvant anaglesics. J Pain Symptom Manag. 1994;9(8):510–4.
16. Wise RA, Bozarth MA. Brain mechanism of drug reward and euphoria. Psychiatr Med. 1985;3(4):445–60.

Part XV

Business of Pain Medication: XV. Research

Informed Consent

91

Olabisi P. Lane

Key Points

- A discussion is required between the patient or legal representative and the healthcare provider regarding proposed medical treatment.
- Informed consent recognizes the patient's right to autonomy and decision-making.
- Full disclosure of all required elements of informed consent including risks, benefits, and alternatives must be provided.
- Must include enough detail to allow a reasonable person to make an informed decision.
- The patient's competence must be assessed and all questions answered.
- For patients over 18 years of age and emancipated minors, parents or legal guardians of minors are able to provide informed consent.
- Communication barriers must be appropriately addressed.
- Documentation of the informed consent process is required.

Introduction

Informed consent is a practice whereby the patient or legal representative and the healthcare provider have a discussion about the proposed medical treatment, alternatives, consequences, risks, and benefits. It is a necessary part of providing health care and recognizes the patient's right to self-determination and decision-making. This process applies to all medical care decisions where one or more alternatives exist, including the option of no treatment at all, and gives the patient the right to make their own decisions. As such, informed consent is needed prior to receiving sedation and anesthesia, undergoing a nonroutine or invasive procedure, receiving blood products or blood components, and participating in IRB to name a few. If informed consent cannot be obtained and there's an emergency situation that is a direct threat to the life or health of the patient, then the provider can proceed with the emergency treatment. In this circumstance a second medical opinion should be obtained and documented.

O.P. Lane, MD, PharmD (✉)
University Hospitals/Case Medical Center, Department of Anesthesiology and Perioperative Medicine,
11000 Euclide Avenue, Cleveland, OH 44106, USA
e-mail: olabisi.lane@uhhospitals.org

Considerations

The disclosure of the following elements is required to ensure the informed consent process is complete:

1. A proper explanation of the condition requiring treatment
2. A description of the proposed treatment
3. The potential risks and benefits of the treatment
4. The probability of success with the proposed treatment
5. Potential consequences of forgoing the treatment
6. An explanation of reasonable alternatives, including associated risks and benefits
7. The material risks of the treatment
8. The role of ancillary service representatives such as vendors in the treatment plan

The physician should assess the patient's mental capacity prior to obtaining informed consent. Patients who are incompetent, incapacitated, or unable to make informed decision still retain their autonomy. It is the responsibility of the medical team to ensure when a patient is not competent that their advance directives are followed or they are represented by their medical power of attorney or authorized legal guardian to provide substituted judgment.

For patients who are competent and over 18 years of age and emancipated minors in some states, parents or legal guardians of minors are able to provide informed consent. At

J.E. Pope, T.R. Deer (eds.), *Treatment of Chronic Pain Conditions*, DOI 10.1007/978-1-4939-6976-0_91

least one parent should be present to sign the consent, although the consent of both is preferred. If either parent or legal guardian is unavailable, then decision is sought in the court of law. If a communication barrier exists (i.e., a patient that speaks a foreign language) is blind or deaf then an interpreter should be utilized. Ideally, family members should not serve as interpreters.

An adequately detailed explanation for a reasonable person to make a decision is required and must be provided during the informed consent process. The patient's understanding and preference must also be assessed. This process may occur at one meeting, or across multiple encounters.

The written consent form must be completed and verified in the patient's medical record prior to the proposed treatment. The documentation should include the date and time, the identity of those who will participate in the process, and the documentation of all the required elements that were discussed. The healthcare provider should document that the patient understood the information provided and was given adequate time to ask questions, all questions were appropriately answered, and an agreement was made to start the proposed treatment planned. The consent expires after the procedure is completed. A new consent must be obtained for future procedures.

Suggested Reading

1. Lennard TA, Vivian DG, Walkowski SD, Singla AK. Medicolegal issues. In: Pain procedures in clinical practice. 3rd ed. Philadelphia, PA: Elsevier; 2011. p. 57–60.
2. Shekelle PG, et al. Making health care safer II: an updated critical analysis of the evidence for patient safety practices. 2013. Available: http://www.ahrq.gov/sites/default/files/wysiwyg/research/findings/evidence-based-reports/services/quality/ptsafetyII-full.pdf. Last Accessed 25 Dec 2015.
3. Warfield C, Zahid B. Principles and practice of pain medicine. 2nd ed. New York: McGraw-Hill; 2004. p. 854–5.

Part XVI

Pain Care and Patient Advocacy/Future Needs XVI

92 Technology and Application Advancement

Steven M. Falowski

Key Points

- The field of pain medicine has seen a paradigm shift away from chronic opioid therapy in favor of sustainable interventional therapies.
- Technology advancement is a multifactorial process that includes physicians, societies, and industry.
- The driving factor for applying technology and advancing the field is a patient-centered approach that is propelled by research and publication.

Introduction

Chronic pain has always been a significant burden to patients, society, and health care. It is associated with rising healthcare costs and a shift onto physicians to alleviate patient suffering. Medications have been a hallmark in the treatment of pain, with opioid therapy being in the forefront. This has fallen short in being an effective therapy and has led the field to look for alternative options. These options largely fall upon interventional therapies. It is because of this paradigm shift that advancement of these therapies through technology and continued research is paramount in the success of the pain management field.

Technology Advancement

Physicians face significant challenges in treating chronic pain. Given the long-term negative effects of chronic opioid therapy, there is more importance on alternative treatment options. This is a paradigm shift from previous practice standards and places an emphasis on the importance of interventional therapies. Although these therapies have existed and been utilized, this shift in our thought process has led to a need for improved technology and research development. The sustainability of the therapy has become just as important as the efficacy. Industry, physicians, and society all play an important role.

Interventional therapies can range in invasiveness and vary from epidural steroid injections, facet blocks, and rhizotomies to the surgical procedures such as spinal cord stimulation. It is well known that earlier intervention in treating chronic pain leads to better success rates. This has been demonstrated in neuromodulation, and in particular with spinal cord stimulation (Fig. 92.1). This has therefore positioned neuromodulation earlier in the treatment paradigm.

Spinal cord stimulation has commonly been used to treat post-laminectomy syndrome, as well as complex regional pain syndrome. It has been based on the premise of paresthesia coverage of the painful area. Technological advancements and progressive research changed this mindset and led to the advancement of waveforms, new targets, and expanding indications. At the forefront of this changing mindset is DeRidder burst stimulation, high frequency stimulation, and dorsal root ganglion stimulation. Each of the novel therapies has been extensively studied and backed by level one evidence for its safety and efficacy.

DeRidder burst stimulation (Fig. 92.2) is based on appropriate spinal mapping, as well as research pertaining to spinal pathways and central nervous system interpretation of pain. It offers paresthesia-free coverage, as well as the ability to utilize tonic stimulation when desired. High-frequency stimulation at 10,000 Hz offers paresthesia-free stimulation with improved patient outcomes compared to traditional tonic stimulation. Dorsal root ganglion stimulation (Fig. 92.3) signifies the change in neural targeting and offers expanded indications for which spinal cord stimulation either had difficulty in delivering pain relief or was not considered.

S.M. Falowski, MD (✉)
St. Lukes University Health Network, Department of Neurosurgery, Ste 302, Bethlehem, PA 18017, USA
e-mail: sfalowski@gmail.com

J.E. Pope, T.R. Deer (eds.), *Treatment of Chronic Pain Conditions*, DOI 10.1007/978-1-4939-6976-0_92

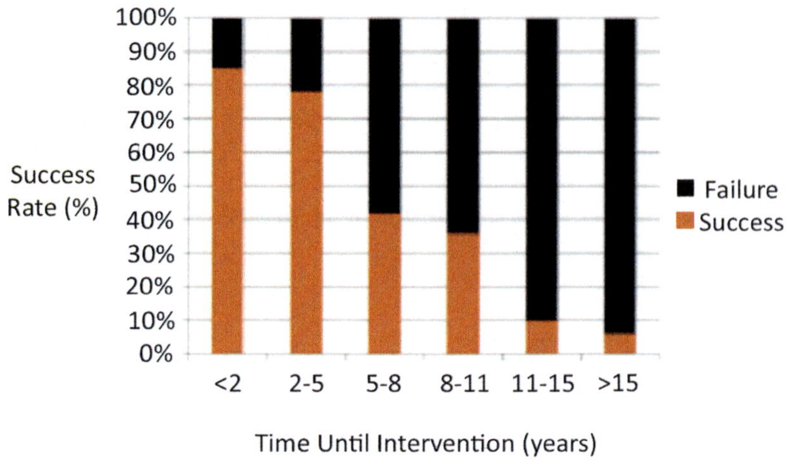

Fig. 92.1 Success of spinal cord stimulation based on time to intervention: duration of pain (With permission from Kumar et al. [5] ©Wolters Kluwer)

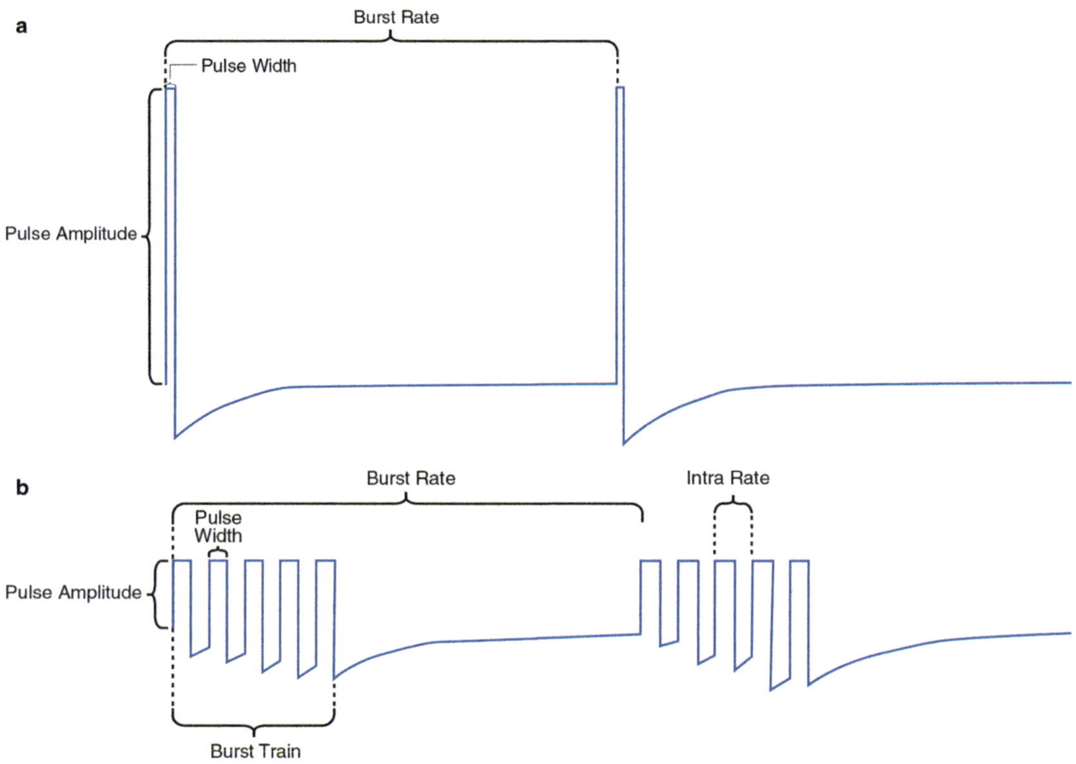

Fig. 92.2 DeRidder burst waveform (With permission from Pope and Deer [8] ©Springer)

The importance of these therapies lies in the advancement of technology leading to improved patient outcomes. They have confirmed the efficacy seen with traditional tonic spinal cord stimulation and opened the door to continue the paradigm shift away from chronic opioid therapy. It signifies the importance of continued level one evidence, a patient-centered approach, and improvements in products.

Conclusion

Technology advancement is a multifactorial process that includes physicians, societies, and industry. The driving factor is a patient-centered approach that is propelled by research and publication. Neuromodulation has seen a paradigm shift

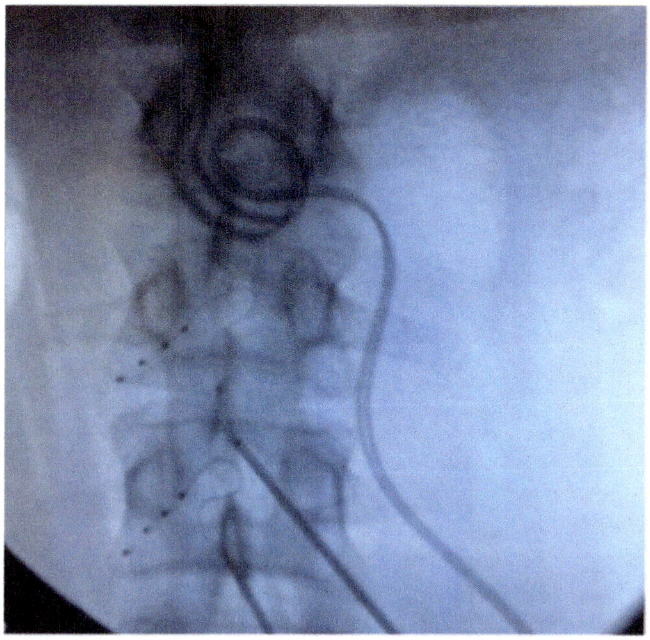

Fig. 92.3 Placement of dorsal root ganglion leads

in its evolution and is being driven by level one evidence. Earlier intervention with these therapies combined with groundbreaking research and technology has and will continue to improve our success.

Suggested Reading

1. A prospective, randomized, multi-center, controlled clinical trial to assess the safety and efficacy of the spinal modulation axium™ neurostimulator system in the treatment of chronic intractable pain. Presented at NANS 2015.
2. De Ridder D, Plaizer M, Kamerling N, Menovsky T, Vanneste S. Burst spinal cord stimulation for limb and back pain. World Neurosurg. 2013;80(5):642–649.e1.
3. Deer TR, Krames E, Mekhail N, Pope J, et al. The appropriate use of neurostimulation: new and evolving neurostimulation therapies and applicable treatment for chronic pain and selected disease states. Neuromodulation. 2014;17(6):599–615. discussion 615. doi:10.1111/ner.12204.
4. Kapural L, Yu C, Doust MW, et al. Novel 10-kHz hi frequency therapy (HF10) is superior to traditional low-frequency spinal cord stimulation for the treatment of chronic back and leg pain. Anesthesiology. 2015;123(4):1–10.
5. Kumar K, Hunter G, Demeria D. Spinal cord stimulation in treatment of chronic benign pain: challenges in treatment planning and present status : a 22 year experience. Neurosurgery. 2006;58:481–96.
6. Liem L, Russo M, Huygen FJ, Van Buyten JP, Smet I, et al. A multicenter, prospective trial to assess the safety and performance of the spinal modulation dorsal root ganglion neurostimulator system in the treatment of chronic pain. Neuromodulation. 2013;16(5):471–82. discussion 482.
7. Manchikanti L, Fellows B, Ailinani H, et al. Therapeutic use, abuse, and nonmedical use of opioids: a ten-year perspective. Pain Physician. 2010;13(5):401–35.
8. Pope JE, Deer TR. Burst stimulation: an innovative waveform strategy for spinal cord stimulation. In: Deer TR, Pope JE, editors. Atlas of implantable therapies for pain management. New York: Springer; 2016. p. 163–7.
9. Sunburst: a prospective, randomized, controlled trial assessing burst stimulation for the treatment of chronic pain. Presented at NANS 2015.

Society Engagement

93

Haroon Hameed

Key Concepts

- Pain medicine and interventional pain management community has a wide array of societies available for its education and support.
- The choice of which societies to choose for involvement should be based on the individual interests of each physician and surgeon.

Introduction

The pain medicine, or for some of us, the interventional pain management community have several national and a multitude of state societies who promote pain-related education, research, and advocacy. The nature, scope, and purpose of each society differ to a degree, while many of their functions and goals overlap significantly. Basic information regarding the history, purpose, and activities of some of the more prominent of these organizations are presented below, as defined at the time of this writing.

International Association for the Study of Pain (IASP)

IASP is the first society that was created specifically with the intent to create a community of physicians and scientists to further the study and knowledge of pain. From its inception in 1973–1974, it had within it the visionary leaders who would shape the landscape of leaders in pain research for decades to come. The name of Dr. John Bonica who engineered its formation, first meetings, its journal "Pain," as well as the first pain medicine fellowship in the United Sates at the University of Washington, has been linked to numerous awards across pain societies bestowed as a mark of excellence and distinction. It has contributed heavily to the advancement of education, and research in pain, and its meeting, conducted once every 4 years remains the premier international pain society meeting.

H. Hameed, MD (✉)
KURE Pain Management,
116 Defense Highway, Ste 403, Annapolis, MD 21401, USA
e-mail: drharoonhameed@yahoo.com

American Pain Society (APS)

This is the American branch of the IASP, founded in 1977 by Dr. John Bonica and other nationally prominent pain physicians, surgeons, and scientists. It is unique among other widely respected national pain societies in that it holds nonphysicians and surgeons, such as psychologists, nurses, pharmacists, and dentists within its active members. It has a strong dedication to the advancement of research, education, and advocacy for the multidisciplinary treatment of pain and has the largest pain-related annual meeting within the United States.

American Academy of Pain Medicine (AAPM)

This society was formed in 1983 initially as the American Academy of Algology. It was founded by prominent members of the APS, and its active members are limited to physicians and surgeons, though it includes nonphysicians within its affiliate member track. It has an interest in both physician and patient education and advocacy and, along with the American Society of Anesthesiologists, has been involved in advocating for pain-related issues within the American Medical Association for decades.

J.E. Pope, T.R. Deer (eds.), *Treatment of Chronic Pain Conditions*, DOI 10.1007/978-1-4939-6976-0_93

Spine Intervention Society (SIS)

This interventional pain and spine society was initially formed in 1988 as the Needle Jockey Club, a society of interventional pain management physicians; following a meeting of the North American Spine Society, a society of primarily spine surgeons. The founding members include Nikolai Bogduk, Charlie Aprill, and others whose research heavily contributed to the advancement of pain intervention-related scientific evidence, standards, and clinical practice. Their annual meeting is still considered one of the main clinically oriented interventional pain meetings. They also offer a number of clinical workshops for those interested in learning or advancing their interventional skills.

American Society of Interventional Pain Physicians (ASIPP)

Laxmaiah Manchikanti and others formed this society in 1998, with the primary intent of advancing scientific evidence and maintaining patient access to Interventional Pain Management procedures. They have a very strong history of advocacy at the state and federal level and were integral in the recognition of the practice designation of "Interventional Pain Management" at the federal level as well as its inclusion on national Carrier Advisory Committees (CACs) thereby increasing the influence of interventional pain physicians on federal and private payment schedules. ASIPP was also integral in the passage of the first electronic prescription reporting legislation known as the National All Schedules Electronic Reporting Act in 2005. They continue to have annual meetings with an emphasis on the advancement of scientific evidence, coupled with a strong lobbying component to their societal activities.

American Society of Regional Anesthesia and Pain Medicine (ASRA)

This is the regional anesthesia and pain medicine division of the American Society of Anesthesiologists. Their annual fall pain meeting remains one of the most academic, comprehensive, and research-based pain meetings in the country. The faculty of ASRA meetings typically consists of highly academic and well-published leaders in the pain medicine community.

North American Neuromodulation Society (NANS)

The North American Neuromodulation Society was formed in 1994 and has among its current and previous faculty and leadership the entire breadth of scientific and advocacy leaders with regard to neuromodulation. Although initially started with a focus on spinal cord and deep brain stimulation and intrathecal therapy, it has grown to encompass physicians and scientists with interests in neuromodulation-based therapies for hearing and visual impairment, bladder dysfunction, and other treatments on the forefront of medical research. Its annual meeting includes faculty and attendees from some of the widest ranges of specialties within medicine.

Suggested Reading

1. http://www.iasp-pain.org/files/Content/ContentFolders/Publications2/FreeBooks/First_Steps_The_Early_Years_of_IASP.pdf
2. http://americanpainsociety.org
3. http://apps.painmed.org
4. https://www.spinalinjection.org
5. https://www.asipp.org
6. https://www.asra.com
7. http://www.neuromodulation.org

Pain Care Advocacy

94

Haroon Hameed

Key Concepts

- Changing political and economic realities are placing increasing pressure on the practice of medicine in general, and pain medicine and interventional pain management in particular.
- Involvement in state medical societies and the American Medical Association is still a relevant approach to influencing the local and national practice of medicine.
- Involvement in pain-related specialty societies with a goal of increasing physician member involvement in health policy initiatives may be an option for those with an interest in influencing their professional destiny

Background

The political and economic setting in which physicians practice medicine has changed dramatically over the last nearly 20 years since the Balanced Budget Act of 1997 was passed, linking increases in Medicare and Medicaid payments to the growth of the US GDP and creating the so called sustainable growth rate (SGR) formula. The SGR was finally repealed in April 2015, but the changes enacted by legislation between 1997 and 2015 gradually intensified the pressure on physician and surgeon practice by decreasing reimbursements and essentially increasing the Medicare cost per patient by non-provider entities. In particular, the Medicare Modernization Act of 2003 increased payments to the pharmaceutical industry through enactment of Medicare Part D and decentralized Medicare by creating Medicare administrators with the primary stated goal of decreasing Medicare expenditure by reducing the centralized inefficiency of the Medicare system and the promise of billions of dollars in savings. On the contrary, the Medicare administrator system ended up costing tens of billions more than expected over the last decade, thereby increasing Medicare costs per patient.

Later, in 2010, the Patient Protection and Affordable Care Act was passed incorporating several provisions that will prove to be challenging for both practicing physicians and surgeons and maintaining patient access to their care. Specifically the Independent Payment Advisory Board, which comes into force in 2015, is thought to place a significant challenge for pain physicians as cuts to payments for specialists are expected. In addition, the Accountable Care Organization (ACO) paradigm enacted in 2010 will come into force over the next few years. The essential principle of which relies on the decreased use of expensive resources such as laboratory data, imaging, and surgical and interventional procedures to create savings, which will be then divided between the various players within the ACO and the Medicare administrators. Despite the fact that the SGR has been repealed, within the bill that repealed it, is a language stating that the formula is being repealed as an interim solution until the full implementation of the Accountable Care Organization paradigm within 5 years.

Inevitably, the changes and challenges mentioned above have created environment of consistently declining physician, and particularly specialist and procedural reimbursements. These declines are often reflected not only in both Medicare and Medicaid reimbursements but also within new and renewal contracts between physician and surgeon private practices and private insurance carriers. These changes have led to a trend of hospital-employed physicians and physician practices, consolidation of smaller groups into large and very large physician practices, and in some case acquisition of physician practices by investors, such as private equity groups. All of these changes can potentially place an increased burden on physicians to produce revenue, over simply providing the best patient care. In order to maintain sovereignty of our clinical practice, it is in the

H. Hameed, MD (✉)
KURE Pain Management,
116 Defense Highway, Ste 403, Annapolis, MD 21401, USA
e-mail: drharoonhameed@yahoo.com

J.E. Pope, T.R. Deer (eds.), *Treatment of Chronic Pain Conditions*, DOI 10.1007/978-1-4939-6976-0_94

interest of physicians to engage all possible media to lobby and advocate on behalf of the pain medicine and interventional pain management community's shared goals of maintaining independent clinical decision making and increased patient access to our care.

American Medical Association (AMA)

The American Medical Association remains the oldest and most important national medical association in the United States. Its primary functions include creating and lobbying for healthcare policies and update and implementation of its correct procedural terminology (CPT) and the related relative value units (RVUs) that each code represents. The values of RVUs are assessed through a committee of primary specialty society delegates by the AMA Specialty and Service Society's (AMA-SSS) Relative Value Scale Update Committee (RUC). Through sale of licensing rights for CPT coding manuals, the AMA generates hundreds of millions of dollars in revenue to fund its various goals and initiatives, which are created by the AMA House of Delegates (HOD) and implemented by the board of trustees and the AMA staff.

State Medical Societies

County and state medical societies are the most common method of becoming more involved in organized medicine at the local and state level. Ideally, through involvement in the state medical society, one can become more involved in the AMA by representing the state in the AMA-HOD, as state societies hold the most numerous delegate seats within the AMA-HOD and are commonly more influential than specialty society with smaller delegations.

American Medical Political Action Committee (AMPAC)

AMPAC is the political arm of the AMA and is responsible for developing relationships with local and national legislators, thereby advocating for priority policies and objectives of the AMA and its House of Delegates. It also provides many resources for physicians and surgeons, including AMPAC campaign and candidate schools for physicians and surgeons interested in more involvement in politics.

Contractor Advisory Committees (CAC)

Contractor Advisory Committees, formerly known as Carrier Advisory Committees, exist in each state and include representatives of all primary specialty designations. In addition to traditional pain-related primary specialties, e.g., anesthesiology, physical medicine and rehabilitation, neurology, etc., they also include interventional pain management. The primary purpose of the CAC is drafting Local Coverage Determinations (LCD) which delineate the necessary indications for the coverage of treatment rendered by federal insurance companies, i.e., Medicare and Medicaid. They do not produce guidelines for coverage by private insurance companies, though often over time their policies significantly influence coverage policies created by private insurers.

Specialty Societies

Many specialty societies are heavily involved in political activities. Within interventional pain management, the American Society of Interventional Pain Physicians (ASIPP) has had a yearly lobbying effort for over 15 years, and the North American Neuromodulation Society (NANS) has recently started a legislative fellowship to place young physicians with an interest in health policy and advocacy in congress members' offices. Other organizations such as the American Society of Anesthesiologists have had many legislative awareness programs and internships that have been available for years.

Direct Political Involvement

Engagement of city, district, county, state, and national legislators is one of the most traditional and reasonable ways to develop personal and working relationships with those in the political sphere that help shape health policy. A link to help guide interested readers to their local, state, and national representatives can be found below.

Suggested Reading

1. http://www.ama-assn.org/ama
2. http://www.ampaconline.org
3. https://med.noridianmedicare.com/web/jeb/policies/lcds/cac
4. https://www.cms.gov/Regulations-and-Guidance/Guidance/Manuals/downloads/pim83c13.pdf
5. https://www.asipp.org
6. http://www.neuromodulation.org
7. http://www.usa.gov/Agencies.shtml

Advanced Practice Practitioners 95

Haroon Hameed

Key Concepts

- Physician extenders are a vital component of the health engagement model.
- Physician extenders can be classified as physician assistants (PAs) or nurse practitioners (NPs).
- Practice autonomy and scope of practice needs to be considered when developing a model that includes physician extender engagement.

Introduction

Health care in the United States is changing. The numbers of patients that need to be served are growing. Estimates suggest a provider shortage of nearly 61,000 physicians and almost 30,000 specialists. As volume pressures mount, along with continued oversight on the development of quality reporting, the reliance on physician extenders (PE), or midlevel providers, is crucial to develop a business model for success.

Physician Assistants (PAs)

PAs are advanced practice clinicians who obtain medical histories, perform examinations, and procedures, order and interpret diagnostic tests, refer patients to appropriate specialists, and diagnose. They may also assist in surgery as a first assist.

Training to become a PA includes a Bachelor of Science and 2000 or more clinical training hours during an accredited program that is typically a 3-year program. Certification is the granted following an exam, and state licensure is required. Mean starting salary at the time of this writing is near $100,000.

Nurse Practitioners (NPs)

NPs treat conditions, perform examinations, procedures, order and interpret diagnostic tests, prescribe and perform procedures for treatment, and refer to other specialties as needed. These providers can serve as a "point of entry" for health care.

Training for NPs includes a Bachelor of Science, a Master of Science, matriculation through an accredited nurse practitioner program, which includes 500–700 clinical hours, and then examination and state licensure. Mean starting salary from $100,000. Further, in some states, NPs can practice autonomously.

Oversight

As an employer, physicians need to appreciate the differences among physician extenders. When an encounter is billed, it can be assigned to the midlevel provider or the physician, based on oversight and the type of the encounter. Under current reimbursement structure, midlevel bill is approximately 80% of what a physician would bill at the same level of encounter. "Incident to" was created to designate a visit which supervision by a physician was performed during the encounter, drawing a distinction from no oversight from a physician and allowing for billing of 100% the physician rate. Each state has different requirements and scope of practice designations, and the reader is directed each state. Generally, PAs require on-campus "direct" supervision when billing "incident to," while an NP does not. Typically, extenders can see new patient encounters and work-up patents with a new condition, but "incident to" cannot be billed.

H. Hameed, MD (✉)
KURE Pain Management,
116 Defense Highway, Ste 403, Annapolis, MD 21401, USA
e-mail: drharoonhameed@yahoo.com

J.E. Pope, T.R. Deer (eds.), *Treatment of Chronic Pain Conditions*, DOI 10.1007/978-1-4939-6976-0_95

Scope of practice and chart audit oversight are recommended on a scheduled basis, along with a clear delineation of duties within the practice. Malpractice coverage is important, and supervision strategies need to be clearly delineated. Liability revolves around inadequate supervision. Study compared claims from 1991–2007, and there was 1 payment per 2.7 physicians as compared to 1 payment for 32.5 PAs and 65.8 NPs, with mean payments higher for claims against physicians. Risk mitigation strategies include written protocols for scope of practice, malpractice crier notification when hiring a midlevel and credential verification, among others.

Pain Practice Engagement Models

Many models exist engaging physician extenders in a multimodal clinic. Models are included in Table 95.1.

Physician Extender Considerations

Literature supports that the level of care provided by PEs and physicians are comparable in the primary care and critical care setting. Some management differences remain, including:

- Midlevel providers are more likely to prescribe a controlled substance in the same clinical setting as compared to a physician, especially in nonmetropolitan areas.
- In complex patients, physician extenders are less likely to institute an appropriate treatment change than physicians, after controlling for additional visit-specific factors, including practice style, measurement, and organizational factors.

Table 95.1 Pain practice engagement models

Resident/fellow staffing model	PE see new and return patients and staff, all of them with the physician on site
Autonomous practice model	NPs manage a patient cohort independently within a practice
Integrated supportive care model	Most common, PE see return visits

- Referrals to a tertiary, academic center scored better from physicians as compared to midlevel.
- Survey of physicians of rural and urban primary care practices reflected that nonphysician providers had the necessary skill to treat patients and improve practice outreach and community needs.
- Patients seen in subspecialty practice where physician extenders are employed had a lower disease activity than those patients that were seen in a practice served by a physician subspecialist only.

Conclusion

PE are a vital component to the subspecialty clinic. Proper scope of practice, supervision, expectation, and designation of patient encounters will allow for creation of patient-centric model that is fulfilling for all those engaged.

Suggested Reading

1. Arthritis Care Res (Hoboken). 2015 Jun 19. doi: 10.1002/acr.22643.
2. Cipher DJ, Hooker RS, Guerra P. Prescribing trends by nurse practitioners and physicians assistants in the United States. J Am Acad Nurse Pract. 2006;18(6):291–6.
3. Crane M. Malpractice risks with NPs and pas in your practice. Medscape Business of Medicine. January, 2013. http://www.medscape.com/viewarticle/775746.
4. Hooker R, Nicholson J, Tuan L. Does the employment of physician assistants and nurse practitioners increase liability? J Med Licensure and Discipline. 2009;9:6–16.
5. Rudy EB, Davidson LJ, Daly B, Clochesy JM, Sereika S, Baldisseri M, Hravnak M, Ross T, Ryan C. Care activities and outcomes of patients cared for by acute care nurse practitioners, physician assistants, and resident physicians: a comparison. Am J Crit Care. 1998;7(4):267–81.
6. Singh B, Parsaik AK, Mielke MM, Roberts RO, Scanlon PD, Geda YE, Shane Pankratz V, Christianson T, Yawn BP, Petersen RC. chronic obstructive pulmonary disease and association with mild cognitive impairment: the mayo clinic study of aging. Mayo Clin Proc. 2013;88(11):1256–71.
7. Subramanian U, Kerr EA, Klamerus ML, Zikmund-Fisher BJ, Holleman RG, Hofer TP. Treatment decisions for complex patients: differences between primary care physicians and mid-level providers. Am J Manag Care. 2009;15(6):373–80.

Current Procedural Terminology

96

Haroon Hameed

Key Concepts

- CPT codes are alphanumeric codes that represent patient care procedures and services.
- CPT codes are divided into three categories, i.e., I, II, and III.
- CPT Category I codes are associated with relative value units, which are directly proportional to their monetary value.

Introduction

Current Procedural Terminology (CPT) codes are a set of alphanumeric character sequences that are used for reporting and billing of patient care evaluation and management services including office visits, procedures, medications, durable medical equipment, diagnostic procedures, vaccines, performance measures, and other emerging technology codes. The American Medical Association (AMA) developed CPT in 1966 and expanded it during the 1970s. In 1983, the Centers for Medicare and Medicaid Services (CMS) mandated the use of CPT in addition to their own coding system which is known as the Healthcare Common Procedure Coding System (HCPCS) for Medicare Part B, i.e., outpatient care services. By 1987, CMS adopted CPT coding for outpatient hospital surgical services as well. The AMA controls the CPT code update process and releases updates in its CPT code manual on a yearly basis and also through updates and clarifications in its "CPT assistant" service. CPT codes are differentiated into three main categories, i.e., Category I, II, and III. Category I codes are divided into six sections, namely, evaluation and management, anesthesiology, surgery, radiology, pathology and laboratory, and medicine. These codes must be reported in conjunction with codes from the tenth edition of the World Health Organization's International Statistical Classification of Diseases and Related Health Problems (ICD-10).

Classification

Category I

Category I CPT codes are five-digit numeric codes that specify distinct services or procedures, medications, vaccines, and durable medical equipment, etc.

Category II

Category II CPT codes are five-digit alphanumeric codes that begin with four numeric characters followed by an alphabetic character and are used for measuring and tracking performance.

Category III

Category III CPT codes are five-digit alphanumeric codes that begin with an alphabetic character followed by a four digit number and are used as temporary codes for emerging technologies, services, or procedures.

CPT Editorial Panel

The CPT editorial panel is a 17-member panel comprised of 11 physicians who are nominated by National Medical Specialty Societies and are confirmed by the AMA Board of Trustees. There is one seat each for physicians representing the American Hospital Association, the Centers for Medicare

H. Hameed, MD (✉)
KURE Pain Management,
116 Defense Highway, Ste 403, Annapolis, MD 21401, USA
e-mail: drharoonhameed@yahoo.com

J.E. Pope, T.R. Deer (eds.), *Treatment of Chronic Pain Conditions*, DOI 10.1007/978-1-4939-6976-0_96

Medicaid Services, the Blue Cross Blue Shield Association, and America's Health Insurance Plans and two seats for CPT Health Care Professionals Advisory Committee. This panel is responsible for maintaining and updating existing CPT codes and designating categories for new or emerging codes.

CPT Code Maintenance and Update Process

A CPT code application has three main components. The first part involves a suggested code designation within a family of Category I CPT codes with a short code descriptor, included services if any (e.g., fluoroscopy), and parentheticals to exclude any similar but either not validated or different services or procedures. The second component is the inclusion of commonly associated ICD-10 diagnoses. And the last component is a vignette describing the service in detail outlining the actual work of the service. Any individual, corporation, or medical society can request CPT code changes. To satisfy inclusion as a Category I CPT code, the interested party is responsible for confirming that the requested code has been cleared by the FDA and must also have data regarding frequency of performance in the United States. They must also prove the requested service is appropriate and consistent with medical practice based on peer-reviewed literature. If these demands are not met, but the procedure or service is performed by and supported by at least one CPT advisor, supported by peer-reviewed literature, or being studied by and institutional review board-approved study in the United States, it will be awarded a Category III CPT code. The AMA CPT committee meets three times per year. Typically, there are winter, spring, and fall meetings. Membership in the CPT committee is dependent on active AMA House of Delegates (HOD) membership by a specialty society though any interested individual or party may attend after obtaining permission from the AMA.

Significance

The major significance of the CPT coding system began with its adoption by the Centers for Medicare and Medicaid Services, which led to its utilization by private payors for reporting and valuation of its component codes. Category I codes are associated with values known as relative value units (RVU), which are estimations of the work or value of the code and determined by the American Medical Association's (AMA) Relative Value Scale Update Committee (RUC). After each CPT meeting, all member societies receive a notice regarding their interest in the codes that have been updated or created in the last meeting. The interested societies send surveys to their members that they then collect and then present this data to the RUC. The assigned RVUs are then multiplied by a conversion factor, which Medicare determines on a yearly basis to create its actual monetary valuation. CMS's monetary valuation is based on compensation for physician labor and costs for services rendered without consideration for profit. This monetary valuation serves as a benchmark for valuation by private payors and has traditionally been associated with a multiplier, which allows for a relative profit margin.

Conclusion

CPT codes are the standard for reporting provider procedures and services. The CPT coding process is a complex process that is overseen by the AMA and its 17-member CPT editorial panel, as well as its constituent advisors that represent Specialty Service Societies that are members of the AMA HOD. The importance of the CPT codes lies in the relative value units that are assigned to each code and the monetary value that each code is associated with.

Suggested Reading

1. Last Accessed 25 Aug 2016: http://www.ama-assn.org/ama/pub/physician-resources/solutions-managing-your-practice/coding-billing-insurance/cpt/cpt-process-faq/code-becomes-cpt.page
2. Last Accessed 25 Aug 2016: http://www.ama-assn.org/ama/pub/physician-resources/solutions-managing-your-practice/coding-billing-insurance/cpt/applying-cpt-codes.page
3. Last Accessed 25 Aug 2016: http://www.ama-assn.org/ama/pub/physician-resources/solutions-managing-your-practice/coding-billing-insurance/cpt/about-cpt/category-i-vaccine-codes.page
4. Last Accessed 25 Aug 2016: http://www.ama-assn.org/ama/pub/physician-resources/solutions-managing-your-practice/coding-billing-insurance/cpt/about-cpt/category-ii-codes.page

Practice Responsibilities Surrounding Opioid Prescribing

97

Ahdev Kuppusamy

Key Concepts

- The development of a comprehensive opioid/treatment agreement is an essential component of a successful pain practice.
- The success of an opioid/treatment agreement relies on excellent communication between physicians and their patients, ensuring a thorough understanding of the goals of such agreement.

Introduction

Approximately 26–36 million people abuse opioids worldwide, with an estimated 2 million people in the United States suffering from substance abuse disorders related to prescription opioid pain relievers in 2012. The number of prescriptions for opioids has escalated dramatically, from 76 million in 1991 to over 207 million in 2013. The United States ranks as the biggest consumer globally, accounting for almost 100% of the world total for hydrocodone and 81% for oxycodone.

Considering these statistics, creating a comprehensive opioid treatment agreement is an essential part in the development of any pain medicine practice. In 1997, the Federation of State Medical Boards (FSMB) undertook an initiative to develop model guidelines and to encourage state medical boards and other healthcare regulatory agencies to adopt policies encouraging the safe and effective treatment of patients with pain. These guidelines were updated in 2003 to reflect the best available evidence. The model guidelines highlight several key points to consider when developing an opiate treatment agreement:

- Goals of treatment, i.e., in terms of pain management, restoration of function, and safety
- Patients' responsibility for safe use of opiate medication (e.g., prohibiting behavior such as self-escalation or using the opioid in combination with alcohol or other substances; storing medications in a secure location and safe disposal of any unused medication)
- Patients' responsibility to obtain prescribed opioids from only one physician or practice
- Periodic drug testing (as of blood, urine, or saliva)
- Periodic review of the state drug monitoring programs, which are now available in 37 states

The development of an *informed consent* with the patient's signature is essential, and one of the most important parts of this process and, in many ways, is complimentary and inclusive of the opioid treatment agreement. This will help to protect physicians and their practices from third party and vicarious litigation. The term "contract" should be avoided.

These consented agreements typically address (Fig. 97.1):

- Potential risks and anticipated benefits of chronic opioid therapy, including potential side effects of pharmacologic treatment
- Risk of drug interactions and side effects, including, but not limited to, constipation, itching, nausea, oversedation, respiratory depression, impaired motor skills (affecting driving, operating heavy machinery, making important decisions, and other tasks)
- Risk of opioid misuse, dependence, addiction, and overdose and the limited evidence as to the benefit of long-term opioid therapy
- The physician's prescribing policies and expectations. For example, clearly delineating the physician's policy on early refills and replacement of lost or stolen medications
- Specific reasons for which drug therapy may be changed or discontinued (including violation of the policies and agreements spelled out in the treatment agreement)

A. Kuppusamy, MD (✉)
LLC, Scottsdale, AZ 85258, USA
e-mail: ahdevkuppusamy@gmail.com

J.E. Pope, T.R. Deer (eds.), *Treatment of Chronic Pain Conditions*, DOI 10.1007/978-1-4939-6976-0_97

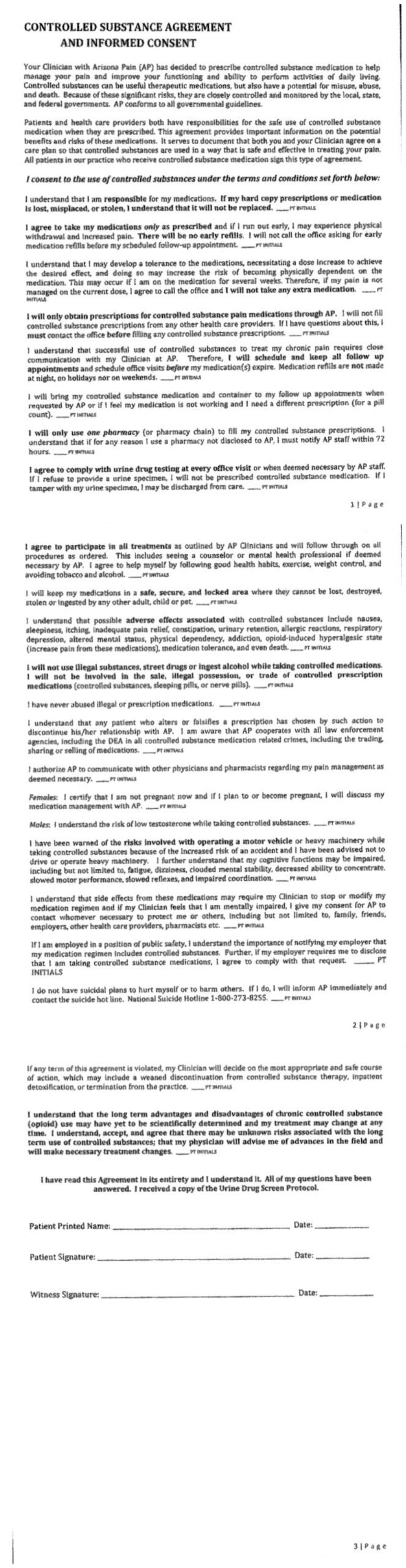

CONTROLLED SUBSTANCE AGREEMENT AND INFORMED CONSENT

Your Clinician with Arizona Pain (AP) has decided to prescribe controlled substance medication to help manage your pain and improve your functioning and ability to perform activities of daily living. Controlled substances can be useful therapeutic medications, but also have a potential for misuse, abuse, and death. Because of these significant risks, they are closely controlled and monitored by the local, state, and federal governments. AP conforms to all governmental guidelines.

Patients and health care providers both have responsibilities for the safe use of controlled substance medication when they are prescribed. This agreement provides important information on the potential benefits and risks of these medications. It serves to document that both you and your Clinician agree on a care plan so that controlled substances are used in a way that is safe and effective in treating your pain. All patients in our practice who receive controlled substance medication sign this type of agreement.

I consent to the use of controlled substances under the terms and conditions set forth below:

I understand that I am **responsible** for my medications. **If my hard copy prescriptions or medication is lost, misplaced, or stolen, I understand that it will not be replaced.** ____PT INITIALS

I agree to take my medications *only* as prescribed and if I run out early, I may experience physical withdrawal and increased pain. **There will be no early refills.** I will not call the office asking for early medication refills before my scheduled follow-up appointment. ____PT INITIALS

I understand that I may develop a tolerance to the medications, necessitating a dose increase to achieve the desired effect, and doing so may increase the risk of becoming physically dependent on the medication. This may occur if I am on the medication for several weeks. Therefore, if my pain is not managed on the current dose, I agree to call the office and **I will not take any extra medication.** ____PT INITIALS

I will only obtain prescriptions for controlled substance pain medications through AP. I will not fill controlled substance prescriptions from any other health care providers. If I have questions about this, I **must** contact the office **before** filling any controlled substance prescriptions. ____PT INITIALS

I understand that successful use of controlled substances to treat my chronic pain requires close communication with my Clinician at AP. Therefore, **I will schedule and keep all follow up appointments** and schedule office visits ***before*** my medication(s) expire. Medication refills are **not** made at night, on holidays nor on weekends. ____PT INITIALS

I will bring my controlled substance medication and container to my follow up appointments when requested by AP or if I feel my medication is not working and I need a different prescription (for a pill count). ____PT INITIALS

I will only use *one pharmacy* (or pharmacy chain) to fill my controlled substance prescriptions. I understand that if for any reason I use a pharmacy not disclosed to AP, I must notify AP staff within 72 hours. ____PT INITIALS

I agree to comply with urine drug testing at every office visit or when deemed necessary by AP staff. If I refuse to provide a urine specimen, I will not be prescribed controlled substance medication. If I tamper with my urine specimen, I may be discharged from care. ____PT INITIALS

1 | Page

I agree to participate in all treatments as outlined by AP Clinicians and will follow through on all procedures as ordered. This includes seeing a counselor or mental health professional if deemed necessary by AP. I agree to help myself by following good health habits, exercise, weight control, and avoiding tobacco and alcohol. ____PT INITIALS

I will keep my medications in a **safe, secure, and locked area** where they cannot be lost, destroyed, stolen or ingested by any other adult, child or pet. ____PT INITIALS

I understand that possible **adverse effects associated** with controlled substances include nausea, sleepiness, itching, inadequate pain relief, constipation, urinary retention, allergic reactions, respiratory depression, altered mental status, physical dependency, addiction, opioid-induced hyperalgesic state (increase pain from these medications), medication tolerance, and even death. ____PT INITIALS

I will not use illegal substances, street drugs or ingest alcohol while taking controlled medications. I will not be involved in the sale, illegal possession, or trade of controlled prescription medications (controlled substances, sleeping pills, or nerve pills). ____PT INITIALS

I have never abused illegal or prescription medications. ____PT INITIALS

I understand that any patient who alters or falsifies a prescription has chosen by such action to discontinue his/her relationship with AP. I am aware that AP cooperates with all law enforcement agencies, including the DEA in all controlled substance medication related crimes, including the trading, sharing or selling of medications. ____PT INITIALS

I authorize AP to communicate with other physicians and pharmacists regarding my pain management as deemed necessary. ____PT INITIALS

Females: I certify that I am not pregnant now and if I plan to or become pregnant, I will discuss my medication management with AP. ____PT INITIALS

Males: I understand the risk of low testosterone while taking controlled substances. ____PT INITIALS

I have been warned of the **risks involved with operating a motor vehicle** or heavy machinery while taking controlled substances because of the increased risk of an accident and I have been advised not to drive or operate heavy machinery. I further understand that my cognitive functions may be impaired, including but not limited to, fatigue, dizziness, clouded mental stability, decreased ability to concentrate, slowed motor performance, slowed reflexes, and impaired coordination. ____PT INITIALS

I understand that side effects from these medications may require my Clinician to stop or modify my medication regimen and if my Clinician feels that I am mentally impaired, I give my consent for AP to contact whomever necessary to protect me or others, including but not limited to, family, friends, employers, other health care providers, pharmacists etc. ____PT INITIALS

If I am employed in a position of public safety, I understand the importance of notifying my employer that my medication regimen includes controlled substances. Further, if my employer requires me to disclose that I am taking controlled substance medications, I agree to comply with that request. ______ PT INITIALS

I do not have suicidal plans to hurt myself or to harm others. If I do, I will inform AP immediately and contact the suicide hot line. National Suicide Hotline 1-800-273-8255. ____PT INITIALS

2 | Page

If any term of this agreement is violated, my Clinician will decide on the most appropriate and safe course of action, which may include a weaned discontinuation from controlled substance therapy, inpatient detoxification, or termination from the practice. ____PT INITIALS

I understand that the long term advantages and disadvantages of chronic controlled substance (opioid) use may have yet to be scientifically determined and my treatment may change at any time. I understand, accept, and agree that there may be unknown risks associated with the long term use of controlled substances; that my physician will advise me of advances in the field and will make necessary treatment changes. ____PT INITIALS

I have read this Agreement in its entirety and I understand it. All of my questions have been answered. I received a copy of the Urine Drug Screen Protocol.

Patient Printed Name: ______________________ Date: ________

Patient Signature: ______________________ Date: ________

Witness Signature: ______________________ Date: ________

3 | Page

Fig. 97.1 Sample treatment agreement provided with the permission of pain doctor

Conclusions

Since the CDC recommendations surrounding opioid use for non-cancer-related pain, there has been an increasing focus on opioid use in the United States. Safe strategies and practice protocols are essential to help ensure safe prescribing for this service line that is an essential component of multimodal pain care.

Suggested Reading

1. Federation of State Medical Boards (FSMB). Model policy on the use of opioid analgesics in the treatment of chronic pain. Washington, DC; 2013.
2. Substance Abuse and Mental Health Services Administration. Results from the 2012 National Survey on Drug Use and Health: Summary of National Findings. NSDUH Series H-46. HHS Publication No. (SMA) 13–4795. Rockville, MD: Substance Abuse and Mental Health Services Administration; 2013.
3. UNODC. World Drug Report 2012. http://www.unodc.org/unodc/en/data-and-analysis/WDR-2012.htmlExternal link, please review our disclaimer.

Surgical Implant Efficiency

98

Brenda Beck

Key Concepts

- Operating room efficiency may save time and money without compromising quality.
- "Lean production" or removing steps that are of little value to the patient can decrease waiting time for patients and improve quality of care.
- Standardized operating room layouts as well as equipment can decrease the likelihood of slowing the procedure or the potential of harming the patient.
- Basic knowledge of operating room surgical equipment, nomenclature, and technique are imperative for the operating physician to master.

Introduction

Due to rising health-care costs, maximizing perioperative efficiency is paramount to reduce waste, decrease personnel cost, and increase financial performance. A lean process strategy (as reflected by the Toyota Production System) eliminates "waste" that may absorb time, personnel, or resources that do not add to the value or efficiency of patient care. On-time starts, eliminating the collection of redundant patient information before the start of a procedure, and reducing operating room turnover times may improve overall efficiency without compromising patient quality of care.

B. Beck, DO (✉)
University Hospitals, Department of Anesthesiology, Division of Pain Management, 11100 Euclid Ave, Cleveland, OH 44106, USA
e-mail: Brenda.beck@uhhospitals.org

Standardized operating room layouts and procedural as well as surgical equipment may help to maintain workflow in the operating room, decrease patient operating room exposure time (which can lead to a lower rate and risk of infection to the patient), and decrease the potential for operating room personnel mistakes or potential errors that may harm the patient.

Having a standard surgical pull sheet for an implant procedure may be helpful in preventing delays and longer surgical exposure time for the patient and can help to maximize efficiency and quality of care.

The physician should have a basic knowledge of the nomenclature of surgical equipment and the basic tools used during a surgical implant procedure (see Appendix 3). A basic minor surgery set should include, but not limited to, instruments designed to cut, grasp, control bleeding, retract, and clamp. Wound care supplies should also be readily available. Different wound dressing techniques can be at the discretion of the physician.

Conclusion

Creating a responsive surgical care delivery is helpful on many fronts; most importantly, it optimizes patient care by reducing surgical site infection. The patient centric strategy associated with the tasking of the personnel during the surgery will reduce costs of the surgery site and improve patient care and physician efficiency.

Suggested Reading

1. Arakelian E, Gunningberg L, Larsson J. How operating room efficiency is understood in a surgical team: a qualitative study. Int J Qual Health Care. 2011;23(1):100–6.
2. Cima RR, Brown MJ, et al. Use of lean and six sigma methodology to improve operating room efficiency in a high-volume tertiary-care academic medical center. Am Coll Surg. 2011;213(1):83–92.

J.E. Pope, T.R. Deer (eds.), *Treatment of Chronic Pain Conditions*, DOI 10.1007/978-1-4939-6976-0_98

Appendix 1
Permanent Implant Targeted Drug Delivery

Procedure reference card	
Procedure: Permanent implant-targeted drug delivery *Anesthesia*: MAC *Preoperative antibiotic*: Vancomycin or weight-dosed Ancef; if penicillin allergic, consider clindamycin *Position of patient*: Left lateral decubitus position *Radiology*: Fluoroscopy with tech for the case	*Skin prep*: Double prep – chlorhexidine sponge prep then Chloraprep stick– wide prep of thoracic and lumbar spine *Nurse notes:* Safety strap around legs and buttocks Grounding pad needed
Medication	**Drapes**
1% lidocaine with epinephrine +/– mixed with 0.25% Marcaine for local skin infiltration 1 gram vancomycin (powdered) which will be spread into wounds before closure Irrigation: Bacitracin 50,000 units Polymyxin B 500,000 units 500 cc of PF normal saline	Basic pack Laparotomy drape C-arm drape Probe cover (needed for interrogation of battery) Half drape
Instruments and equipment	**Sterile supplies**
Mini set Weitlaner retractor (small and large) Adson tissue forceps (rat tooth pick ups) Debakey vascular forceps Needle driver (2) Senn retractor/army navy (hold) Medication cup (2) Kidney basin Suture scissors Metzenbaum scissors Tenotomy scissors Mosquito clamps (4) Spinal cord stimulator lead kit (supplied by preferred vendor) Spinal cord stimulator internal pulsed generator – SCS battery (supplied by preferred vendor)	Bovie – unipolar vs. bipolar Ioban antimicrobial incise drape: 23″ × 17″ Towel packs Raytec sponges Suction tubing Yankauer Skin marker Light handles Needle mat Bulb syringe Loss of resistance syringe 10 cc syringe (2) 25 gauge needle (for local infiltration) Dermabond 4 × 4's Telfa (2) Tegaderm (large) Gown Gloves Abdominal binder
Closure	
O Ethibond pop offs 2–0 Vicryl CT2 pop offs (1–2 needed) 3–0 Monocryl (1–2 needed) Skin stapler (if desired)	

J.E. Pope, T.R. Deer (eds.), *Treatment of Chronic Pain Conditions*, DOI 10.1007/978-1-4939-6976-0

Appendix 2
Spinal Cord Stimulator û Permanent Implant

Procedure reference card	
Procedure: Spinal cord stimulator – permanent implant *Anesthesia*: MAC *Preoperative antibiotic*: Vancomycin or weight-dosed Ancef; if penicillin allergic, consider clindamycin *Position of patient*: Prone with arms above head on plexiglass board or hanging from sides; 1–2 pillows underneath patient's abdomen to mildly flex the spine *Radiology*: Fluoroscopy with tech for the case	*Skin prep*: Double prep – chlorhexidine sponge prep then Chloraprep stick – wide prep of thoracic and lumbar spine *Nurse notes:* Safety strap around legs and buttocks Grounding pad needed
Medications	**Drapes**
1% lidocaine with epinephrine +/– mixed with 0.25% Marcaine for local skin infiltration 1 gram vancomycin (powdered) which will be spread into wounds before closure Irrigation: Bacitracin 50,000 units Polymyxin B 500,000 units 500 cc of PF normal saline	Basic pack Laparotomy drape C-arm drape Probe cover (needed for interrogation of battery) Half drape
Instruments and equipment	**Sterile supplies**
Mini set Weitlaner retractor (small and large) Adson tissue forceps (rat tooth pick ups) Debakey vascular forceps Needle driver (2) Senn retractor/army navy (hold) Medication cup (2) Kidney basin Suture scissors Metzenbaum scissors Tenotomy scissors Mosquito clamps (4) Spinal cord stimulator lead kit (supplied by preferred vendor) Spinal cord stimulator internal pulsed generator – SCS battery (supplied by preferred vendor)	Bovie – unipolar vs. bipolar Ioban antimicrobial incise drape: 23″ × 17″ Towel packs Raytec sponges Suction tubing Yankauer Skin marker Light handles Needle mat Bulb syringe Loss of resistance syringe 10 cc syringe (2) 25 gauge needle (for local infiltration) Dermabond 4×4's Telfa (2) Tegaderm (large) Gown Gloves Abdominal binder
Closure	
O Ethibond pop offs 2–0 Vicryl CT2 pop offs (1–2 needed) 3–0 Monocryl (1–2 needed) Skin stapler (if desired)	

J.E. Pope, T.R. Deer (eds.), *Treatment of Chronic Pain Conditions*, DOI 10.1007/978-1-4939-6976-0

Appendix 3
Sample Pull Sheet for Intrathecal Pump Insertion

Medications	Equipment/preparation	Room setup	Positioning
Nonionic contrast (Omnipaque)	Bean bag	Fluoroscopy available	Patient laterally (nonsurgical side down)
Triple antibiotic ointment	Bovie	Standard anesthesia equipment	Axillary role in place
Bacitracin 50,000 units (in 1000 mL sodium chloride*)	Alcohol and 2 large Chloroprep (26 mL)		Blankets and safety strap for the lower extremities
Lidocaine 2% with epinephrine and 0.5% bupivacaine plain	Sterile gloves and gown		
Dermabond for dressing	Axillary roll		
Bac-neo-poly ointment 28.4 grams	Yankauer suction with tubing		
*Sodium chloride 0.9% 1000 mL Irrigation	Sponges (10 pack), drapes, towels, ioban		
	Surgical 10 blade, spinal 25 gauge needle, syringes (10 mL and 20 mL)		
Intrathecal pump equipment and medication	Sterile cover for the fluoroscopy		
	Kidney basin		
	Mastisol, suture		

Adapted from "Intrathecal Pump Insertion Pull Sheet, Permanent." Dr. Salim Hayek, MD, PhD. University Hospitals Case Medical Center, Cleveland, OH (used with permission)

J.E. Pope, T.R. Deer (eds.), *Treatment of Chronic Pain Conditions*, DOI 10.1007/978-1-4939-6976-0

Appendix 4 Example of Opioid Agreement

Opioid medications are used to treat moderate-to-severe pain. This sheet is meant to inform you of the more serious risks of opioid medications that your doctor is prescribing to be certain you are informed of them. This list is not all inclusive.

There are short-acting formulations and extended-release formulations of opioid medication. The extended release formulations should NEVER be broken, crushed, chewed, or damaged and are meant to be time-release formulations.

Risks

1. The most important risk of opioid includes death due to overdose which is often associated with respiratory depression. Overdose symptoms may include extreme drowsiness, confusion, pinpoint pupils, weak pulse, cold and clammy skin, shallow breathing, fainting, or breathing that stops. If these symptoms occur, the medication should be discontinued immediately, and emergency medical attention needs to be sought immediately.
2. The risk of overdose is significantly increased when the medications are taken in larger doses than prescribed, or the opioid medications are combined with other central nervous system depressants such as ALCOHOL or BENZODIAZEPINES (such as Valium, Ativan, Xanax, clonazepam, or similar medications). It is very important and strongly recommended that ALCOHOL BE AVOIDED when taking opioid medications. Benzodiazepines and similar medications, such as muscle relaxants or sleeping medications, must be prescribed with great caution , and all prescribing doctors need to be informed of the addition of any medications in these classes.
3. Certain medical conditions, such as sleep apnea, asthma, chronic obstructive pulmonary disease (COPD), or other breathing disorders, can also put a patient at increased risk of respiratory depression with opioids. These conditions need to be brought to the prescribing doctor's attention as they can increase risk of death with opioids due to respiratory depression.
4. Other more unusual life-threatening issues with opioids can occur if opioids are combined with certain MAOI class antidepressants. Also certain opioids can have effects on the heart, such as methadone, affecting the heart in certain cases, and this can also lead to sudden death. These effects can be avoided by monitoring current medications from all prescribers and monitoring EKG studies if on methadone or a similar opioid medication.
5. Other side effects that can become quite serious and need to be brought to medical attention include urinary retention which can rapidly become significant, constipation which can become severe and needs to be addressed with the prescribing physician quickly, decreased testosterone, dizziness, confusion, altered mental status, itching, rash, allergic reaction, nausea, drowsiness, double vision, dry mouth, changes in mood or mental status, or dry mouth which can lead to tooth decay.
6. Also keep in mind that these medications can be habit-forming. If the medication is craved for any reason other than pain control, this must be brought to the attention of your physician immediately. Again, these medications may be habit forming.
7. Opioid medications may have unpleasant withdrawal symptoms. This can generally be avoided by discussing with your doctor how to withdraw these medications appropriately.

Driving While on Opiods This is generally not recommended. It is especially dangerous if there is a feeling of mental impairment. Driving or operating other heavy machinery must be absolutely avoided with any feeling of mental impairment, confusion, or drowsiness from these medications. We also recommend avoidance of large financial decisions if there is any feeling of mental impairment present. A particularly dangerous period for driving or operating heavy machinery is the first few weeks, while an opioid is being started or the dosage increased.

J.E. Pope, T.R. Deer (eds.), *Treatment of Chronic Pain Conditions*, DOI 10.1007/978-1-4939-6976-0

By signing this list, you are acknowledging that you understand the risks of opioid medications and understand that there are other risks not listed on this sheet and that you have discussed any questions that you have with your prescribing physician.

____

____

Patient Signature Date

____

____

Physician Signature Date

Appendix 5
Example of an Opioid Monograph

Your doctor and this pain management center are considering prescribing an opiate medication to help reduce your pain. Before your physician does this, you will be asked to adhere to the attached medication contract. Part of the contract involves understanding what opiate medications are.

Opiates are pain medications that resemble opium. Opium is a chemical that has been used for thousands of years to control pain. It is found in Asian poppy plants. Most patients have taken some opiates to control their pain. Opiates include Vicodin, Percocet, Darvocet, Hydrocodone, Demerol, Methadone, Heroin, Morphine, Levo-Dromoran, Oxycodone, Dilaudid, and others.

Opiates work by binding the receptor sites on cells in the brain and spinal cord. The human brain actually makes its own chemicals that bind these receptors. These chemicals are called endorphins and enkephalins. Opiates bind to the same receptor sites and change the way your brain and spinal cord process pain signals. Your pain is then reduced.

There are many effects to opiates. The most common two are sedation and constipation. Other side effects are nausea, difficulty urinating, sweating, dizziness, difficulty swallowing, wheezing, decreased appetite, and itching. You may have side effects with one type of opiate but not with a different one.

The biggest fear for patients and physicians with opiate use is addiction. Most people don't realize that addiction is a mental problem. Very few patients treated for medical problems become addicts unless they have had problems controlling their drug or alcohol usage.

Addiction is the continued use of a substance (drug) despite physical, social, or psychological harm to oneself or others. Addiction is characterized by craving, compulsive use, an inability to control use, and an obsession with maintaining supply. Addiction is different than withdrawal, which is a physical phenomenon initiated by abstinence.

The vast majority of the patients who take opiates will not become addicted. They will become physically dependent. Physical dependency means that if you stop the drug suddenly, you will suffer an abstinence syndrome. This may include diarrhea, cramping, flu-like symptoms, muscle aches, rapid heartbeat, and sweating. This withdrawal can be avoided by weaning (reducing the dose a little each day) over a 2-week period.

Using opiates to control pain is controversial. Many physicians believe it is better to suffer than to take morphine. Some physicians believe you can be taught to live with your pain. Others feel that pain is in your mind, and you can be taught to ignore it. We have been more impressed with how narcotics have made many patients more functional and comfortable.

If you cannot adhere to our contract or if we feel the drugs are harming you, we will stop prescribing them after weaning you off. This happens less than 10% of the time with our patients. Not everyone is helped, but many patients are.

J.E. Pope, T.R. Deer (eds.), *Treatment of Chronic Pain Conditions*, DOI 10.1007/978-1-4939-6976-0

Index

J.E. Pope, T.R. Deer (eds.), *Treatment of Chronic Pain Conditions*, DOI 10.1007/978-1-4939-6976-0

R

S

Printed by Printforce, the Netherlands